Progress in Pain Research and Management
Volume 23

Spinal Cord Injury Pain: Assessment, Mechanisms, Management

Mission Statement of IASP Press®

The International Association for the Study of Pain (IASP) is a nonprofit, interdisciplinary organization devoted to understanding the mechanisms of pain and improving the care of patients with pain through research, education, and communication. The organization includes scientists and health care professionals dedicated to these goals. The IASP sponsors scientific meetings and publishes newsletters, technical bulletins, the journal *Pain,* and books.

The goal of IASP Press is to provide the IASP membership with timely, high-quality, attractive, low-cost publications relevant to the problem of pain. These publications are also intended to appeal to a wider audience of scientists and clinicians interested in the problem of pain.

Progress in Pain Research and Management
Volume 23

Spinal Cord Injury Pain: Assessment, Mechanisms, Management

Editors

Robert P. Yezierski, PhD

Departments of Orthodontics and Neuroscience
College of Dentistry, and the McKnight Brain Institute
University of Florida, Gainesville, Florida, USA

Kim J. Burchiel, MD

Department of Neurological Surgery
Oregon Health Sciences University
Portland, Oregon, USA

IASP PRESS® • SEATTLE

Library of Congress Cataloging in Publication Data

International Association for the Study of Pain. Research Symposium (3rd : 2001 : Phoenix, Ariz.)
Spinal cord injury pain : assessment, mechanisms, management / editors, Robert P. Yezierski, Kim J. Burchiel.
p. ; cm. -- (Progress in pain research and management ; v. 23)
Proceedings of the 3rd IASP Research Symposium held April 16-19, 2001.
Includes bibliographical references and index.
ISBN 0-931092-43-4 (alk. paper)
1. Spinal cord--Wounds and injuries-- Congresses. 2. Pain--Etiology--Congresses. I. Yezierski, Robert P., 1949- . II. Burchiel, Kim. III. Title. IV. Series.
[DNLM: 1. Pain--etiology--Congresses. 2. Pain--therapy--Congresses. 3. Spinal Cord Injuries--complications--Congresses. WI PR677BL v.23 2002/WE 725 I615 2002]
RD594.3 .I576 2001
617.4'82044--dc21

2002024071

Published by:

IASP Press
International Association for the Study of Pain
909 NE 43rd St., Suite 306
Seattle, WA 98105 USA
Fax: 206-547-1703
www.iasp-pain.org
www.painbooks.org

Printed in the United States of America

Contents

Contributing Authors

Antonio J. Acosta-Rua *Department of Neuroscience and McKnight Brain Institute, University of Florida College of Medicine, Gainesville, Florida, USA*

Douglas K. Anderson, PhD *Departments of Neuroscience and Neurological Surgery, College of Medicine, and McKnight Brain Institute, University of Florida; and Malcom Randall Veterans Affairs Medical Center, Gainesville, Florida, USA*

A. Vania Apkarian, PhD *Department of Physiology and Neuroscience Institute, Department of Surgery, and Department of Anesthesia, Northwestern University Medical School, Chicago, Illinois, USA*

Flemming W. Bach, MD, PhD *Department of Neurology and Danish Pain Research Center, Aarhus University Hospital, Aarhus, Denmark*

Brian C. Bowen, PhD *Department of Radiology, University of Miami School of Medicine, Miami, Florida, USA*

Ephraim Brenman, MD *Spine and Rehabilitation Center, Austin, Texas, USA*

Kim J. Burchiel, MD *Department of Neurological Surgery, Oregon Health Sciences University, Portland, Oregon, USA*

Richard L. Cannon, PhD *Department of Neuroscience and McKnight Brain Institute, University of Florida College of Medicine, Gainesville, Florida, USA*

Kenneth L. Casey, MD *Neurology Research Laboratories, Veterans Affairs Hospital, Ann Arbor, Michigan, USA*

Arthur D. (Bud) Craig, PhD *Atkinson Pain Research Laboratory, Division of Neurosurgery, Barrow Neurological Institute, Phoenix, Arizona, USA*

Ernesto Cuevo, MS *The Miami Project to Cure Paralysis, University of Miami School of Medicine, Miami, Florida, USA*

Richard G. Fessler, MD, PhD *Departments of Neuroscience and Neurological Surgery, College of Medicine, and McKnight Brain Institute, University of Florida, Gainesville, Florida, USA; currently Chicago Institute of Neurosurgery and Neuroresearch, Chicago, Illinois, USA*

Nanna B. Finnerup, MD *Department of Neurology and Danish Pain Research Center, Aarhus University Hospital, Aarhus, Denmark*

Bernardo R. Garcia, RT *Department of Radiology, University of Miami School of Medicine, Miami, Florida, USA*

Ira Garonzik, MD *Department of Neurosurgery, Johns Hopkins Hospital, Baltimore, Maryland, USA*

John P. Gorecki, MD, FRCSC, FACS *Wichita Surgical Specialists, Wichita, Kansas, USA*

R. Norman Harden, MD *Center for Pain Studies, Rehabilitation Institute of Chicago, Chicago, Illinois, USA*

Jin-Xia Hao, MD, PhD *Department of Medical Laboratory Sciences and Technology, Division of Clinical Neurophysiology, Karolinska Institute, Huddinge University Hospital, Huddinge, Sweden*

Jennifer A. Haythornthwaite, PhD *Department of Psychiatry and Behavioral Sciences, Johns Hopkins University, Baltimore, Maryland, USA*

Bret L. Hicken, MA *Department of Physical Medicine and Rehabilitation, University of Alabama at Birmingham, Birmingham, Alabama, USA*

Timothy T. Houle, BA *Illinois Institute of Technology, Illinois, USA*

Sherwin Hua, MD, PhD *Department of Neurosurgery, Johns Hopkins Hospital, Baltimore, Maryland, USA*

Charles H. Hubscher, PhD *Department of Physiological Sciences and McKnight Brain Institute, University of Florida, Gainesville, Florida, USA; currently Department of Anatomical Sciences and Neurobiology, University of Louisville, Louisville, Kentucky, USA*

Claire E. Hulsebosch, PhD *Department of Anatomy and Neurosciences, University of Texas Medical Branch, Galveston, Texas, USA*

Troels S. Jensen, MD, PhD *Department of Neurology and Danish Pain Research Center, Aarhus University, Aarhus, Denmark*

Inger L. Johannesen, MD *Department of Rheumatology, Viborg Hospital, Viborg, Denmark*

Richard D. Johnson, PhD *Department of Physiological Sciences and McKnight Brain Institute, University of Florida, Gainesville, Florida, USA*

Ellen Jørum, MD, PhD *Laboratory of Clinical Neurophysiology, Department of Neurology, The National Hospital, Oslo, Norway*

Frederick A. Lenz, MD, PhD, FRCS(C) *Department of Neurosurgery, Johns Hopkins Hospital, Baltimore, Maryland, USA*

Alan R. Light, PhD *Department of Cell and Molecular Physiology, University of North Carolina School of Medicine, Chapel Hill, North Carolina, USA*

Hong-Gang Liu, MS *Division of Nuclear Medicine, Department of Radiology, University of Alabama at Birmingham, Birmingham, Alabama, USA*

John D. Loeser, MD *Departments of Neurological Surgery and Anesthesiology, University of Washington, Seattle, Washington, USA*

Alberto Martinez-Arizala, MD *Department of Neurology, University of Miami School of Medicine, Miami, Florida, USA*

Thomas J. Morrow, PhD *Neurology Research Laboratories, Veterans Affairs Hospital, Ann Arbor, Michigan, USA*

James M. Mountz, MD, PhD *Division of Nuclear Medicine, Department of Radiology, University of Alabama at Birmingham, Birmingham, Alabama, USA*

Timothy J. Ness, MD, PhD *Department of Anesthesiology, Pain Treatment Center, University of Alabama at Birmingham, Birmingham, Alabama, USA*

Shinji Ohara, MD, PhD *Department of Neurosurgery, Johns Hopkins Hospital, Baltimore, Maryland, USA*

Pradip M. Pattany, PhD *Department of Radiology, University of Miami School of Medicine, Miami, Florida, USA*

John D. Putzke, PhD *Department of Physical Medicine and Rehabilitation, University of Alabama at Birmingham, Birmingham, Alabama, USA*

Robert M. Quencer, MD *Department of Radiology, University of Miami School of Medicine, Miami, Florida, USA*

Paul J. Reier, PhD *Departments of Neuroscience and Neurological Surgery, College of Medicine, and McKnight Brain Institute, University of Florida, Gainesville, Florida, USA*

J. Scott Richards, PhD *Department of Physical Medicine and Rehabilitation, University of Alabama at Birmingham, Birmingham, Alabama, USA*

Samuel Saltz, BA *Center for Pain Studies, Rehabilitation Institute of Chicago, Chicago, Illinois, USA*

Christine N. Sang, MD, MPH *Clinical Trials Program, MGH Pain Center, and Department of Anesthesia and Critical Care, Massachusetts General Hospital, Boston, Massachusetts, USA; and Department of Anesthesia, Harvard Medical School, Boston, Massachusetts, USA*

Philip J. Siddall, MBBS, PhD *Pain Management and Research Centre, University of Sydney, Royal North Shore Hospital, Sydney, Australia*

Søren H. Sindrup, MD, PhD *Department of Neurology, Odense University Hospital, Odense, Denmark*

Kristin A. Stevens *Department of Neuroscience and McKnight Brain Institute, University of Florida College of Medicine, Gainesville, Florida, USA*

Xiao-Jun Xu, PhD *Department of Medical Laboratory Sciences and Technology, Division of Clinical Neurophysiology, Karolinska Institute, Huddinge University Hospital, Huddinge, Sweden*

Charles J. Vierck, Jr., PhD *Department of Neuroscience and McKnight Brain Institute, University of Florida College of Medicine, Gainesville, Florida, USA; and Department of Cell and Molecular Physiology, University of North Carolina School of Medicine, Chapel Hill, North Carolina, USA*

Stephen Wegener, PhD *Department of Physical Medicine and Rehabilitation, Johns Hopkins University, Baltimore, Maryland, USA*

Eva Widerström-Noga, DDS, PhD *Miami Project to Cure Paralysis, Department of Neurological Surgery, University of Miami School of Medicine, Miami, Florida, USA*

Zsuzsanna Wiesenfeld-Hallin, PhD *Department of Medical Laboratory Sciences and Technology, Division of Clinical Neurophysiology, Karolinska Institute, Huddinge University Hospital, Huddinge, Sweden*

William D. Willis, Jr., MD, PhD *Department of Anatomy and Neurosciences, University of Texas Medical Branch, Galveston, Texas, USA*

Edward D. Wirth III, MD, PhD *Department of Neuroscience, College of Medicine, and McKnight Brain Institute, University of Florida, Gainesville, Florida, USA; currently Department of Neurosurgery, Rush-Presbyterian-St. Luke's Medical Center, Chicago, Illinois, USA*

Robert P. Yezierski, PhD *Departments of Orthodontics and Neuroscience, College of Dentistry, and the McKnight Brain Institute, University of Florida, Gainesville, Florida, USA*

Foreword

Having been actively involved for many years in studying different aspects of the physiology and pharmacology of nociception at the level of the spinal cord, I am struck by the small number of experimental studies focused on pain in spinal cord trauma. The existing research has significant gaps, not only due to the complex mechanisms brought into play by spinal injury but also because of methodological issues, notably the difficulty in creating reproducible experimental models. Finally, the concept of being able to perform a "clinical examination" of an animal is dubious. These problems have long prevented researchers from fully entering into this field.

My participation over the years in many congresses and symposia has made me aware of the difficulties faced by clinicians who treat pain that occurs after lesions of the spinal cord. Spinal trauma is often associated with moderate to severe pain. The frequency of these types of pain is still poorly documented, with estimates varying from 18% to 63% of patients.

Paraplegic patients may endure osteoarthritic pain, visceral pain, pain associated with spasticity, radicular pain, and central neuropathic pain. These pains, most often found in peroneal or leg areas, at first appear paradoxical as they can be associated with reduced sensitivity or even anesthesia. Spontaneous pains include poorly localized burning, needling, viselike, and crushing pains. Some paraplegics also complain of electrical discharges, lancinating pains, pins and needles, and unpleasant prickling pains. In the case of complete section of the spinal cord, the sensation may resemble the phantom pain that can occur after an amputation. Finally, certain patients exhibit hypersensitivity to cold or to the lightest touch, the very disabling allodynias.

These pains are often difficult to treat, and the available treatments often are only partially effective. Results of studies on the effectiveness of pharmacological treatments (antidepressants, anticonvulsants, and opioids) vary considerably. Nevertheless, the prospects are promising for improved treatments using NMDA-receptor antagonists, cannabinoids, and calcium channel blockers. More and more research groups are researching pain associated with traumatic injuries of the spinal cord, and animal studies have started to reveal the multiple underlying mechanisms. Clinicians have started to tackle the problem in a rigorous manner with regard to taxonomy, epidemiology, evaluation, pharmacological treatments, and behavioral approaches to therapy. New imaging techniques should lead to new insights into the mechanisms of pain after spinal trauma.

Inspired by a suggestion from Robert Yezierski, I created a task force on pain following spinal cord injury (SCI) during my tenure as president of the International Association for the Study of Pain (IASP). Drs. Kim J. Burchiel and Robert P. Yezierski assumed responsibility of chairing the task force. Its long-range objectives were divided into two general areas. First, the task force sought to initiate programs directed toward improving clinical assessment strategies for different spinal injury pain syndromes, developing a standardized taxonomy, evaluating different treatment strategies, and developing education programs for patients and health care professionals. Where appropriate, the task force would facilitate interactions with other professional societies whose members shared the responsibility of providing health care to SCI patients with acute or chronic pain. Second, in the area of basic research the task force was to identify research areas important to understanding the mechanisms of acute and chronic pain associated with SCI and list priority areas for the development of novel therapeutic strategies. The work represented by this volume leaves little doubt that new research will narrow the gap between laboratory research and clinical realities.

JEAN-MARIE BESSON, PHD
INSERM, Paris, France

Preface

Pain following spinal cord injury (SCI) severely compromises the quality of life in nearly 70% of individuals with SCI, yet for nearly half a century little progress has been made in developing effective long-term treatments for this condition. Evidence from assessment studies showing that nearly one-third of all SCI patients have severe pain provides added motivation to begin a comprehensive evaluation of SCI pain.

This volume, the first of its kind, provides a state-of-the-art assessment of the clinical characteristics, central mechanisms, and treatment strategies of the most common pain states associated with SCI. It recommends areas of clinical and basic research that will continue to improve our understanding and treatment of SCI pain syndromes.

One of the most pressing challenges in SCI pain research is to improve the quality of life of those with SCI. Although it would be greatly satisfying if our research efforts could help our patients shed their wheelchairs, we must not ignore the importance of efforts that will enable those with SCI to return to work, re-establish connections with families and friends, and reduce their need for debilitating pharmacotherapy.

An important step in evaluating the clinical characteristics and prevalence of SCI pain syndromes is the development of a unified taxonomy of SCI-related pain. At present there are nearly as many descriptions of different pain categories associated with spinal injury as there are papers dealing with this topic. For nearly 20 years authors have been inventing new ways to describe abnormal sensory conditions related to spinal injury. Part I, Clinical Characteristics and Assessment, reviews the evolution of a taxonomy of SCI pain in the context of the terminology presented in *Classification of Chronic Pain: Descriptions of Chronic Pain Syndromes and Definitions of Pain Terms* (2nd ed., H. Merskey and N. Bogduk, Eds., Seattle: IASP Press, 1994). The newly proposed taxonomy for SCI pain, described fully in Chapter 2, is based on the location or region of pain, source of pain or presumed site of pathology, and on general descriptors of pain and putative mechanisms. Part I also reviews current methods used in the clinical assessment of SCI pain, including quantitative sensory testing and the evaluation of psychosocial factors.

Another aspect of understanding SCI pain is to correlate the onset of different pain syndromes with pathophysiology (central and peripheral). Part II, Experimental Studies, evaluates the clinical pathophysiology of SCI, attempting to determine the relationships between pathological and physiological findings in different SCI pain syndromes. Efforts to determine the critical factors responsible for different pain syndromes, for example the contribution of peripheral tissue damage as well as spinal cord changes, are important if we are to develop effective therapeutic strategies.

Proposed mechanisms for different SCI pain syndromes have been controversial. Part II also reviews putative central mechanisms (spinal and supraspinal) that may contribute to the onset and maintenance of different pain syndromes. Contributors evaluate different experimental models of spinal injury (including spinal lesions, contusion injury, photochemical and excitotoxic models) along with clinical findings in order to determine the anatomical, neurochemical, molecular, and functional changes responsible for different SCI pain syndromes. Most experimental work related to SCI pain has focused on the condition of central pain rather than on pain associated with injury to peripheral tissue. However, because spinal and peripheral nerve damage as well as soft tissue damage are associated with spinal injury, in the future efforts must be made to address the interaction of pain states associated with peripheral tissue damage as well as those of central origin.

Part III, Imaging, evaluates new insights from radiology and spectroscopy. The development of new technology as well as the novel application of existing methods to study the anatomical, neurochemical, and functional changes at different levels of the neuraxis are providing a better understanding of potential mechanisms responsible for at-level and below-level pain states.

Part IV provides a critical evaluation of past and present treatment strategies and makes recommendations for future treatment protocols for pain syndromes associated with SCI. Currently used strategies include psychological/behavioral, surgical, pharmacological, and physical therapy approaches. These chapters also introduce novel strategies of SCI pain management.

Expansion of knowledge related to the mechanisms of SCI pain should improve the design of future studies. Existing work shows a continuing need for large-scale epidemiological studies to define better the public health impact of different types of pain as well as a need for longitudinal studies designed to identify the critical pathophysiological changes occurring in the spinal cord during the evolution of different pain states. The differential effect of selective drug classes on different components of central and peripheral neuropathic pain and on the distributions of SCI pain (at-level and below-level pain) invites further investigation. More information is also needed on the central mechanisms and potential therapeutic targets of different types of SCI pain and on the involvement of spinal and supraspinal mechanisms in the onset and progression of these pain states. Moreover, the potential therapeutic contributions of surgical interventions, of combined pharmacological strategies, and of alternative or complementary approaches in SCI pain remain to be elucidated. It will also be important to determine the effect that regenerative therapies aimed at restoring function in the injured spinal cord will have on the development of pain conditions or in altering ongoing pain levels. Part V, The Future, discusses these new directions in SCI pain research.

This volume represents the proceedings of the 3rd IASP Research Symposium, entitled *Spinal Cord Injury Pain: Clinical Characteristics and Experimental Studies,* held April 16–19, 2001, in Phoenix, Arizona, USA. The symposium was organized by the International Association for the Study of Pain (IASP) Task Force on Pain following Spinal Cord Injury, chaired by Drs. Kim J. Burchiel and Robert P. Yezierski. The contributors to this volume include basic and clinical investigators from the United States, Canada, Australia, Denmark, Sweden, and Norway. They reflect a cross-section of members of the task force as well as distinguished members of the spinal cord injury and pain communities. We would especially like to recognize and thank Drs. John D. Loeser, Philip J. Siddall, Charles J. Vierck, and Troels S. Jensen for their enthusiastic, committed, and thoughtful involvement in the work of the task force.

ROBERT P. YEZIERSKI, PHD

KIM J. BURCHIEL, MD

Acknowledgments

The editors wish to thank the following organizations and pharmaceutical companies for their support and sponsorship of the 3rd IASP Research Symposium, Spinal Cord Injury Pain: Clinical Characteristics and Experimental Studies, held April 16–19, 2001, in Phoenix, Arizona, USA:

INTERNATIONAL ASSOCIATION FOR THE STUDY OF PAIN

BARROW NEUROLOGICAL FOUNDATION

ELAN PHARMACEUTICALS

ENDO PHARMACEUTICALS

JANSSEN PHARMACEUTICALS

KENT WALDREP NATIONAL PARALYSIS FOUNDATION

MEDTRONIC CORPORATION

PARALYZED VETERANS OF AMERICA

PFIZER PHARMACEUTICALS

PHARMACIA CORPORATION

PURDUE FREDERICK

THE MIAMI PROJECT

Part I

Clinical Characteristics and Assessment

Spinal Cord Injury Pain: Assessment, Mechanisms, Management. Progress in Pain Research and Management, Vol. 23, edited by Robert P. Yezierski and Kim J. Burchiel, IASP Press, Seattle, © 2002.

1

Pain after Spinal Cord Injury

John D. Loeser

Departments of Neurological Surgery and Anesthesiology, University of Washington, Seattle, Washington, USA

Thirty-three-year-old D.R. was an elite skier until she fell 30 feet from a cliff 8 years ago. She felt immediate neck pain and was unable to feel or move her legs. At the regional trauma center, she was found to have a C7–T1 fracture dislocation and a spinal cord transection. She was given an early posterior spinal fusion with instrumentation and was quickly transferred to the spinal cord injury service. Within 3 months she was fully acclimated to wheelchair mobilization and was capable of self-care in her modified home. She resumed her work as an administrative assistant and engaged in vigorous wheelchair athletic competitions. Except for her bowel program, she takes no medications on a regular basis. Although she is sometimes saddened by her loss of function and mobility for the past 8 years, she enjoys a fulfilling life with many activities, including para-skiing. She denies having had any pain since her initial wounds healed.

Forty-two-year-old S.R. sustained a T8 spinal cord transection in a motorcycle accident when he was 26. He was taken from a local hospital to a spinal cord injury center within 2 days of his injury and had a posterior fusion with Harrington rods to stabilize a complex T5–T6 ligamentous and bony injury. He has been flaccid and anesthetic below the level of his injury from the onset of his trauma. Within 2 years of his injury, he developed severe spasticity that did not adequately respond to oral medications. He also developed pain in the anesthetic lower half of his body, most prominently in the buttocks and rectum. Low doses of oral opioids were tried, and he found that oxycodone at a dose of 20 mg p.o. q.i.d. provided moderate pain relief. His insurance company would not let him have sustained-release opioids of any type because of their cost. Methadone was tried in an equivalent dose, but it made him very drowsy. An intrathecal (i.t.) catheter and subcutaneous pump were placed 9 years after his injury. His spasticity was controlled with a daily dose of 355 μg of baclofen. I.t. morphine at doses up to 25 mg per day did not improve his pain relief. He continues to take 80 mg of oxycodone every day and reports fair pain relief. He has not responded favorably to anticonvulsants, antidepressants, or any other drugs tried for pain relief. He uses a wheelchair, takes good care of his skin and bladder, and rarely has medical issues related to his paraplegia. Although he would like better pain relief, he remains functional, although unemployed, on his current regimen.

J.J. is a 53-year-old male who was driving his car through an intersection when a drunk driver struck his vehicle, causing it to roll over. When he regained consciousness, he felt pain in his neck and was unable to move his legs or feel anything beneath his nipples. The regional trauma center diagnosed a C6–C7 fracture dislocation, with magnetic resonance imaging (MRI) evidence of a contused spinal cord. He was promptly stabilized with a posterior fusion of C5–T1 and was immediately started on an intensive rehabilitation program. He had complete motor and sensory loss at the C7 level. He was a cooperative and motivated patient in the early phases of his rehabilitation, but began to complain of pain in his buttocks, genitalia, and legs about 3 weeks after injury. He gradually became depressed and failed to meet his goals for rehabilitation. Severe spasticity of the legs and torso developed that was not controlled with oral medications. He tried antidepressant and anticonvulsant medication, oral opioids in large doses, and other pain medicines and treatments. He had an i.t. catheter and subcutaneous pump placed to deliver baclofen, with dramatic relief of his spasticity. A trial of i.t. morphine did not alleviate his pain at the highest dose he could tolerate without unacceptable side effects. His lower body pain has persisted in spite of every treatment offered by a wide array of health care providers. J.J. spends most of his days in his motorized wheelchair, watching television. He takes high doses of anticonvulsants, opioids, and antidepressants without obvious beneficial effect. Sometimes he consumes excessive alcohol to "deaden his pain." He has had several decubiti. When this patient comes to see me in consultation, I have no meaningful medical treatments to offer him. He and I both leave our meeting feeling depressed. He is seeing a psychologist, thus far without clear benefit.

These three vignettes, based on patients in my practice, demonstrate the wide variety of painful experiences after spinal cord injury (SCI). The patients are typical of those found in an SCI service. We have no idea why pain follows SCI in some patients (Siddall et al. 1999). Nor do we know why some of those with pain after SCI respond to antidepressants, anticonvulsants, or opioids. Clearly, what appear to be identical spinal cord transections can cause pain in some patients and not in others. The mechanisms underlying such pain must vary, even when we focus on the neurological pain syndromes characterized by pain in anesthetic areas of the body. Perhaps genetic differences in persons who sustain SCI determine whether pain occurs and by what mechanisms.

Clinicians are frustrated by the lack of meaningful diagnostic procedures and the paucity of useful treatment options. Other than a description of symptoms by the patient, a description of signs by the physician, and radiological and MRI studies to define anatomical abnormalities, there are no diagnostic procedures or strategies that permit us to categorize types of pain and define potentially useful treatments. Clinical neurophysiology may help define the completeness of the spinal cord injury or associated nerve root injuries, but it does not delineate pain types or predict the likelihood of successful treatments with various strategies. Physicians can describe the type of pain in broad categories, but not on the basis of the underlying mechanisms (Loeser 2000). We do not know whether the presence of SCI pain in one patient and its absence in another is due to the substrate of the injury (pre-existing characteristics of an apparently normal person) or to subtle differences in the qualities of injuries that are grossly similar. Until we can ascertain this critical distinction, our attempts to categorize pain types and establish logical treatments are unlikely to move forward.

Physicians are also frustrated by the absence of outcome data on different types of treatment for SCI pain. We have a significant body of literature on this topic, but it can be characterized, in the main, as small convenience case series from which it is hazardous to generalize to the population of patients. Systematic approaches to treatment are rarely described; instead, the author's approach is described as the treatment of choice. A few well-conducted prospective, randomized controlled studies have been reported, and some are presented in this volume.

Injury of the spinal cord is a disaster that leads to dramatic loss of function. Paraplegics and quadriplegics require major resource allocation and complex health care if their impairments are not to lead to catastrophic disability. Clinicians in SCI units labor to teach their patients methods of adapting to their loss of neural control so as to permit independent functioning and gainful employment. Years of experience permit such clinicians to predict a patient's ultimate functional capacities based solely upon the level of SCI. Only one thing routinely prevents the attainment of the predicted level of functioning—pain (Mariano 1992).

Of course, pain interferes with anyone's ability to engage in gainful employment or to enjoy life. In this sense, the pain seen after SCI is not unique. Millions of the citizens of developed countries claim an inability to work because of back pain, but most of them do not have significant neurological deficits. Repetitive strain injury, neck pain, arthritis, and headaches all cause people to miss work and reduce their social and recreational activities. Some clinicians believe that such patients do have something wrong in their backs or peripheral nerves or, perhaps, that their spinal cord serves as the generator of their pain and suffering. Others consider that such patients may have something different about their brains or may be influenced by environmental factors. The same issues may apply to patients who develop pain after SCI. Is the cause of the pain to be found at the site of injury? Alternatively, are there factors related to past experience, brain development, or current environmental contingencies that perpetuate the patient's complaint of pain?

Chapter 2 classifies the types of pain that can follow SCI. Some of these pain syndromes are mechanical: either instability of the spine at the region of injury or overuse of the upper extremities in a paraplegic. These pain syndromes do not reflect injury to the nervous system; they represent, instead, the normal functioning of nerves in innervated tissues that have sustained trauma. Compression of nerve roots and dorsal root ganglia can also produce pain, not only after a fractured spine, but also with much simpler and less threatening injuries such as herniation of a nucleus pulposus. Again, the pain syndrome due to nerve root or dorsal root ganglion compression is not unique to SCI and can be explained by what we know of the effects of external compression and scarring on a nerve root (Howe et al. 1977). Most patients with SCI have a transitional zone from normal skin sensation to complete loss of sensation. Some of these patients report painful sensations in this girdle zone that are evoked by non-noxious stimulation. We know that such a perversion of sensation, known as allodynia, is related to changes in the spinal cord at the segments that have been traumatized and partially denervated. Transecting the cord above the level of partial sensation, cutting the dorsal roots, or making dorsal root entry zone lesions usually will stop this type of pain. Present evidence supports the idea that the generator of painful sensations lies in the segments just rostral to the transected spinal cord. SCI pain ascribed to the anesthetic segments below a complete cord transection is unique in that the brain is not connected to the neural segments from which the pain is thought to originate. A patient with a thoracic cord transection may complain bitterly of burning pain in his buttocks, genitalia, and legs. The genesis of this pain syndrome cannot lie in the part of the body that hurts, in its peripheral innervation, or in the spinal cord segments that contain the central connections of the nerves from this region (Melzack and Loeser 1978). This type of SCI pain must use different mechanisms than all other types of pain. We have few clues as to its genesis and no good treatment strategies.

Unfortunately for those who wish to study different types of SCI, the anatomical delineation of injury to the spinal cord in clinical settings is not as clear as in experimental models or in the small number of patients who have had direct visualization of their injured spinal cord. More commonly, an incomplete lesion occurs in association with a contusion of the spinal cord. The status of long tracts and local circuitry is indeterminable. The alterations in function, both at the level of injury and in segments above and below, are unclear. Mechanisms are largely unknown, and treatment is often ineffective.

This volume describes what is known about the basic and clinical sciences relevant to pain after SCI, and presents new research findings. It discusses neuropathic pain syndromes and their treatment, but does not delve into the treatment for mechanical causes of pain, as these are well described in standard neurosurgical, orthopedic, and physical medicine textbooks. Studies of SCI are presented, for there is the hope that if the effects of trauma upon the spinal cord can be minimized, the development of chronic pain can be curtailed. Most of the basic science studies and clinical research relate to the pain of SCI itself, as we have no routinely effective treatments for those who complain of pain in the anesthetic parts of their body. As is true for so many chronic pain conditions, few properly conducted clinical trials have studied treatments of the various types of pain that can follow SCI. As Finnerup and colleagues argue in Chapter 20, we need large randomized clinical trials for all types of treatments for the various pain syndromes that occur after SCI. Almost all of the existing clinical reports are case series, on which we cannot base rational treatment strategies. There are no consensus treatment guidelines, no proven algorithms, no standards for diagnosis or treatment of any of the chronic pains that follow SCI. Although many claims have been made for the importance of a mechanisms-based classification system of chronic pain, we are just taking the first steps toward this goal in SCI pain.

Research must solve the puzzle of pain after spinal cord injury. That is what this book is all about. We have a long way to go, but it is time to start.

REFERENCES

Howe JF, Loeser JD, Calvin WH. Mechanosensitivity of dorsal root ganglia and chronically injured axons: a physiological basis for the radicular pain of nerve root compression. *Pain* 1977; 3:25–41.

Loeser JD. Generalized pain syndromes: pain in spinal cord injury patients. In: Loeser JD (Ed). *Bonica's Management of Pain,* 3rd ed. Philadelphia: Lippincott, 2000, pp 613–620.

Mariano AJ. Chronic pain and spinal cord injury. *Clin J Pain* 1992; 8:87–92.

Melzack R, Loeser JD. Phantom body pain in paraplegics: evidence for a central "pattern generating mechanism" for pain. *Pain* 1978, 4:195–210.

Siddall PJ, Taylor DA, McClelland JM, Rutkowski SB, Cousins MJ. Pain report and the relationship of pain to physical factors in the first six months following spinal cord injury. *Pain* 1999; 81:187–197.

Correspondence to: John D. Loeser, MD, Department of Neurological Surgery, University of Washington, Box 356470, Seattle, WA 98195, USA. Tel: 206-543-3570; Fax: 206-543-8315; email: jdloeser@u.washington.edu.

Spinal Cord Injury Pain: Assessment, Mechanisms, Management. Progress in Pain Research and Management, Vol. 23, edited by Robert P. Yezierski and Kim J. Burchiel, IASP Press, Seattle, © 2002.

2

Taxonomy and Epidemiology of Spinal Cord Injury Pain[1]

Philip J. Siddall,[a] Robert P. Yezierski,[b] and John D. Loeser[c]

[a]Pain Management and Research Centre, University of Sydney, Royal North Shore Hospital, Sydney, Australia; [b]Departments of Orthodontics and Neuroscience, College of Dentistry, and the McKnight Brain Institute, University of Florida, Gainesville, Florida, USA; [c]Department of Neurological Surgery, University of Washington, Seattle, Washington, USA

Pain is a debilitating consequence of spinal cord injury (SCI). Although loss of function is considered the most significant consequence of SCI, pain itself has a direct bearing on the patient's ability to regain his or her optimal level of activity. Results from a postal survey in Britain indicated that for 11% of those responding, it was pain rather than loss of function that stopped them from working (Rose et al. 1988). Another study demonstrating the impact of SCI pain reported that 37% of SCI patients with high thoracic and cervical lesions and 23% of patients with low thoracic or lumbosacral lesions would be willing to trade pain relief for loss of bladder, bowel, or sexual function (Nepomuceno et al. 1979). Another survey examined how persons with SCI rated their perceived difficulty in dealing with the consequences of their injury. Chronic pain's high ratings were only surpassed by those for decreased ability to walk or move, loss of sexual function, and diminished ability to control bowel or bladder function (Widerström-Noga et al. 1999).

---

[1] This chapter is modified with permission of IASP from the article, "Pain following spinal cord injury: clinical features, prevalence, and taxonomy," by P.J. Siddall, R.P. Yezierski, and J.D. Loeser, published in the *IASP Newsletter* (2000, Issue 3).

EPIDEMIOLOGY

PREVALENCE OF PAIN

Many studies have reported the prevalence of pain in SCI patients (Davis and Martin 1947; Munro 1950; Botterell et al. 1953; Kaplan et al. 1962; Burke 1973; Nepomuceno et al. 1979; Richards et al. 1980; Lamid et al. 1985; Woolsey 1986; Rose et al. 1988; Berić 1990; Britell and Mariano 1991; Mariano 1992). A summary of the results from 10 of these earlier studies indicates that an average of 69% of patients with SCI experience pain and that nearly one-third of these patients rate their pain as severe (Bonica 1991). Although postal and community surveys have generally reported a slightly higher prevalence of around 75–80% (Rintala et al. 1999; Widerström-Noga et al. 1999; Ravenscroft et al. 2000), most recent studies have confirmed Bonica's figures, showing a prevalence of chronic pain of around 65%, with approximately one-third of these patients reporting severe pain (Levi et al. 1995; New 1997; Störmer et al. 1997; Demirel et al. 1998; Siddall et al. 1999).

Although many studies have reported the prevalence of pain after SCI, few have investigated the prevalence of specific *types* of pain. Types of pain that can accompany SCI include musculoskeletal pain, visceral pain, and two distinct types of neuropathic pain, either at or below the level of injury. A study identifying these specific types of pain reported that musculoskeletal pain is the most common category (affecting 40% of patients 6 months after their injury), but 36% had at-level neuropathic pain and 19% had below-level neuropathic pain (Siddall et al. 1999). Below-level neuropathic pain is the most likely to be described as severe or excruciating (Siddall et al. 1999), and many patients develop this type of pain months and even years following their initial injury.

RELATIONSHIP OF PAIN TO OTHER FACTORS

Although pain is a relatively common problem for patients with SCI (Bonica 1991; Nashold 1991; Mariano 1992), the various contributing factors are unclear. Several factors may be important, including level of SCI, cause of injury, completeness of SCI, and psychosocial issues.

Some authors consider that pain is most likely to be associated with injury at specific spinal cord levels, including cervical (Holmes 1919) and thoracolumbar levels (Davis and Martin 1947) and the conus medullaris and cauda equina (Botterell et al. 1953; Burke 1973; Nashold 1991), but their suggestions lack supporting evidence. Others have stated that spinal cord injuries from gunshot wounds are more likely to result in pain (Richards et al. 1990; Nashold 1991). Clinical observations that neuropathic pain is more common in those with incomplete lesions (Davidoff et al. 1987; Berić et al. 1988) have been supported by findings at autopsy (Kakulas et al. 1990).

Despite these studies, which suggest that physical factors determine pain following SCI, other authors have found no significant relationship between the presence or severity of pain and the level or completeness of SCI (Richards et al. 1980; Summers et al. 1991; Störmer et al. 1997). These authors concluded that psychosocial rather than physical factors were more closely associated with the experience or severity of SCI pain. Chronic pain in SCI patients is associated with more depressive symptoms and more perceived stress (Rintala et al. 1999). Cluster analysis of data obtained from questionnaires in another study revealed a relationship between pain, spasticity, "abnormal nonpainful sensations," and sadness (Widerström-Noga et al. 1999).

CLASSIFICATION OF PAIN TYPES

The wide disparity in reported prevalence and in the relationship of pain to various factors may stem from the inherent variability associated with the design of studies (postal survey, interviews, time following injury, severity of pain, etc.). However, the inconsistency may also be due to the lack of a clear consensus about which types of pain are included and how they are classified. The need for a taxonomy of SCI pain has been cited many times. Lack of consensus regarding terminology has hindered effective communication in the research and treatment of this problem. Therefore, one of our aims as members of the Task Force on Pain following Spinal Cord Injury of the International Association for the Study of Pain (IASP) has been to develop a taxonomy that can be used generally by practitioners and researchers in this field.

WHY A NEW TAXONOMY?

Several classification systems have been used by various authors (Michaelis 1970; Davis 1975; Burke and Woodward 1976; Maury 1978; Donovan et al. 1982; Waisbrod et al. 1984; Frisbie and Aguilera 1990; Segatore 1992; Berić 1997; Siddall et al. 1997). At present, there is no universally accepted classification system and little consistency of terminology among studies. Although there are some similarities, many studies refer to types of pain not included by others. Furthermore, although several broad categories can be identified that have features in common, the terminology varies. This lack of consistency in inclusion criteria and terminology has had negative implications for both SCI research and the evaluation of treatments.

EPIDEMIOLOGICAL STUDIES

Epidemiological studies have been hampered by lack of a universally approved taxonomy. This problem was highlighted by Bonica (1991), who found widely disparate reports of the prevalence of SCI pain. Although this observed variation in prevalence may be partly due to methodological issues regarding the way the data were collected, it is likely to be mainly due to variability in the definition and classification of pain types.

BASIC RESEARCH

The need for a taxonomy is apparent in basic research. Numerous animal models of neuropathic pain after SCI present slightly different features (Levitt and Levitt 1981; Hao et al. 1991; Siddall et al. 1995; Christensen et al. 1996; Yezierski et al. 1998; Vierck and Light 1999). The aim of studies using these models is to understand the pathophysiological mechanisms responsible for the development of pain following SCI and to identify possible therapeutic targets for novel treatment strategies. However, if there are several distinct types of pain following SCI, a clear, consistent, and generally accepted taxonomy is necessary to identify consistently the different types of pain that are being investigated. Such a system will enable more effective application of research findings to the clinical setting.

CLINICAL RESEARCH

Clinical treatment studies and patient management have been hampered by the lack of a consistent taxonomy. SCI pain treatment studies often rely on descriptors to indicate pain type and use terms that are ambiguous and impede interpretation of results. Even when a particular taxonomy is used, variation in terminology across studies can often impair comparison and application of the findings. A standardized taxonomy will enhance communication among clinicians and enable more accurate evaluations of specific therapies for different types of pain associated with SCI.

PAIN TYPES

In developing a taxonomy that meets the desirable criteria described above, IASP's task force had to address several issues. A comprehensive system must include most, if not all, types of pain that are generally recognized as being associated with SCI. The terms that have been used in the past are too numerous to list here. Many authors have used different words to describe the same types of pain. A summary of the different types of pain that can accompany SCI is presented below.

MECHANICAL INSTABILITY OF THE SPINE

This musculoskeletal pain is due to disruption of ligaments or fracture of bones with resultant instability, although it does not require an injury to the spinal cord itself. Pain may be present from the time of injury or, rarely, may develop later. Pain occurs in the region of the spine and may radiate toward the extremities, but it is not radicular. It is characterized by movement of osseous structures in abnormal planes or with unusual range of motion and is therefore related to position, is increased by activity, and is relieved by immobilization. Radiographs or computed tomography (CT) or magnetic resonance (MR) imaging will help demonstrate instability. The pain is usually sensitive to opioids and non-steroidal anti-inflammatory drugs (NSAIDs). Immobilization pending spontaneous healing or surgical fusion is an effective treatment in almost all patients.

MUSCLE SPASM PAIN

Muscle spasm pain is observed in some cases of complete and incomplete SCI. It usually starts well after the injury and is best relieved by alleviating the muscle spasms with antispasmodic medications. Analgesics are rarely helpful.

SECONDARY OVERUSE OR PRESSURE SYNDROMES

Chronic musculoskeletal pain can occur with overuse or "abnormal" use of structures such as the arm and shoulder (Dalyan et al. 1999). This type of nociceptive pain is very common in paraplegics but much less common in tetraplegics. The pain occurs in normally innervated regions rostral to the level of the SCI. The pain is described as aching in the area of pressure or overuse and worsens with use of involved joints or pressure on the affected area. It is typically seen in the shoulders of those who use wheelchairs (Nichols et al. 1979), and as many as 72% of paraplegics have evidence of degenerative changes in the shoulder joint (Lal 1998). Resting the painful part or protecting it from trauma can alleviate this type of pain; NSAIDs or opioids are also helpful.

VISCERAL PAIN

Visceral pain usually has delayed onset following SCI and is indicated by burning, cramping, and constant but fluctuating pain in the abdomen. It may be due to normal afferent input via the sympathetic or vagal nerves in paraplegics and via the vagus in tetraplegics (Kuhn 1950; Komisaruk et al. 1997). Visceral pain is often poorly defined and may occur in the absence of any demonstrable visceral pathology. However, such pain should initially be considered as nociceptive, as it may be arising from stimulation of visceral nociceptive afferents. Treatment is directed at addressing any pathology thought to be responsible for the pain.

If investigations fail to find evidence of visceral pathology, and if treatment or blockade of peripheral inputs from visceral structures fails to alleviate pain, then consideration must be given to classifying the pain as neuropathic rather than visceral and treatments appropriate to this type of pain should be used. Visceral nociceptive inputs may also trigger neuropathic pain in some individuals.

ABOVE-LEVEL NEUROPATHIC PAIN

Neuropathic pain can occur above the level of injury and includes pains that are not specific to SCI. Pain occurs with peripheral nerve compression (Davidoff et al. 1991). Although not always due to nerve injury, complex regional pain syndromes (CRPS types I and II, sometimes referred to as reflex sympathetic dystrophy and causalgia, respectively) may also occur and are associated with vasomotor and sudomotor disturbances in the affected region (Stanton-Hicks et al. 1995). Although peripheral nerve compression and CRPS occur in the general population, individuals with SCI may be more susceptible because of the activity associated with wheelchair use or transfers. Patients with SCI, particularly those with cervical injuries, are at risk of developing CRPS in the upper limbs (Cremer et al. 1989; Philip et al. 1990; Aisen and Aisen 1994). One retrospective study has indicated that 63% of patients with cervical SCI had CRPS-like features affecting the shoulder and arm, with a mean time of onset of 24 days (Aisen and Aisen 1994). Patients received a range of therapies including exercises, heat, NSAIDs, systemic corticosteroids, and stellate ganglion block. Medications such as tricyclic antidepressants and anticonvulsants may also be useful. If the pain is due to nerve compression in affected extremities, electrophysiological tests as well as MR and nerve conduction studies can aid in diagnosis. Peripheral nerve compression can, when necessary, be alleviated by surgical decompression.

NERVE ROOT ENTRAPMENT

Nerve root entrapment may result in lancinating, burning, stabbing pain in the distribution of a single nerve root, although pain may be bilateral. Pain occurs at the level of spinal trauma and is usually present from the time of injury. If the affected nerve root contributes to the brachial or lumbosacral plexus, there may be electromyographic and evoked potential abnormalities. Radiographic, CT, or MR scans often show evidence of compression of a nerve root in the intervertebral foramen by bone or disk, although the same findings can sometimes be seen in the absence of pain. If the pain is associated with vertebral instability it should be relieved by stabilization. The pain may be relieved by opioids or by neuropathic pain-relieving drugs. If there is bone or disk material in the foramen, surgical decompression is usually effective.

Pain arising from damage to the cauda equina is a type of nerve root pain with a burning quality that affects the legs, feet, perineum, genitals, and rectum. There are several potential etiologies for pain after such an injury. First, the spinal cord may be significantly deafferented, leading to changes in central connectivity and neuronal activity that could cause pain. Second, the damaged roots of the cauda equina could be spontaneously active and generate signals that are interpreted as pain. The arachnoiditis that follows major injury to the cauda equina may limit the normal movement of the nerve roots and lead to mechanical irritation of the roots with very slight movements (Howe et al. 1977). Third, peripheral stimuli could lead to abnormal activity at the site of axonal injury. The pain is reported in the lower lumbar and sacral dermatomes and is usually described as burning, stabbing, and hot. It is constant but may fluctuate with activity or autonomic activation. Spinal cord stimulation has sometimes been successful in relieving the pain.

SEGMENTAL DEAFFERENTATION PAIN

Neuropathic pain often occurs at the border of normal sensation and anesthetic skin and is referred to as girdle, end zone, border zone, or transitional zone pain. The pain occurs within a band of two to four segments and can be unilateral or bilateral and circumferential. Allodynia and hyperalgesia often occur within the painful region. Segmental pain usually develops during the first few months after injury. It does not usually respond to opioids but may respond to neuropathic pain-relieving medications. The pain may also be relieved by a number of interventions including epidural or somatic root blocks, dorsal root entry zone lesions, dorsal rhizotomy, spinal cord stimulation, or distal cordectomy that raises the sensory level to the top of the painful region.

In the past, pain that occurs at the level of the lesion and has features of nerve root pain in the absence of definitive evidence of nerve root damage has often been classified as radicular. However, segmental neuropathic pain may occur in the absence of nerve root damage and may be due to spinal cord rather than nerve root pathology. Animal models of SCI that have damage confined to the spinal cord without root involvement exhibit pain behaviors that are similar to those seen in patients with at-level neuropathic pain. The only distinguishing feature of at-level neuropathic pain arising from spinal cord damage appears to be that the pain is usually bilateral in distribution (Riddoch 1938; Burke and Woodward 1976). Although this type of pain may be difficult to distinguish from nerve root pain on the basis of descriptors, the distinction is important because the underlying mechanisms and therefore the recommended treatment may be different.

SYRINGOMYELIA

Syringomyelia must always be considered in the patient who has delayed onset of neuropathic pain, especially where there is a rising level of sensory loss (Frisbie and Aguilera 1990; Milhorat et al. 1996). A loss of pain and temperature sensation is typical, but all sensory and motor functions can be affected. Nashold (1991) reports that 65% of a group of paraplegics who had a delayed onset of pain exhibited syringomyelia, with an average onset 6 years after the initial spinal injury. Patients describe a constant, burning pain that may be associated with allodynia. Diagnosis is established by MR scan. The most effective treatment for the syrinx is surgical decompression of the arachnoid scar at the level of injury so that there is free flow of spinal fluid around the spinal cord. Treating the syrinx by inserting a drainage tube that goes either to the subarachnoid space or the peritoneal cavity provides less satisfactory long-term results. Even though the syrinx may collapse, the pain is not always relieved. Medications used for neuropathic pain may be helpful when syringomyelic pain persists after collapse of the syrinx.

BELOW-LEVEL NEUROPATHIC PAIN

This type of SCI pain is perceived more diffusely in anesthetic regions below the level of injury and is usually bilateral. It is often referred to as deafferentation pain, dysesthetic pain, or central dysesthesia syndrome (Davis and Martin 1947; Davidoff et al. 1987; Berić et al. 1988; Segatore 1992). Common descriptors are burning, tingling, numbness, aching, and throbbing. The pain is usually constant and is unrelated to position or activity, but may worsen with concurrent infections and may be triggered by sudden noises or jarring movements. Although it is difficult to allocate pain types described in the literature to specific categories, it appears that of all types of SCI pain, below-level neuropathic pain is the most common and the most difficult to treat successfully (Davis 1954; Bonica 1991). It is found in about 15–40% of SCI patients who complain of chronic pain (Berić 1997; Siddall et al. 1999). A double lesion phenomenon occurring in patients with cervical or thoracic cord injuries who developed lower motor neuron signs in the lumbosacral segments has also been described (Berić 1987). This type of pain usually responds poorly to opioids, but it may be relieved by neuropathic pain-relieving drugs. It may also respond to intrathecal opioids and clonidine when the systemic route is ineffective (Chapter 21). It does not usually respond to cordectomy or any other ablative procedure and only rarely responds to spinal cord or brain stimulation.

COGNITIVE, AFFECTIVE, AND ENVIRONMENTAL FACTORS

As would be expected, SCI results in significant psychological disruption. However, the prevalence and severity of disruption are not as high as many clinicians predict. Many patients who exhibit psychological morbidity return to normal limits within the first year following injury. Several authors mention "psychological" or "psychogenic" as a specific type of pain (Kaplan et al. 1962; Bedbrook 1981; Donovan et al. 1982; Davidoff and Roth 1991; Summers et al. 1991), while others specifically exclude this category (Bonica 1991; Britell and Mariano 1991; Mariano 1992). There is no doubt that psychological issues have tremendous importance in the experience and expression of pain (Craig 1994). Indeed, the disability ascribed to chronic pain is highly likely to be primarily related to psychosocial issues. It is also possible that the entirety of a patient's pain behaviors can be related to affective or environmental factors, but this is certainly not common. Therefore, while psychological factors may contribute to any of these pain types, "psychogenic pain" should not be considered an entity in its own right.

Of course, pain itself may also affect psychological status. Lundqvist et al. (1991) found that pain was the only complication of SCI that lowered quality of life scores, and Westgren and Levi (1998) reported that pain had more effect upon quality of life scores than did the extent of SCI. All pain syndromes related to SCI can benefit from the application of psychological management strategies (Summers et al. 1991).

A SYSTEM FOR CLASSIFICATION

A MECHANISMS-BASED TAXONOMY

The above description of pain types provides a comprehensive list of the different types of pain that are commonly seen following SCI. However, as mentioned above, one of the other desirable characteristics of a taxonomy is that it should be systematic. Several systems have been proposed based on location, descriptors, and pathology, or on a combination of these factors (Donovan et al. 1982; Siddall et al. 1997; Berić 1999; Bryce and Ragnarsson 2000). In common with the IASP taxonomy, some of these have several tiers to allow further definition. Dividing a taxonomy into tiers provides a structure that may aid clinical assessment, identification of mechanisms, and treatment. Our proposed taxonomy includes the pain types described above within a three-tier structure.

Each tier of the proposed taxonomy is broadly mechanisms based in that it aims to define the structure and pathology responsible for the pain. The first tier is very broad and simply divides pain into *nociceptive* and *neuropathic* types. This division is based on the presumed location of primary pathology that gives rise to the generation of afferent impulses rather than on the location of pathophysiology that may occur secondary to any change. We recognize that this is sometimes a difficult distinction to make both conceptually and clinically and that both of these types of pain have shared features and mechanisms. However, even though the clinical determination of nociceptive versus neuropathic pain is not always certain, these categories may be distinguishable on the basis of location and patient descriptors and have the strongest implications for any management approaches. Nociceptive pain is usually described as dull, aching, and cramping and occurs in a region of sensory preservation; it is presumably due to signals arising from somatic or visceral nociceptors. Neuropathic pain is usually described as sharp, shooting, electric, or burning, occurs in a region of sensory disturbance (increased or decreased sensibility), and is due to generation of impulses following damage to neural structures.

The second tier of classification provides further definition of these broad pain types and offers further direction for treatment. Nociceptive pain is divided into *musculoskeletal* and *visceral* pain types. Neuropathic pain is divided into *above-level*, *at-level,* and *below-level* neuropathic pain types, where level refers to the segmental level at which the spinal cord is damaged. Thus, below-level neuropathic pain will be present in the dermatomes below the level of neurological injury. The exception to this general rule is pain in the lower limbs that arises from damage to the cauda equina following lumbar vertebral injury. In this case the pain would be classified as at-level neuropathic pain. The second-tier grouping of SCI pain is shown in Table I.

The third tier of classification provides further refinement in terms of a specific structure and pathology and therefore more closely identifies a possible mechanism with implications for treatment. For example, musculoskeletal pain includes pain that may be due to muscle spasm, bone trauma, or inflammation around a joint. At-level neuropathic pain includes pain due to nerve root damage (including damage to the cauda equina), syringomyelia, or spinal cord trauma.

Psychological factors are not included in the taxonomy as a type of pain. Cognitive, affective, and environmental factors are often superimposed upon any of the pain types following SCI and should always be considered as contributing factors. As discussed above, psychological factors should be considered as part of any pain syndrome and not as a specific pain type.

TERMINOLOGY

Once the pain types to be included are identified, the next step is to decide on terminology. The choice of terms is influenced by several factors, including previous use, familiarity, "correctness," and the system that is to be used.

In the tier one division, the terms *nociceptive* and *neuropathic* are recommended. This familiar "first pass" classification is consistent with clinical use, simplifies assessment, and indicates treatment. Nociceptive pain is pain arising from stimulation of somatic or visceral nociceptors, and neuropathic pain is pain initiated or caused by a primary lesion or dysfunction in the nervous system (Merskey and Bogduk 1994). The term *neuropathic* is suggested rather than *neurogenic* to be consistent with the IASP taxonomy that limits the use of *neurogenic* to pain due to a *transitory* perturbation of the nervous system.

Table I
Tier two groupings

Term	Distinguishing Features
Musculoskeletal	Dull, aching, movement related, eased by rest, opioid and NSAID responsive, located in musculoskeletal structures
Visceral	Dull, cramping, located in abdominal region with preserved innervation, includes dysreflexic headache (vascular)
Neuropathic	Sharp, shooting, burning, electric, abnormal responsiveness (hyperesthesia, hyperalgesia)
Above-level	Located in the region of sensory preservation
At-level	Located in a segmental pattern at the level of injury
Below-level	Located diffusely below the level of injury

In the tier two division, nociceptive pain is divided into *musculoskeletal* and *visceral* pains, terms that are also in common use. Neuropathic pain is divided into types based on site (*above-*, *at-*, and *below-level* pain). Defining these types of pain relative to the level of SCI may be the best available option for further division, based on our current understanding of mechanisms. At-level neuropathic pain is located in dermatomes adjacent to the level of injury and may be due to specific pathology such as nerve root injury or syringomyelia. However, it may be present without any identifiable pathology other than spinal cord damage. SCI may also give rise to below-level neuropathic pain in the dermatomes below the level of injury. Therefore, there may be no distinction in terms of pathology, but only in location. If it is difficult to distinguish these types of pain on the basis of specific pathology (third tier), we suggest that they simply be referred to as *at-level* and *below-level* neuropathic pain.

In the tier three division, the primary objective is to identify a specific structure and pathology that may be acting as a pain generator. We have avoided using syndromes as terminology as much as possible. This division is often difficult because of the gaps in our understanding of mechanisms and the limitations of current diagnostic techniques. However, we feel that identification of a specific structure and pathology is an important step toward a mechanisms-based classification that will permit correct diagnosis and enable more effective treatment. Any limitations at this level may be an important guide in directing research into both understanding mechanisms and developing diagnostic tools.

USE OF THE PROPOSED TAXONOMY

The three tiers provide a structure for grouping different types of pain and provide some direction in assessment and management of SCI pain. The first tier provides a general direction in assessment and treatment, but we expect that most SCI pains will be classified at least at the second tier. We hope that with progress it will be increasingly possible to identify the structure and pathology (third tier) responsible for the generation of pain.

If it is possible to make a tier three diagnosis, then the tier two diagnosis becomes redundant. For example, if a patient has pain due to muscle spasm it would be referred to as muscle spasm pain rather than nociceptive/musculoskeletal/muscle spasm pain. In a situation where it is not possible to accurately identify a structure, then a second-tier term such as visceral or at-level neuropathic pain can be used.

Table II
Proposed taxonomy

Broad Type (Tier One)	Broad System (Tier Two)	Specific Structures and Pathology (Tier Three)
Nociceptive	Musculoskeletal	Bone, joint, muscle trauma or inflammation Mechanical instability Muscle spasm Secondary overuse syndromes
	Visceral	Renal calculus, bowel dysfunction, sphincter dysfunction, etc. Dysreflexic headache
Neuropathic	Above-level	Compressive mononeuropathies Complex regional pain syndromes
	At-level	Nerve root compression (including cauda equina) Syringomyelia Spinal cord trauma/ischemia (transitional zone, etc.) Dual-level cord and root trauma (double lesion syndrome)
	Below-level	Spinal cord trauma/ischemia (central dysesthesia syndrome, etc.)

Although we have taken a hierarchical approach in classifying tier two and three diagnoses (Table II), they are not meant to be exclusive or definitive. For example, visceral pain is classified as a nociceptive pain, which holds true if the evidence suggests that the pain is due to stimulation of visceral nociceptors. However, if it appears that there is no nociceptive generator then the pain may be reclassified as neuropathic. Similarly, CRPS is listed under above-level neuropathic pain, but it may occur below the level of injury. Syringomyelia may also produce pain above, at, and below the level of injury. Therefore, the taxonomy is not meant to indicate that these pathologies will only occur or only produce pain within these categories. It is only meant to indicate possible tier three diagnoses that may be responsible for this type of pain.

On behalf of the task force, we hope the proposed taxonomy will result in improved communication that will ultimately benefit both research and treatment. Further knowledge about the clinical characteristics and mechanisms of SCI pain should in turn lead to further improvements in the way this type of pain is classified.

ACKNOWLEDGMENTS

The authors would like to acknowledge the helpful contributions from members of the IASP Task Force on Pain following Spinal Cord Injury as well as the helpful suggestions and comments of Prof. Michael Cousins and Drs. David Taylor, James Middleton, Sue Rutkowski, William Donovan, and Elliot Roth.

REFERENCES

Aisen ML, Aisen PS. Shoulder-hand syndrome in cervical spinal cord injury. *Paraplegia* 1994; 32:588–592.

Bedbrook GM. Pain and phantom sensation. In: Bedbrook GM (Ed). *The Care and Management of Spinal Cord Injuries.* New York: Springer-Verlag, 1981, pp 224–229.

Berić A. A clinical syndrome of rostral and caudal spinal injury: neurological, neurophysiological and urodynamic evidence for occult sacral lesion. *J Neurol Neurosurg Psychiatry* 1987; 50:600–606.

Berić A. Altered sensation and pain in spinal cord injury. In: Dimitrijevic MR, Wall PD, Lindblom U (Eds). *Altered Sensation and Pain,* Recent Achievements in Restorative Neurology, Vol. 3. Basel: Karger, 1990, pp 27–36.

Berić A. Post-spinal cord injury pain states. *Pain* 1997; 72:295–298.

Berić A. Spinal cord damage: injury. In: Wall PD, Melzack R (Eds). *Textbook of Pain,* 4th ed. London: Churchill Livingstone, 1999, pp 915–927.

Berić A, Dimitrijevic MR, Lindblom U. Central dysesthesia syndrome in spinal cord injury patients. *Pain* 1988; 34:109–116.

Bonica JJ. Introduction: semantic, epidemiologic, and educational issues. In: Casey KL (Ed). *Pain and Central Nervous System Disease: The Central Pain Syndromes.* New York: Raven Press, 1991, pp 13–29.

Botterell EH, Callaghan JC, Jousse AT. Pain in paraplegia: clinical management and surgical treatment. *Proc R Soc Med* 1953; 47:281–288.

Britell CW, Mariano AJ. Chronic pain in spinal cord injury. *Phys Med Rehabil: State of the Art Reviews* 1991; 5:71–82.

Bryce TN, Ragnarsson KT. Pain after spinal cord injury. *Phys Med Rehabil Clin N Am* 2000; 11:157–168.

Burke DC. Pain in paraplegia. *Paraplegia* 1973; 10:297–313.

Burke DC, Woodward JM. Pain and phantom sensation in spinal paralysis. In: Vinken PJ, Bruyn GW (Eds). *Handbook of Clinical Neurology.* New York: Elsevier, 1976, pp 489–499.

Christensen MD, Everhart AW, Pickelman JT, Hulsebosch CE. Mechanical and thermal allodynia in chronic central pain following spinal cord injury. *Pain* 1996; 68:97–107.

Craig KD. Emotional aspects of pain. In: Wall PD, Melzack R (Eds). *Textbook of Pain,* 3rd ed. Edinburgh: Churchill Livingstone, 1994, pp 261–274.

Cremer S, Maynard F, Davidoff G. The reflex sympathetic dystrophy syndrome associated with traumatic myelopathy: report of 5 cases. *Pain* 1989; 37:187–192.

Dalyan M, Cardenas DD, Gerard B. Upper extremity pain after spinal cord injury. *Spinal Cord* 1999; 37:191–195.

Davidoff G, Roth EJ. Clinical characteristics of central (dysaesthetic) pain in spinal cord injury patients. In: Casey KL (Ed). *Pain and Central Nervous System Disease: The Central Pain Syndromes.* New York: Raven Press, 1991, pp 77–83.

Davidoff G, Roth E, Guarracini M, Sliwa J, Yarkony G. Function-limiting dysesthetic pain syndrome among traumatic spinal cord injury patients: a cross-sectional study. *Pain* 1987; 29:39–48.

Davidoff G, Werner RA, Waring WP. Compression mononeuropathies of the upper extremities in chronic paraplegia. *Paraplegia* 1991; 29:17–24.

Davis L. Treatment of spinal cord injuries. *AMA Arch Surg* 1954; 69:488–495.

Davis L, Martin J. Studies upon spinal cord injuries. *J Neurosurg* 1947; 4:483–491.

Davis R. Pain and suffering following spinal cord injury. *Clin Orthop* 1975; 112:76–80.

Demirel G, Yllmaz H, Gencosmanoglu B, Kesiktas N. Pain following spinal cord injury. *Spinal Cord* 1998; 36:25–28.

Donovan WH, Dimitrijevic MR, Dahm L, Dimitrijevic M. Neurophysiological approaches to chronic pain following spinal cord injury. *Paraplegia* 1982; 20:135–146.

Frisbie JH, Aguilera EJ. Chronic pain after spinal cord injury: an expedient diagnostic approach. *Paraplegia* 1990; 28:460–465.

Hao JX, Xu XJ, Aldskogius H, Seiger A, Wiesenfeld-Hallin Z. Allodynia-like effects in rat after ischaemic spinal cord injury photochemically induced by laser irradiation. *Pain* 1991; 45:175–185.

Holmes G. Pain of central origin. In: *Contributions to Medical and Biological Research,* Vol. 1. New York: P.B. Hoeber, 1919, pp 235–246.

Howe JF, Loeser JD, Calvin WH. Mechanosensitivity of dorsal root ganglia and chronically injured axons: a physiological basis for the radicular pain of nerve root compression. *Pain* 1977; 3:25–41.

Kakulas BA, Smith E, Gaekwad U, Kaelan C, Jacobsen PF. The neuropathology of pain and abnormal sensations in human spinal cord injury derived from the clinicopathological data base at the Royal Perth Hospital. In: Dimitrijevic MR, Wall PD, Lindblom U (Eds). *Altered Sensation and Pain,* Recent Achievements in Restorative Neurology, Vol. 3. Basel: Karger, 1990, pp 37–41.

Kaplan LI, Grynbaum BB, Lloyd KE, Rusk HA. Pain and spasticity in patients with spinal cord dysfunction. *JAMA* 1962; 182:918–925.

Komisaruk BR, Gerdes CA, Whipple B. "Complete" spinal cord injury does not block perceptual responses to genital self-stimulation in women. *Arch Neurol* 1997; 54:1513–1520.

Kuhn RA. Functional capacity of the isolated human spinal cord. *Brain* 1950; 73:1–51.

Lal S. Premature degenerative shoulder changes in spinal cord injury patients. *Spinal Cord* 1998; 36:186–189.

Lamid S, Chia JK, Kohli A, Cid E. Chronic pain in spinal cord injury: comparison between inpatients and outpatients. *Arch Phys Med Rehabil* 1985; 66:777–778.

Levi R, Hultling C, Nash MS, Seiger A. The Stockholm spinal cord injury study: 1. Medical problems in a regional SCI population. *Paraplegia* 1995; 33:308–315.

Levitt M, Levitt JH. The deafferentation syndrome in monkeys: dysaesthesias of spinal origin. *Pain* 1981; 10:129–147.

Lundqvist C, Siosteen A, Blomstrand C, Lind B, Sullivan M. Spinal cord injuries: clinical, functional, and emotional status. *Spine* 1991; 16:78–83.

Mariano AJ. Chronic pain and spinal cord injury. *Clin J Pain* 1992; 8:87–92.

Maury M. About pain and its treatment in paraplegics. *Paraplegia* 1978; 15:349–352.

Merskey H, Bogduk N. *Classification of Chronic Pain: Descriptions of Chronic Pain Syndromes and Definitions of Pain Terms.* Seattle: IASP Press, 1994.

Michaelis LS. The problem of pain in paraplegia and tetraplegia. *Bull NY Acad Med* 1970; 46:88–96.

Milhorat TH, Kotzen RM, Mu HTM, Capocelli AL, Milhorat RH. Dysesthetic pain in patients with syringomyelia. *Neurosurgery* 1996; 38:940–946.

Munro D. Two-year end-results in the total rehabilitation of veterans with spinal-cord and cauda-equina injuries. *N Engl J Med* 1950; 242:1–10.

Nashold BS. Paraplegia and pain. In: Nashold BS, Ovelmen-Levitt J (Eds). *Deafferentation Pain Syndromes: Pathophysiology and Treatment.* New York: Raven Press, 1991, pp 301–319.

Nepomuceno C, Fine PR, Richards JS, et al. Pain in patients with spinal cord injury. *Arch Phys Med Rehabil* 1979; 60:605–609.

New P. A survey of pain during rehabilitation after acute spinal cord injury. *Spinal Cord* 1997; 35:658–663.
Nichols PJ, Norman PA, Ennis JR. Wheelchair user's shoulder? Shoulder pain in patients with spinal cord lesion. *Scand J Rehabil Med* 1979; 11:29–32.
Philip PA, Philip M, Monga TN. Reflex sympathetic dystrophy in central cord syndrome: case report and review of the literature. *Paraplegia* 1990; 28:48–54.
Ravenscroft A, Ahmed YS, Burnside IG. Chronic pain after SCI: a patient survey. *Spinal Cord* 2000; 38:611–614.
Richards JS, Meredith RL, Nepomuceno C, Fine PR, Bennett G. Psycho-social aspects of chronic pain in spinal cord injury. *Pain* 1980; 8:355–366.
Richards JS, Stover SL, Jaworski T. Effect of bullet removal on subsequent pain in persons with spinal cord injury secondary to gunshot wound. *J Neurosurg* 1990; 73:401–404.
Riddoch G. The clinical features of central pain. *Lancet* 1938; 234:1150–1156.
Rintala D, Loubser PG, Castro J, Hart KA, Fuhrer MJ. Chronic pain in a community-based sample of men with spinal cord injury: prevalence, severity, and relationship with impairment, disability, handicap, and subjective well-being. *Arch Phys Med Rehabil* 1999; 79:604–614.
Rose M, Robinson JE, Ells P, Cole JD. Pain following spinal cord injury: results from a postal survey. *Pain* 1988; 34:101–102.
Segatore M. Deafferentation pain after spinal cord injury. Part 1. Theoretical aspects. *SCI Nursing* 1992; 9:46–50.
Siddall PJ, Xu CL, Cousins MJ. Allodynia following traumatic spinal cord injury in the rat. *Neuroreport* 1995; 6:1241–1244.
Siddall PJ, Taylor DA, Cousins MJ. Classification of pain following spinal cord injury. *Spinal Cord* 1997; 35:69–75.
Siddall PJ, Taylor DA, McClelland JM, Rutkowski SB, Cousins MJ. Pain report and the relationship of pain to physical factors in the first six months following spinal cord injury. *Pain* 1999; 81:187–197.
Stanton-Hicks M, Jänig W, Hassenbusch S, et al. Reflex sympathetic dystrophy: changing concepts and taxonomy. *Pain* 1995; 63:127–133.
Störmer S, Gerner HJ, Grüninger W, et al. Chronic pain/dysaesthesiae in spinal cord injury patients: results of a multicentre study. *Spinal Cord* 1997; 35:446–455.
Summers JD, Rapoff MA, Varghese G, Porter K, Palmer RE. Psychosocial factors in chronic spinal cord injury pain. *Pain* 1991; 47:183–189.
Vierck CJ, Light AR. Effects of combined hemotoxic and anterolateral spinal lesions on nociceptive sensitivity. *Pain* 1999; 83:447–457.
Waisbrod H, Hansen D, Gerbeshagen HV. Chronic pain in paraplegics. *Neurosurgery* 1984; 15:933–934.
Westgren N, Levi R. Quality of life and traumatic spinal cord injury. *Arch Phys Med Rehabil* 1998; 79:1433–1439.
Widerström-Noga EG, Felipe-Cuervo E, Broton JG, Duncan RC, Yezierski RP. Perceived difficulty in dealing with consequences of spinal cord injury. *Arch Phys Med Rehabil* 1999; 80:580–586.
Woolsey RM. Chronic pain following spinal cord injury. *J Am Paraplegia Soc* 1986; 9:39–41.
Yezierski RP, Liu S, Ruenes GL, Kajander KJ, Brewer KL. Excitotoxic spinal cord injury: behavioural and morphological characteristics of a central pain model. *Pain* 1998; 75:141–155.

Correspondence to: Philip Siddall, MBBS, PhD, Pain Management and Research Centre, Royal North Shore Hospital, St. Leonards, NSW 2065, Australia. Fax: 61-2-9926-6548; email: phils@med.usyd.edu.au.

Spinal Cord Injury Pain: Assessment, Mechanisms, Management. Progress in Pain Research and Management, Vol. 23, edited by Robert P. Yezierski and Kim J. Burchiel, IASP Press, Seattle, © 2002.

3

Classification of Spinal Cord Injury Pain: Literature Review and Future Directions

Bret L. Hicken, John D. Putzke, and J. Scott Richards

Department of Physical Medicine and Rehabilitation, University of Alabama at Birmingham, Birmingham, Alabama, USA

Pain is a common problem in persons with spinal cord injury (SCI). The prevalence of pain is well documented, but varies widely from 18% to 96% (Anson and Shepherd 1996; Demirel et al. 1998; Johnson et al. 1998; Siddall et al. 1999; Putzke et al., in press). The experience of chronic pain can have a substantial negative impact on many dimensions of quality of life, often causing decreased emotional well-being, impaired social functioning, and lower overall life satisfaction (Putzke et al., in press). Progress in the treatment of pain has been slow, and chronic pain continues to be a major problem for many individuals with SCI. One reason for the slow progress is the lack of a reliable, widely accepted system for the classification of SCI pain. Accurate classification of pain is important for communication among health professionals and for meaningful interpretations of research findings. Likewise, if the underlying pathology is distinct for individual pain subtypes, then accurate classification of pain will be essential for maximal treatment response.

This chapter focuses on the challenging task of categorizing SCI pain into meaningful subtypes. First, we review SCI pain classification systems published in the literature over the last 50 years, discuss the numerous pain subtypes and criteria proposed in these schemes, and review some of their limitations. We then review psychometric issues related to classification schemes and methods of measuring reliability and validity. Finally, we discuss ongoing psychometric research on existing pain classification systems and outline future directions for classification of SCI pain.

CLASSIFICATION SCHEMES

We reviewed the pain and rehabilitation literature to find articles that classified SCI-associated pain into distinct subtypes and reported criteria associated with those subtypes. We identified 28 such classification schemes published between 1947 and 2000 (Davis and Martin 1947; Freeman and Heimburger 1947; Pollock et al. 1951; Davis 1954; Krueger 1960; Kaplan et al. 1962; Michaelis 1970; Burke 1973; Guttmann 1973; Davis 1975; Hohmann 1975; Melzack and Loeser 1978; Donovan et al. 1982; Bedbrook 1985; Tunks 1986; Woolsey 1986; Frisbie and Aguilera 1990; Bonica 1991; Nashold Jr. 1991; Britell and Mariano 1991; Segatore 1994; Anke et al. 1995; Beric 1997; Christensen and Hulsebosch 1997; Siddall et al. 1997, 1999; Demirel et al. 1998; Bryce and Ragnarsson 2000).[1]

A few of these classification schemes are formalized systems for classifying SCI pain that were described in articles that specifically focused on this topic (Donovan et al. 1982; Tunks 1986; Siddall et al. 1997, 1999; Bryce and Ragnarsson 2000). More often, however, pain subtypes and criteria were reported within the methods section of an empirical paper that described the procedure for classifying pain prior to intervention. In a few cases, pain subtypes and criteria were discussed briefly in a review article about SCI but were not the specific focus of that review. Consequently, some classification schemes included in our review provided relatively little information beyond listing subtypes and a few simple criteria for classification. Regardless of the criteria provided, however, we included in our review any article that reported distinct SCI pain categories. The recent SCI pain classification system sponsored by the International Association for the Study of Pain (IASP; Siddall et al. 2000), which was not included in our review, is discussed in detail in Chapter 2.

There was substantial variability in the number of pain types included in each of the 28 schemes and in the number of criteria used to classify pain. Five pain subtypes were included on average per scheme (range = 2–15 subtypes). This average decreased to four subtypes, however, when three systems with a large number of pain types were excluded from the total (Beric 1997, 12 types; Bryce and Ragnarsson 2000, 15 types; Tunks 1986, 9 types). We identified 44 different labels for pain types across the different schemes, many of which were probably used to describe the same underlying type of pain. Variability was also considerable in the type and number of criteria used to define types of pain. Despite this heterogeneity, however,

[1] A table summarizing these classification schemes is too lengthy to appear in this volume but is available from the authors of this chapter on request.

classification of pain following SCI appears to follow two basic approaches—etiological and descriptive.

ETIOLOGICAL APPROACH

This approach focuses on physiological or physical mechanisms that precede or cause the pain. These mechanisms distinguish pain types from each other. While other pain criteria may also be included in the scheme, they are of secondary importance to etiology. Most authors who described visceral pain, for example, focused mainly on etiological factors such as bowel and bladder distension rather than on other criteria such as verbal pain descriptors. Pain types for which there is limited understanding of the physiological or physical sequelae leading to pain (e.g., central pain) generally rely on other criteria such as verbal descriptors to describe the pain. For other pain types, such as musculoskeletal pain, for which there is general agreement as to etiology (e.g., tissue damage), other criteria received less emphasis.

DESCRIPTIVE APPROACH

Descriptive systems, in contrast, focus on pain factors that tend to cluster together and seem to be associated with certain pain types. These factors often include location of the pain site, duration of painful episodes, time of onset of pain after SCI, verbal descriptors of the pain, and factors that aggravate and mitigate the pain. Theoretically, each pain subtype within a descriptive scheme would have a unique set of descriptors that distinguish it from other subtypes. Descriptive systems may also include information about etiology, but this criterion is not central to the classification of pain. For example, the classification scheme proposed by Donovan et al. (1982), while containing information about the possible etiology of each pain subtype, relies mainly on descriptive criteria to classify pain.

COMPARISON OF UTILITY OF ETIOLOGICAL AND DESCRIPTIVE SCHEMES

A scheme based primarily on etiology would ultimately be the most useful and psychometrically sound method of classifying pain because it would be less susceptible to bias from patient memory, pain tolerance, psychological history, and physician experience, factors that may have a substantial impact on reporting of descriptive criteria. Few schemes rely exclusively on etiology to distinguish among pain types, however, and the utility of such a system is limited by two factors. First, the etiology of some of the types of SCI pain has not been completely determined. Second, even in situations in which pain etiology is well understood, it would probably be expensive and time consuming to determine the etiology for each pain type experienced by a person with SCI. Thus, systems based solely on etiological criteria are likely to be cost-prohibitive. Etiology may be more important in defining treatment options and in understanding mechanisms of pain relief. Thus, descriptive factors may be a more cost-effective method for classifying pain into subtypes, with some exceptions, and etiology may be better suited for guiding treatment decisions and the development of new treatments.

While some classification schemes place greater emphasis on either etiological or descriptive factors in describing pain types, most systems utilize both etiological and descriptive criteria to classify pain. Many schemes "mix and match" by applying descriptive and etiological criteria to different pain types within the scheme. For example, Bonica (1991) used a single descriptive criterion to classify central pain, with the verbal descriptors "burning," "lancinating," and "dysesthetic"). However, he described visceral pain mainly in terms of etiological criteria such as full bladder or fecal impaction. The 28 schemes varied considerably in terms of how consistently diagnostic criteria were applied to pain types. Only Donovan et al. (1982) applied the same criteria to all five subtypes in their system. For each pain subtype, the authors described a unique set of verbal pain descriptors, onset, duration, and mitigating or aggravating factors. In contrast, many other schemes relied on only one or two criteria to define a pain type and did not uniformly apply these criteria to other pain types within the scheme.

CLASSIFICATION CRITERIA

In the 28 published classification schemes reviewed for this chapter, seven criteria were most commonly used to classify pain. These criteria were location of the pain site, verbal descriptors of pain character, duration of pain episodes, time between injury and onset of pain, factors that aggravate pain, factors that mitigate pain, and etiology of the pain. All classification schemes included at least one of these seven criteria. However, our labels for these criteria represent our conceptualization of the authors' descriptions and may differ somewhat from the authors' original intent.

Character (verbal descriptors). This criterion refers to terms that patients and physicians use to describe how the pain feels. Twenty-six (93%) of the classification schemes included verbal descriptors of the pain to classify at least one pain type. However, only eight of the schemes reported verbal descriptors for every pain type within the scheme (Davis and Martin 1947; Freeman and Heimburger 1947; Donovan et al. 1982; Frisbie and

Aguilera 1990; Britell and Mariano 1991; Anke et al. 1995; Siddall et al. 1997; Demirel et al. 1998). More often, the different schemes described a few types using verbal descriptors while other subtypes were classified using other criteria. Neuropathic pains such as central pain and nerve root pain generally included verbal pain descriptors as one of the classification criteria, while visceral pain was generally described in terms of etiology. The one pain type that was never described by any author with specific verbal descriptors was "psychic" pain.

Location. Twenty-six schemes utilized some type of information regarding somatic location of the pain to classify pain subtype. *Location* in this context is intended to mean any terms used to describe the distribution of pain across the body. Thus, while some scales assigned a specific body location to a pain type, for example, the abdomen as the site of visceral pain, other scales described pain location in terms of its position relative to the lesion level. Davis (1975), for example, describes central pain as occurring in areas below the lesion level. A few scales used lesion level as a means of further classifying pain using "above-level," "at-level," and "below-level" to describe pain location. For example, while many scales included central pain as a subtype, a few systems (e.g., Bryce and Ragnarsson 2000) labeled central pain in terms of its position relative to the lesion level (e.g., "at-level central pain," "below-level central pain").

Other common uses of location information included describing the pain site as being either "localized," "diffuse," "radiating," "asymmetric," "symmetric," "bilateral," "in areas of sensory loss," "the site of injury," and "segmental." A few pain types associated with a specific body location were included (e.g., visceral pain, fracture site pain, headache). Guttmann (1973) described musculoskeletal pain as being located in the shoulders and arms and Beric (1997) described phantom pain as being located in the rectal area, feet, legs, and perineum. Bryce and Ragnarsson (2000) located neuropathic-at level-complex regional pain syndrome in the upper extremities and Michaelis (1970) described root pain as radiating to the arms, legs, and abdomen, depending on the lesion level.

Etiology. Another commonly used criterion, etiology, was included in 90% of schemes and refers to any physical, physiological, or psychological factors that are thought to precede the onset of pain. This criterion also includes references to specific aspects of the neurological injury (e.g., central pain is more common with cauda equina injuries; Segatore 1994). As with the other criteria, etiology was not universally applied to every pain type. The pain types that most frequently included etiological criteria were visceral pain (due to distended bowel or bladder), musculoskeletal pain (due to muscle overuse), and syringomyelia pain (due to a syrinx).

Onset and duration. *Onset* refers to the time span (in days, weeks, months, or years) between the time of injury and the onset of pain at a particular site. *Duration* refers to the length in time of painful episodes (minutes, hours, constant) and to the likelihood that pain will cease over time. These were some of the least utilized criteria. Of the 28 schemes reviewed, only 41% used information about onset, and 48% included duration of painful episodes.

Mitigating and aggravating factors. These variables were also used less frequently than location, character, and etiology; 41% of the schemes included mitigating factors and 69% included aggravating factors.

Validity of classification criteria. The percentages presented above may be somewhat misleading because they refer to schemes that included that criterion in the classification of at least one pain subtype in the scheme. Aside from Donovan et al. (1982), none of the schemes incorporated every criterion universally across the different pain types. It could be inferred, however, that having only three or four of the seven criteria commonly used is evidence that the other criteria may be less important for classification. Unfortunately, no empirical data exist to support that assumption.

More problematic, however, is the substantial disagreement among schemes about the nature of the criteria included. For example, several authors report that central pain gradually recedes over time (Davis and Martin 1947; Michaelis 1970; Guttmann 1973; Davis 1975), while others indicate that it is experienced chronically (Freeman and Heimburger 1947; Tunks 1986; Demirel et al. 1998). However, there is less disagreement among the schemes on location, etiology, character, and aggravating factors, suggesting that these criteria may be more reliable than the other ones used. Again no data exist to support or reject this claim. Additional research is needed to examine the validity and reliability of these and other potential classification criteria.

In many cases, criteria are not mutually exclusive to a particular pain type within a scheme. For example, many scales used "burning" as an indicator of both segmental and central pain. However, one would assume that each pain type would have a unique combination of criteria. More problematic, however, is that a patient's description of pain may not match the unique combination of criteria delineated for a specific pain type (i.e., the patient may provide information that conflicts with all established pain types). For example, a patient may describe pain as "crushing," a term that does not appear in most schemes. Unfortunately, none of the classification schemes provides information on how to prioritize the criteria for a specific pain type when inconsistencies occur. Both quantitative scaling and qualitative signs may be used to help resolve conflicting criteria. For instance, quantitative severity or intensity ratings could be used to more specifically determine which pain type best fits the criterion (e.g., severe "burning" may typify segmental pain, as opposed to mild "burning" with visceral pain). Relatedly, qualitative criteria may also be helpful for resolving conflicting criteria to the extent that a qualitative pathognomic sign can be identified that is specific to a particular pain type.

A second issue relates to the number of pain types included in each scheme. Some authors restricted the number of subtypes to pain exclusive to, or most commonly found in, persons with SCI. Thus, pain types also experienced by non-SCI populations were not included in these schemes. For example, some schemes did not include above-lesion musculoskeletal pains in their classification because such pains are not unique to persons with SCI. Conversely, other schemes attempted to be all-inclusive, incorporating and classifying all possible pain types that might be experienced by persons with SCI, including acute pains associated with recovery from tissue damage (Beric 1997) and headaches.

A third limitation relates to the data on which classification schemes are based. These data are mainly derived from three different sources. First, several schemes appear to be mainly based on clinical experience rather than on systematically collected data (e.g., interviews with patients regarding their pain). Data based on anecdotal clinical experience are obviously limited by the patient population to which the authors are exposed, a population that may not be representative of individuals with SCI in other geographic locations. Similarly, systems based on clinician experience are more subject to personal bias because categories are not based on an objective standard. Several schemes fit this description, including those of Guttmann (1973), Anke et al. (1995), and Christensen and Hulsebosch (1997).

Second, several classification schemes were derived from data obtained from an empirical study of a population of persons with SCI. These descriptive studies measured the prevalence of different types of pain and assessed other criteria associated with each particular pain type including location, character, pain onset, duration, and aggravating and mitigating factors (see Woolsey 1986 and Frisbie and Aguilera 1990 for an example of schemes based on a study of SCI patients). A major limitation to this data source is small sample size, which limits the generalizability of these classification categories to other SCI populations and also limits the number of pain types and criteria that might be seen in a larger population. Also, many of these studies attempted to fit patients' pain into predefined categories that were created, most often, from clinical experience, the limitations of which have been discussed, or from a review of the literature.

Classification schemes based on a review of existing literature also have inherent limitations. A few schemes were created based on careful review of existing schemes and other literature on pain associated with SCI (Bryce and Ragnarsson 2000). This approach synthesizes criteria and subtypes across many different schemes to create additional criteria and pain subtypes. The approach is limited, however, by the fact that any literature review is based on schemes that were derived from personal clinical experience or from data obtained from a small sample of patients. Thus, any classification scheme based solely on a review and synthesis of previous schemes will suffer from the same weaknesses as the systems on which it is based.

We do not suggest that it is inappropriate to use any of these data sources. On the contrary, they are an important part of the design process of a classification system. However, none of the published classification schemes, to our knowledge, is accompanied by reliability or validity data. An examination of the psychometric characteristics of any rating scheme is essential if it is to become a useful tool for research and treatment.

PSYCHOMETRIC ISSUES

Reliability refers to the consistency or stability of a score or rating or the likelihood that the rating will remain the same over time (e.g., likelihood that a particular pain classification will remain unchanged). Reliability is of fundamental importance to classification schemes because it is a necessary component of validity and clinical utility. In other words, for a scale to be valid it must first be shown to be reliable. *Validity,* more difficult to define and measure, refers to the degree to which a scale measures what it is intended to measure or the degree to which scores or classifications reflect an underlying construct or variable (e.g., the degree to which a label of visceral pain reflects a distinct phenomenon). Both reliability and validity must be established before a scale can be useful in clinical and research settings. Several approaches to estimation of reliability and validity that are particularly applicable to classification schemes are described below.

Inter-rater reliability. This type of reliability refers to agreement between two observers on independent measurements of the same variable. High inter-rater reliability is obtained when two or more clinicians with similar experience classify the same pain with an identical pain subtype. This agreement suggests that the classification categories are clearly distinguishable from one another and that any experienced SCI clinician would be likely to make the same classification decision. Conversely, low inter-rater reliability suggests that the pain subtypes in the scheme may not be mutually exclusive phenomena or that the classification criteria do not clearly rule out competing subtypes. To estimate inter-rater reliability of a classification scheme, two or more independent raters must classify a set of pain sites according to the criteria of the chosen classification scheme. The percentage of agreement among the raters is then calculated as a rough indication of inter-rater reliability. Kappa statistics may be computed as a statistical indicator of whether the observed inter-rater agreement is greater than what would be expected by chance.

Test-retest reliability. Conceptually the simplest approach to estimating reliability, test-retest reliability refers to the consistency or stability of scores (or classifications) over time (Pedhazur and Schmelkin 1991). In the context of pain following SCI, one would expect that a pain site classified with a given pain type (e.g., musculoskeletal pain) would be assigned the same pain type if it were re-evaluated at some future date (provided no additional information had been added that might be pertinent to classification). Thus, high test-retest reliability would be obtained when pain classifications remain consistent over time. An estimate of test-retest reliability is simply a correlation among repeated observations (separated by a reasonable time interval) of the same factor (Pedhazur and Schmelkin 1991). High positive correlations suggest good test-retest reliability.

Predictive (or criterion-referenced) validity. This type of validity refers to the degree to which ratings predict a specified outcome (e.g., response to targeted pain treatments). To conduct a study of the predictive validity of a given classification scheme, researchers would systematically classify a set of persons with SCI who are experiencing pain. All individuals, regardless of pain type, would receive a targeted treatment and would then be evaluated on a predetermined outcome. If the classification scheme has predictive validity, persons with the pain type to which the treatment is targeted will show the best response. For example, to determine whether a classification of central pain predicts response to a targeted medication, a group of persons with SCI-related pain would be classified based on a scheme that includes a central pain category. All individuals would then receive a medication hypothesized to be effective in treating central pain. If the scale has predictive validity, then individuals with central pain will exhibit the most favorable response to the medication relative to individuals with other pain classifications.

Concurrent validity. Concurrent validity is the degree to which ratings from one scheme correlate with those from another scheme that measures the same factor. In other words, individuals with central pain according to one scheme should be classified with central pain on another scheme. Unfortunately, concurrent validity assumes a gold standard of measurement to which other scales could be compared. Obviously, in the case of classification of SCI pain, no gold standard exists, and none of the schemes appears to have been universally accepted and used in clinical research and practice. Thus, the usefulness of this type of validity is somewhat limited in this context.

Construct validity. This type of validity is "concerned with the validity of inferences about unobserved variables (constructs) on the basis of observed variables (construct indicators)" (Pedhazur and Schmelkin 1991). *Construct validity* refers to the degree to which observable or measurable criteria reflect an underlying unobservable factor, or construct. In the case of classification of SCI pain, pain subtype would be the unobservable construct, and the different classification criteria (e.g., location, etiology) would be observed variables. As with other types of validity, construct validity can only be inferred because the variable in question cannot be directly measured. One method of inferring construct validity is through statistical analyses such as factor or cluster analysis that group criteria together independent of any classification scheme. If criteria are grouped according to the pain types described in the scheme, construct validity can be inferred.

RECOMMENDATIONS AND FUTURE DIRECTIONS

The importance of accurate pain classification and the need for assessment of reliability and validity cannot be underestimated. We lack published information regarding the reliability, validity, and utility of the pain classification schemes described in this chapter. Studies examining the psychometric properties of these classification schemes are needed.

We have initiated several studies to examine the psychometric properties of several pain classification schemes. In a recent study of the interrater reliability of the scheme published by Donovan et al. (1982), three experienced SCI clinicians rated 60 pain sites according to the proposed criteria (Richards et al., in press). Disagreement across the three raters on pain classification was observed on 40–50% of the pain sites evaluated. Even when using less stringent criteria for agreement, such as agreement between paired raters, clinicians still disagreed on about 30–40% of the pain sites. These results are even more disappointing considering that the vast majority of the pain sites were categorized by all three raters into only three of the five Donovan pain types (i.e., over 97% of the pain sites were either mechanical pain, SCI pain, or segmental pain). Kappa statistics for three-way and paired agreement were below traditional cutoffs considered to be at the low end of the acceptable range. A second study currently underway

(J.S. Richards et al., unpublished data) examines the inter-rater reliability of an early version of the IASP classification system (Siddall et al. 2000) and another system described by Tunks (1986).

We have also examined (J.D. Putzke, unpublished manuscript) the utility of verbal descriptors taken from the short form of the McGill Pain Questionnaire (MPQ) in the classification of pain according to the classification schemes of Donovan et al. (1982), Tunks (1986), and IASP (Siddall et al. 2000). Within each classification scheme, none of the verbal descriptors was specific to a particular type of pain. That is, every verbal descriptor from the MPQ was endorsed at least 8% of the time by our sample for each of the three most common pain types across classification schemes (except that none of the participants endorsed "sickening" for Tunks' myofascial pain). Even when considering endorsement only within the "moderate to severe" intensity range, there was considerable overlap across the three most common pain types for each of the MPQ descriptors. Thus, there does not appear to be a pathognomic verbal descriptor that can be used to identify a specific pain type. However, cluster analysis revealed that, in general, "aching" tended to be associated with mechanical pain and "tingling" and "sickening" with neuropathic pain (J.D. Putzke, unpublished manuscript). This finding is consistent with our earlier review of SCI pain classification literature that indicated that 78% of SCI pain classification schemes considered "aching" to be characteristic of mechanical pain, whereas 54% of schemes used "tingling" to describe neuropathic pain.

One question that remains unresolved concerns whether narrowly defined pain types are clinically useful. Will different pain types be differentially responsive to targeted treatments? If assigning a pain type does not imply a unique therapeutic aim, then the clinical utility of that pain category is in doubt. Obviously, a great deal of research is needed to examine the clinical utility of pain types. However, a recently published study suggests some progress in this area. Sindou and colleagues (2001), examining the dorsal root entry zone (DREZ) coagulation procedure in SCI patients, suggested that certain treatments are more effective with certain pain types. In that study, patients with segmental pain reported significantly greater pain relief relative to individuals with diffuse pain.

Another issue to be resolved concerns whether scales should be inclusive and incorporate all types of pain experienced by persons with SCI, even those not uniquely or commonly associated with SCI. A related question is whether many pain subtypes should be used to reflect the many nuances of pain experienced by persons with SCI or whether pain categories should be broader and include only general classes of pain (e.g., neuropathic pain instead of central or nerve root pain). All-inclusive systems will, as a consequence, have numerous pain categories. Unfortunately, as more categories are included in a scale, reliability, especially inter-rater reliability, tends to decrease. Thus, the detailed classification provided by such schemes would most likely come at the cost of reliability and, consequently, validity. Conversely, classification schemes with broadly defined categories that include only those pain types most commonly experienced by persons with SCI would probably be much more reliable. Increased reliability would, of course, come at a cost with regard to diagnostic specificity.

This issue could be resolved through studies that collect numerous predictor variables (e.g., location, onset, verbal descriptors, and lesion level) from a large population of persons with SCI who report pain. Cluster analysis could then be performed to statistically group predictors into specific pain types independently of any predetermined classification scheme. These pain types and their corresponding predictors (criteria) would constitute a new classification scheme that would also need to be evaluated psychometrically.

A classification scheme is needed for pain following SCI that is psychometrically sound, universally accepted, and easily applied, similar to the American Spinal Injury Association's neurological standards, which have become the standard method of classifying the severity of SCI and are accepted and endorsed by clinicians and professional groups and used almost universally in research on and treatment of SCI. The proposed IASP classification scheme described in Chapter 2 is a good start toward creating a standard classification system for SCI pain. However, the psychometric properties of this system must also be carefully evaluated. If the classification system demonstrates adequate reliability and validity, it will become an important tool in the diagnosis and treatment of SCI pain.

ACKNOWLEDGMENTS

Resources for the production of this manuscript were provided by the University of Alabama at Birmingham Model Spinal Cord Injury System of Care grant #H133N50009 from the National Institute on Disability and Rehabilitation Research, Office of Special Education and Rehabilitation Services; by the National Institutes of Health, National Research Service Award T32 HD07420-10; by the National Center for Medical Rehabilitation Research; and by Rehabilitation Research Training Center grant #H133B980016-00 from the National Institute on Disability and Rehabilitation Research, Office of Special Education and Rehabilitation Services.

REFERENCES

Anke AG, Stenehjem AE, Stanghelle JK. Pain and life quality within 2 years of spinal cord injury. *Paraplegia* 1995; 33:555–559.

Anson CA, Shepherd C. Incidence of secondary complications in spinal cord injury. *Int J Rehabil Res* 1996; 19:55–66.

Bedbrook G. Pain in paraplegia and tetraplegia. In: Bedbrook GM (Ed). *Lifetime Care of the Paraplegic Patient.* New York: Churchill Livingstone, 1985, pp 245–248.

Beric A. Post-spinal cord injury pain states. *Pain* 1997; 72:295–298.

Bonica J. Introduction: semantic, epidemiologic, and educational issues. In: Casey K (Ed). *Pain and Central Nervous System Disease: The Central Pain Syndromes.* New York: Raven Press, 1991, pp 13–29.

Britell C, Mariano A. Chronic pain in spinal cord injury. *Phys Med Rehabil: State of the Art Rev* 1991; 5:71–82.

Bryce TN, Ragnarsson KT. Pain after spinal cord injury. *Phys Med Rehabil Clin N Am* 2000; 11:157–168.

Burke DC. Pain in paraplegia. *Paraplegia* 1973; 10:297–313.

Christensen MD, Hulsebosch CE. Chronic central pain after spinal cord injury. *J Neurotrauma* 1997; 14:517–537.

Davis L. Treatment of spinal cord injuries. *Arch Surg* 1954; 69:488–495.

Davis L, Martin J. Studies upon spinal cord injuries. II. The nature and treatment of pain. *J Neurosurg* 1947; 4:483–491.

Davis R. Pain and suffering following spinal cord injury. *Clin Orthop* 1975; 112:76–80.

Demirel G, Yllmaz H, Gencosmanoglu B, Kesiktas N. Pain following spinal cord injury. *Spinal Cord* 1998; 36:25–28.

Donovan WH, Dimitrijevic MR, Dahm L, Dimitrijevic M. Neurophysiological approaches to chronic pain following spinal cord injury. *Paraplegia* 1982; 20:135–146.

Freeman L, Heimburger R. Surgical relief of pain in paraplegic patients. *Arch Surg* 1947; 55:433–440.

Frisbie JH, Aguilera EJ. Chronic pain after spinal cord injury: an expedient diagnostic approach. *Paraplegia* 1990; 28:460–465.

Guttmann L. *Spinal Cord Injuries: Comprehensive Management and Research.* Oxford: Blackwell Scientific, 1973.

Hohmann GW. Psychological aspects of treatment and rehabilitation of the spinal cord injured person. *Clin Orthop* 1975; 112:81–88.

Johnson R, Gerhart K, McCray J, Menconi J, Whiteneck G. Secondary conditions following spinal cord injury in a population-based sample. *Spinal Cord* 1998; 36:45–50.

Kaplan L, Brynbaum B, Lloyd E, Rusk H. Pain and spasticity in patients with spinal cord dysfunction. *JAMA* 1962; 182:918–925.

Krueger E. Management of painful states in injuries of the spinal cord and cauda equina. *Am J Phys Med* 1960; 39:103–110.

Melzack R, Loeser JD. Phantom body pain in paraplegics: evidence for a central "pattern generating mechanism" for pain. *Spinal Cord* 1978; 4:195–210.

Michaelis LS. The problem of pain in paraplegia and tetraplegia. *Bull NY Acad Med* 1970; 46:88–96.

Nashold B Jr. Paraplegia and pain. In: Nashold Jr B, Ovelmen-Levitt J (Eds). *Deafferentation Pain Syndromes: Pathophysiology and Treatment.* New York: Raven Press, 1991, pp 301–319.

Pedhazur E, Schmelkin L. *Measurement, Design, and Analysis: An Integrated Approach.* Hillsdale, NJ: Lawrence Erlbaum, 1991.

Pollock L, Brown M, Boshes B, et al. Pain below the level of injury of the spinal cord. *Arch Neurol* 1951; 65:319–322.

Putzke J, Richards J, Hicken B, DeVivo M. Pain following spinal cord injury: important predictors and impact on quality of life. *Pain;* in press.

Richards JS, Hicken B, Putzke JD, Ness TJ, Kazar L. Classification of pain following spinal cord injury: inter-rater reliability of the Donovan pain classification scheme. *Arch Phys Med Rehabil;* in press.

Segatore M. Understanding chronic pain after spinal cord injury. *J Neurosci Nurs* 1994; 26:230–236.

Siddall PJ, Taylor DA, Cousins MJ. Classification of pain following spinal cord injury. *Spinal Cord* 1997; 35:69–75.

Siddall PJ, Taylor DA, McClelland JM, Rutkowski SB, Cousins MJ. Pain report and the relationship of pain to physical factors in the first 6 months following spinal cord injury. *Pain* 1999; 81:187–197.

Siddall P, Yezierski R, Loeser J. Pain following spinal cord injury: clinical features, prevalence, and taxonomy. *IASP Newsletter* 2000; 3:3–7.

Sindou M, Mertens P, Wael M. Microsurgical DREZotomy for pain due to spinal cord and/or cauda equina injuries: long-term results in a series of 44 patients. *Pain* 2001; 92:159–171.

Tunks E. Pain in spinal cord injured patients. In: Bloch R, Basbaum M (Eds). *Management of Spinal Cord Injuries.* Baltimore: Williams and Wilkins, 1986, pp 180–211.

Woolsey RM. Chronic pain following spinal cord injury. *J Am Paraplegia Soc* 1986; 9:39–41.

Correspondence to: J. Scott Richards, PhD, Spain Rehabilitation Center, 1717 6th Avenue South, Room 529, Birmingham, AL 35233-7330, USA. Tel: 205-934-3450; Fax: 205-975-4691; email: richard@sun.rehabam.uab.edu.

Spinal Cord Injury Pain: Assessment, Mechanisms, Management. Progress in Pain Research and Management, Vol. 23, edited by Robert P. Yezierski and Kim J. Burchiel, IASP Press, Seattle, © 2002.

4

Assessment of Pain and Sensory Abnormalities in Patients with Spinal Cord Injury

Ellen Jørum

Laboratory of Clinical Neurophysiology, Department of Neurology, The National Hospital, Oslo, Norway

This chapter reviews the assessment of pain and sensory abnormalities in patients with spinal cord injury (SCI), describing quantitative sensory testing (QST) and its results in patients with SCI. Studies report a high prevalence of pain following SCI of around 65% (Bonica 1991; Störmer et al. 1997). Neuropathic pain is especially problematic due to limitations of treatment. This chapter focuses on the evaluation of neuropathic pain, which, according to the International Association for the Study of Pain (IASP) is "pain initiated or caused by a primary lesion or dysfunction in the nervous system" (Merskey and Bogduk 1994). Neuropathic pain following SCI may occur in segments above, at, and below the level of injury and may be caused by compressive mononeuropathies, nerve root compression, or injury to the spinal cord (Siddall et al. 1997, 2000). Few studies present results from QST in the evaluation of SCI pain, and information is limited about findings at different spinal cord levels caused by various lesions.

Nociceptive pain is also accompanied by sensory abnormalities (Hansson and Lindblom 1993). Both muscle pain (Graven-Nielsen et al. 1997) and visceral pain referred to skin (Vecchiet et al. 1989) may also show sensory abnormalities. Thus, sensory abnormalities are not restricted to neuropathic pain conditions, and may reflect the involvement of common neurophysiological mechanisms (mainly involving central sensitization). Nociceptive pain with secondary involvement of central sensitization mechanisms may be difficult to differentiate from neuropathic pain. Although the use of QST may be of great value, the results of such tests are difficult to interpret unless they are correlated with the patient's overall clinical picture.

That picture includes the patient's history and symptoms, the results of clinical neurological testing, and in many cases supplementary testing to determine nerve injury (computed tomography, magnetic resonance, or clinical neurophysiological testing).

Recently, Woolf et al. (1998) proposed a mechanism-based pain classification of pain. In a broad sense, this view implies that instead of classifying a painful condition according to its etiology, we should try to identify and classify the various pathophysiological mechanisms involved. Neuropathic pains of different etiologies may involve similar pathophysiological mechanisms. The general idea is that treatment can be targeted against the different underlying mechanisms. The challenge for both basic and clinical researchers will be to identify these neurophysiological mechanisms and to develop appropriate clinical testing procedures. At this stage, we are far from a full understanding of the basic mechanisms. We are still at the starting point in this process and do not yet know whether it will be possible to identify relevant pathophysiological mechanisms by examining patients. QST and tests of central hyperexcitability are of value in the clinical evaluation of patients.

CLINICAL CHARACTERISTICS OF NEUROPATHIC PAIN

Neuropathic pain following SCI will in many respects have the same clinical characteristics as neuropathic pain of other origin. Typically, the patient with neuropathic pain will complain of several types of pain, but interindividual variability is substantial. Most patients will complain of constant pain, of which the quality may vary, with typical descriptions including "burning," "aching," or "sore." This constant pain may vary spontaneously in intensity, but will typically be intensified by physical activity and by exposure to cold. Many patients will suffer from paroxysmal pain lasting from a few seconds to several minutes, both within the painful area and radiating from it. The frequency may vary from a few times a week to several times a day. Paroxysmal pain may be described as "shooting," "intense," and "sharp." Typically the patient also complains of evoked pain, mostly pain evoked by lightly touching the skin or by exposure to wind. The painful condition may worsen over time, often resulting in an increase in the area of pain or an intensification of constant pain.

NEUROPATHIC PAIN FOLLOWING SPINAL CORD INJURY

Much of the information available on neuropathic pain following SCI is based on interviews rather than on clinical testing. Many patients report neuropathic pain starting at the time of injury or shortly afterwards (New et al. 1997; Störmer et al. 1997) and sometimes intensifying over time. Neuropathic pain occurs mostly below the level of injury. Data about above-level neuropathic pain are scarce, although the literature describes cases of syringomyelia (New et al. 1997), and there is little information as to whether such pain is derived from injury to the cord or to nerve roots.

In a large study of 901 SCI patients, Störmer et al. (1997) found that a total of 66% of patients suffered from pain and/or dysesthesia, with pain alone in 50%, painful dysesthesia in 11%, and distressing dysesthesia without pain in 5%. Of a total of 591 patients with pain and/or dysesthesia, the onset of pain was within the first year in 58% of cases, and the pain had started immediately in 34% of cases. The intensity of the pain decreased over time in 7%, but increased in 47% of patients. Pain was localized below or within the transition zone in 86% of patients, with 47% of the pain below the lesion, 22% both below the lesion and in the transition zone, and 17% in the transition zone alone. Patients experiencing pain and/or dysesthesia described the sensation as "burning" (24.4%), "tingling" (23%), "stabbing" (23%), "tight" (21%), "cramping" (13.4%), "pulling" (14.7%), and "other" (23.2%). These data indicate a high proportion of below-level neuropathic pain, but the study did not include any further differentiation as to the level of pain.

In a study of acute pain following SCI, New et al. (1997) assessed the type of pain experienced by 24 patients. Neuropathic pain was the most common category. Most injuries resulted from trauma, and most patients had an incomplete injury. Neuropathic pain was diagnosed on the basis of pain quality: "burning," "stabbing," "pins and needles," or "numbness," and was located at or below the level of paralysis. Neuropathic pain was present in 67% of patients at the time of their admission to the rehabilitation ward. Pain frequency decreased to around 65% at discharge, but returned to the inpatient frequency 1 year later. Of the patients with neuropathic pain, 79% reported greater than 50% reduction in pain intensity at the time of discharge from the inpatient ward, but 1 year later, 37% reported pain of equal or greater intensity. The patients in this study were assessed according to the type of pain present: neuropathic, myofascial, or orthopedic. Of the patients reporting pain during inpatient rehabilitation, 48% had multiple pain conditions, compared to only 10% at a 1-year follow-up review.

CLINICAL EXAMINATION

In most cases, neuropathic pain is characterized by sensory abnormalities (Lindblom and Verrillo 1979; Lindblom 1985) due to lesions of sensory nerve fibers or sensory pathways within the central nervous system (Boivie et al. 1989). The large variety of sensory disturbances is presented in Table I.

Routine neurological sensory examination (testing of light touch with a cotton swab or pin-prick) can often detect these disturbances. However, hypoesthesia is often masked by allodynia to light mechanical stimulation, although some patients report reduced sensibility to light touch. Hyperalgesia to pin-prick is often reported as a different, more painful sensation, often with radiation and an unpleasant aftersensation.

The diagnosis of neuropathic pain can in most cases be made by a careful interview of the patient and a routine neurological examination. QST provides further diagnostic and descriptive characterization through quantitative evaluation of sensory qualities.

SENSORY QUALITIES

The sensations of touch, pressure, and vibration are all mechanosensitive modalities transmitted in thick, myelinated Aβ fibers, dorsal columns, and medial lemniscal pathways, and are accessible to testing through conventional neurophysiological techniques such as neurography and electrically induced sensory evoked potentials (SEP). For testing the modalities of fast pain (Aδ fibers), dull, burning, aching pain (C fibers), heat and heat pain (C fibers), cold (Aδ fibers) and cold pain (Aδ and C fibers), neurography and conventional SEP testing (with electrical stimulation) are of no value. SEP

Table I
Sensory abnormalities in neuropathic pain

Quantitative	Hypoesthesia Hyperesthesia Hyperalgesia Hypoalgesia
Qualitative	Allodynia Paresthesia Dysesthesia
Spatial	Dyslocalization Radiation
Temporal	Abnormal latency Abnormal aftersensation Abnormal summation

following CO_2 laser stimulation relates to pain and nociceptive impulses projected in the spinothalamic tract. The high interindividual variation in the amplitude of laser evoked potentials suggests that they may not be suitable for routine examinations in clinical practice, but they can provide useful information that is not accessible by conventional electrophysiological techniques. Central pain syndromes could be caused by disinhibition of spinothalamic excitability or by reduction of spinothalamic function due to other central changes or disease. Casey et al. (1996) found that central pain patients with cerebral or brainstem infarctions who retained normal tactile sensation had significantly smaller laser evoked potentials on the affected side compared with the unaffected side. This study supports a deficit in spinothalamic tract function but does not suggest excessive central responses to the activation of cutaneous nociceptive pathways.

In recent years sensory testing has become a valuable supplement to routine neurological testing, which is inadequate for a quantitative, modality-specific assessment of sensory disturbance. Sensory testing can be applied in the laboratory for basic studies and in the clinic to characterize patients with dysfunction within the pain pathways. Electrical, thermal, and mechanical techniques are available in the laboratory setting, and some are commercially available.

QUANTITATIVE SENSORY TESTING

Quantitative sensory tests are used to measure the intensity of stimuli needed to produce specific sensory perceptions. Tests are developed to determine sensory thresholds for tactile, vibratory, pressure, and temperature stimulation. Various laboratories have used different approaches and different paradigms. Few laboratories offer QST as a routine investigation to evaluate pain patients. All quantitative sensory tests are psychophysical tests requiring awake and alert patients who fully understand the instructions given and who are fully capable of cooperating.

Qualitative changes may be as important as quantitative changes. There may be large interindividual differences, which must be taken into consideration in clinical research. QST methods have been mainly used for research purposes in the classification of neuropathic pain, in studies of pathophysiological mechanisms, and in pharmacological trials. For a purely clinical evaluation of the individual patient, the diagnosis of neuropathic pain may be made without using these time-consuming methods.

ESTIMATION OF TACTILE SENSIBILITY BY VON FREY NYLON FILAMENTS

For quantitative testing of tactile sensibility, many researchers use von Frey nylon filaments, a series of filaments of varying thickness, calibrated according to the force required to make them bend. Hairs with low bending pressures are applied to the skin to stimulate the rapidly adapting cutaneous receptors. One way to assess tactile sensation is to apply the hairs in an ascending and descending order of magnitude and to record the threshold for both appearance and disappearance of sensation. In neuropathic pain, tactile sensibility as measured by von Frey hairs may be reduced in affected skin areas (Eide et al. 1994). This finding may be overlooked in a routine neurological examination, where testing for tactile sensibility with a cotton swab may only give a sensation of hyperesthesia that constitutes allodynia to light mechanical stimulation, masking a reduced tactile sensibility. Another way to assess the tactile threshold is to determine the value of the bending force of the filament that the patient can detect 50% of the time.

With increasing bending force, von Frey hairs will excite skin nociceptors and may be used to determine tactile pain detection thresholds. Von Frey hairs may also be used to map areas of secondary hyperalgesia to punctate stimuli (due to central sensitization), either in experimental models of pain (Warncke et al. 1997) or in a clinical context (Stubhaug et al. 1997). Secondary hyperalgesia to punctate stimuli (due to central sensitization) is mediated by conduction in Aδ nociceptive fibers (Ziegler et al. 1999), in contrast to the Aβ-fiber-mediated secondary hyperalgesia to light brushing.

THE THERMOTEST

Neuropathic pain and other pain syndromes are often characterized by alteration in sensations mediated by thin nerve fibers that are not accessible to electrophysiological tests such as neurography or conventional SEP. The thermotest allows testing of qualities such as heat, cold, and both heat and cold pain sensations (Fig. 1). Whereas neurography tests for dysfunction of peripheral nerve fibers, the thermotest describes the status of temperature-sensitive somatosensory afferents all the way from the cutaneous receptors to the brain. However, it is not possible to draw conclusions about the level of injury. Various thermotest devices are commercially available with different technical parameters. Testing for thermal sensory abnormalities is useful in the evaluation of pain patients and of patients with thermal sensory abnormalities in general, such as thin-fiber neuropathies. Some devices are designed primarily to evaluate sensory deficits to heat, cold, and heat pain.

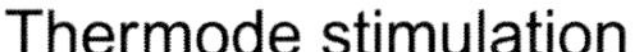

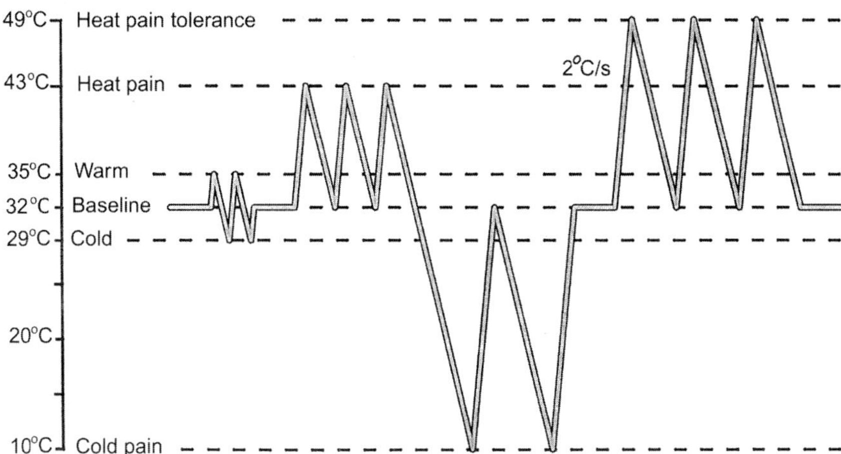

Fig. 1. Normal thermal thresholds measured by thermotest from a baseline of 32°C. From Lars Arendt-Nielsen, with permission.

Prominent findings in neuropathic pain conditions are heat and cold hyperalgesia. The mechanisms of thermal hyperalgesia are unclear, but many indications suggest that this condition is also mediated by central sensitization. Testing only for heat and cold functions in patients with neuropathic pain may give inconclusive results because heat and cold hyperalgesia may occur despite normal heat and cold thresholds. In evaluating neuropathic pain patients, researchers should test all four thermal qualities: heat, cold, heat pain, and cold pain (Verdugo and Ochoa 1992). In addition to determining the threshold values, it is equally important to ask the patient about the quality of the sensation. Paradoxical sensations are frequently reported, most often that cold pain is perceived as heat. Heat and cold pain are often described as occurring suddenly, with radiation and aftersensations; this information is of value in the evaluation of hyperalgesia. Interindividual variability in sensory abnormality is substantial.

Two methods of thermotest are available, the forced-choice method and the method of limits. The forced-choice method reduces response bias and therefore seems better suited for a psychophysical examination. However, the method is time-consuming, and it has mainly been used to evaluate neurological patients with sensory deficits in general and not pain patients in particular. For evaluating pain patients, the method of limits is best suited from an ethical standpoint because a suprathreshold stimulus may evoke excruciating and often long-lasting pain. For the same reason, it is desirable to determine a threshold using as few stimuli as possible. Tolerance threshold may also be assessed, but for some patients, the detection threshold itself will represent the level of tolerance. For cold and heat detection thresholds, 5–10 repeated tests are adequate, while for cold and heat pain, three repeated measurements are typically used.

Many variables can influence test results. Baseline temperature is an important factor that can influence the subject's ability to sense a rise or fall in temperature. In many laboratories, the contact probe is applied at a standard temperature of 32°C, thereby reducing interindividual variability in thresholds. Sometimes the contact probe is set at a different temperature. When the baseline temperature is higher, heat thresholds are assessed at the baseline temperature itself or at a very short interval from the baseline. At a lower baseline temperature the cold threshold is assessed at a short interval from the baseline. Heating the patient's skin before testing is not recommended. Another possibility is to adjust the temperature to the patient's skin temperature. Due to autonomic dysfunction in patients with complex regional pain syndromes, the skin temperature may be lowered by 1–3°C in the affected part. It may be difficult to compare sensory thresholds in affected and normal skin areas in these patients if the baseline temperature of the contact probe is set at different levels for different parts of the body, so baseline temperature should be kept constant for each individual. To avoid injury to the skin, the recommended upper temperature limit is 50°C and the lower limit is 5°C.

The rate of stimulus rise may also influence the sensory threshold. The most commonly employed change of temperature is 1°C. Quicker rates may induce large reaction time artefacts, while slower changes make over-long stimuli. Due to the influence of spatial summation of sensory modalities, the size of the contact probe may also influence the sensory thresholds, in the sense that recruitment of more receptors will lower the threshold. For practical reasons, thresholds are not comparable when probes of different sizes are used. Surface areas tested may vary from 9 to 12.5 cm^2, and smaller contact probes are needed for testing the face or fingertip.

TESTS OF CENTRAL HYPEREXCITABILITY

Temporal summation of neural impulses in nociceptive nerve fibers is a physiologically important mechanism that can intensify the sensation of pain (Lundberg et al. 1992). Clinical practice has shown that repetitive stimulation of a painful skin area in a patient suffering from neuropathic pain may produce an intense and long-lasting pain in a phenomenon referred to as abnormal temporal summation or sometimes as "wind-up-like pain" (Eide et al. 1994). The abnormal temporal summation seen in patients may be assessed roughly by repetitive skin stimulation (usually with a frequency of 2–3 Hz) with a von Frey hair for up to 20–30 seconds. If temporal summation is abnormal, the patient will report a sudden intense pain in the stimulated area, often occurring within a few seconds, with aftersensation and radiation. Abnormal temporal summation may be regarded as a sign of central hyperexcitability and can be quantified by measuring latency, duration of aftersensation, and area of radiation. For scientific purposes, more elegant techniques are available, including von Frey application with standardized pressure and frequencies and electrical skin stimulation.

ALLODYNIA/HYPERALGESIA TO MECHANICAL STIMULI

There are two types of allodynia/hyperalgesia to tactile stimuli, one to light touch (the dynamic type) and one to punctate stimuli (the static type). Although both are caused by central sensitization mechanisms, they are mediated by different peripheral nerve fibers. The dynamic type is mediated by peripheral Aβ fibers, whereas the punctate type has recently been shown to be mediated by Aδ fibers (Ziegler et al 1999). Mapping of the area may be recommended for both types. Punctate allodynia/hyperalgesia can be mapped by the use of von Frey hairs as described previously, while dynamic allodynia is usually mapped by lightly brushing the skin. Areas of punctate allodynia/hyperalgesia are in general larger than areas of dynamic allodynia.

RESULTS OF QST IN PATIENTS WITH SPINAL CORD INJURY PAIN

Future studies of SCI pain (Siddall et al. 1997, 2000) should test cutaneous sensitivity above, at, and below the level of the lesion. Prior studies of SCI pain have not done so systematically; those using QST to evaluate SCI pain have mainly dealt with the pathophysiology of central neuropathic pain.

Beric et al. (1988) studied below-level pain in 13 patients with central dysesthesia syndrome. Of a total of 102 patients, 13 developed spontaneous diffuse and unpleasant sensations distal to the level of the lesion, which began during the first year after injury. All patients were evaluated by neurological examination, a pain interview, and assessment of pain intensity on a visual analogue scale. QST and conventional neurophysiological investigations were performed on the legs. Light touch was tested by von Frey hairs, vibratory threshold with a vibrameter, and thermal thresholds with the

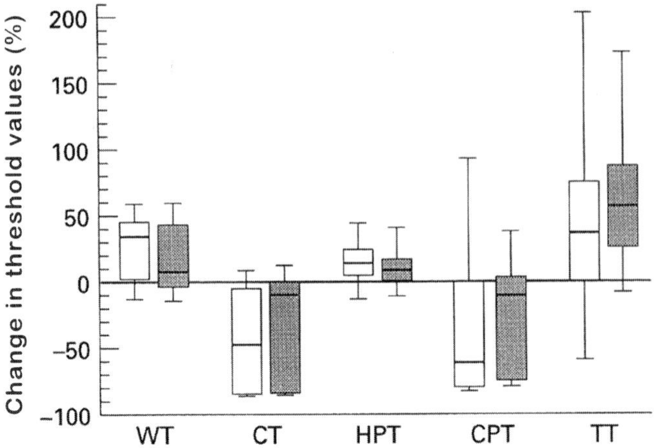

Fig. 2. Comparison of changes in sensory thresholds in nonpainful (open boxes) and painful (cross-hatched boxes) denervated skin areas. The different sensory thresholds (WT = warm thresholds; CT = cold thresholds; HPT = heat pain thresholds; CPT = cold pain thresholds; TT = tactile thresholds) are not increased in painful compared to nonpainful denervated skin areas ($P > 0.10$, Wilcoxon signed-rank test). Data are derived from Eide et al. (1998), with permission.

thermotest. Nine of the 13 patients had dysesthesias at the level of the lesion and caudally, while four patients had a free zone caudally and had dysesthesias only from the waist down. All complained of a burning sensation. Two patients had no sensation below the level of the lesion, while 11 had incomplete preservation of sensation. QST of thermal thresholds and thermal pain revealed absence of sensation in 10 patients. Vibratory sensibility and touch were reduced in 10 and 9 patients, respectively. There were significant differences between the temperature and thermal pain thresholds and those for vibration and touch. These results suggest a relative preservation of dorsal column function along with an abolition of spinothalamic system function.

Beric's study indicates that a high proportion of patients with below-level pain have this specific sensory profile, which is consistent with studies of central poststroke pain by Boivie et al. (1989) indicating that an imbalance between the temperature and pain system and the large-fiber touch system can contribute to abnormal spontaneous sensation. These authors proposed that the pain-producing dysfunction is located rostral to the spinal cord at the level of the lower brainstem or thalamus. Their speculation was that the dysesthesias may result from central misinterpretation of residual dorsal column system input in the absence of suppression via integrated spinothalamic system activity. The results of this study show how QST may differentiate between sensibility changes due to dorsal column and spinothalamic tract function.

In a study of 16 patients with traumatic SCI and below-level pain (Eide et al. 1996), we compared somatosensory abnormalities in painful denervated skin areas below the level of the lesion as well as in nonpainful denervated skin areas at the level of the lesion. Central dysesthesia pain is also characterized by evoked pain (pain due to central sensitization mechanisms), so we included tests of central hyperexcitability, such as "wind-up-like pain" and allodynia to brush as described previously. The patients complained of spontaneous pain, paroxysmal pain, and evoked pain, mostly to light touching of the skin. In the painful denervated area, we found a highly significant reduction of sensibility to heat and cold, indicating reduced function in the spinothalamic tract system and supporting the results of Beric et al. (1988) (Table II). We found no significant cold allodynia. An important observation was that there was no significant difference in sensory thresholds in the *painful* denervated skin areas compared with the *nonpainful* denervated skin areas (at level) (Fig. 2). Thus, in these patients, deafferentation of spinothalamic pathways was not a sufficient condition for development of central neuropathic pain. One of the main findings was the demonstration of evoked pain, both allodynia to brush and "wind-up-like pain" (Fig. 3) in the painful denervated area alone. Our data show that sensory loss must be coupled with abnormal pain responsiveness to reach a diagnosis of neuropathic pain (Eide et al. 1996; Eide 1998).

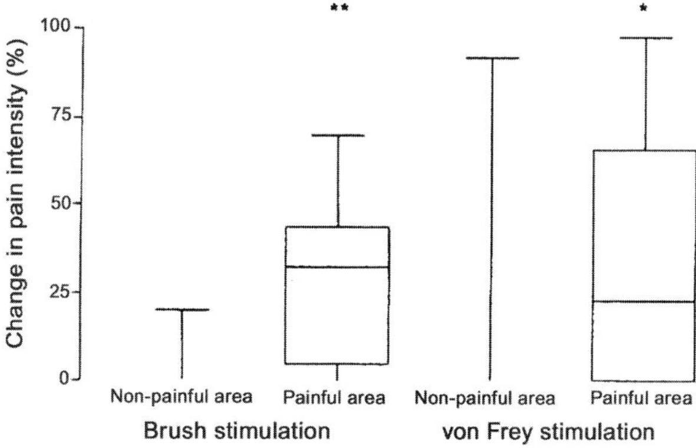

Fig. 3. Comparisons of brush allodynia and abnormal temporal summation (wind-up like pain) in nonpainful and painful denervated skin areas. Significant differences are indicated by asterisks (* $P < 0.05$, ** $P < 0.001$; Wilcoxon signed-rank test). Data are derived from Eide et al. (1996), with permission.

Table II
Threshold medians (and range) in normal skin area and in nonpainful and painful denervated skin areas

Somatosensory Threshold	Normal Skin Area	Nonpainful Denervated Skin Area	Painful Denervated Skin Area
Warm threshold (°C)	35.7 (33.0–42.6)	39.8 (34.1–52.0)*	49.2 (34.4–52.0)***
Cold threshold (°C)	31.2 (26.4–32.7)	27.9 (5.0–31.2)**	16.4 (5.0–31.2)***
Heat pain threshold (°C)	42.1 (36.2–51.6)	47.2 (38.6–52.0)*	50.5 (39.4–52.0)**
Cold pain threshold (°C)	22.3 (5.0–28.7)	16.4 (5.0–29.1)	5.0 (5.0–27.6)*
Tactile threshold ($\log_{10}$ 0.1 mg)	33.2 (1.65–4.44)	4.93 (3.84–6.45)***	4.19 (1.65–6.65)

Source: Data are derived from Eide et al. (1996), with permission.
$*P < 0.5$; $**P < 0.01$; $***P < 0.005$; significant differences compared with measurements in normal skin area (Wilcoxon signed rank test).

QST has also been used in pharmacological studies of SCI pain to test sensory abnormalities before and after administration of drugs (Eide et al. 1995; Attal et al. 2000; see Chapter 20 for review).

In summary, the inclusion of QST and tests of central hyperexcitability in future studies of SCI pain may contribute to a further understanding of the complicated neurophysiological mechanisms of pain above, at, and below the SCI level, caused by injury to nerves, nerve roots, and the spinal cord.

REFERENCES

Attal N, Gaude V, Brasseur L, et al. Intravenous lidocaine in central pain: a double-blind, placebo-controlled, psychophysical study. *Neurology* 2000; 54:564–574.

Beric A, Dimitrijevic MR, Lindblom U. Central dysthesia syndrome in spinal cord injury patients. *Pain* 1988; 34:109–116.

Bonica JJ. Semantic, epidemiologic and educational issues. In: Casey KL (Ed). *Pain and Central Nervous System Disease: The Central Pain Syndrome. New York: Raven Press,* 1991, pp 13–29.

Boivie J, Leijon G, Johansson I. Central post-stroke pain—a study of the mechanisms through analyses of the sensory abnormalities. *Pain* 1989; 37:173–185.

Casey K, Beydoun A, Boivie J, et al. Laser-evoked cerebral potentials and sensory function in patients with central pain. *Pain* 1996; 64:485–491.

Eide PK. Pathophysiological mechanisms of central neuropathic pain after spinal cord injury. *Spinal Cord* 1998; 36:601–612.

Eide PK, Jørum E, Stubhaug A, Bremnes J, Breivik H. Relief of post-herpetic neuralgia with the *N*-methyl-D-aspartic acid receptor antagonist ketamine: a double-blind, cross-over comparison with morphine and placebo. *Pain* 1994; 58:347–354.

Eide PK, Stubhaug A, Stenehjem AE. Central dysesthesia pain after traumatic spinal cord injury is dependent on N-methyl-D-aspartate receptor activation. *Neurosurgery* 1995; 37:1080–1087.

Eide, PK, Jørum E, Stenehjem AE. Somatosensory findings in patients with spinal cord injury and central dysesthesia pain. *J Neurol Neurosurg Psychiatry* 1996; 60:411–415.

Hansson P, Lindblom U. Quantitative evaluation of sensory disturbances accompanying focal or referred nociceptive pain. In: Vecchiet L, Albé-Fessard D, Lindblom U (Eds). *New Trends in Referred Pain and Hyperalgesia.* Amsterdam: Elsevier Science, 1993, pp 251–258.

Graven-Nielsen T, Arendt-Nielsen L, Svensson P, Jensen TS. Stimulus-response functions in areas with experimentally induced referred muscle pain: a psychophysical study. *Brain Res* 1997; 744:121–128.

Lindblom U. Assessment of abnormal evoked pain in neurological pain patients and its relation to spontaneous pain: a descriptive and conceptual model with some analytical results. In: Fields HL, Dubner R, Cervero F (Eds). *Proceedings of the Fourth World Congress on Pain,* Advances in Pain Research and Therapy, Vol. 9. New York: Raven Press, 1985; pp 409–423.

Lindblom U, Verrillo RT. Sensory functions in chronic neuralgia. *J Neurol Neurosurg Psychiatry* 1979; 42:422–435.

Lundberg LER, Jørum E, Holm E, Torebjörk HE. Intraneural electrical stimulation of cutaneous nociceptive fibres in humans: effects of different pulse patterns on magnitude of pain. *Acta Physiol Scand* 1992; 51:207–219.

Merskey H, Bogduk N (Eds). *Classification of Chronic Pain: Descriptions of Chronic Pain Syndromes and Definitions of Pain Terms,* 2nd ed. Seattle: IASP Press, 1994.

New PW, Lim TC, Hill ST, Brown DJ. A survey of pain during rehabilitation after acute spinal cord injury. *Spinal Cord* 1997; 35:658–663.

Siddall PJ, Taylor DA, Cousins MJ. Classification of pain following spinal cord injury. *Spinal Cord* 1997; 35:69–75.

Siddall PJ, Yezierski RP, Loeser JD. Pain following spinal cord injury: clinical features, prevalence and taxonomy. *IASP Newsletter* 2000; 3:3–7.

Stubhaug A, Breivik H, Eide PK, Kreunen M, Foss A. Mapping of punctate hyperalgesia around a surgical incision demonstrates that ketamine is a powerful suppressor of central sensitisation to pain following surgery. *Acta Anaesthesiol Scand* 1997; 41:1124–1132.

Störmer S, Gerner HJ , Grüninger W, et al. Chronic pain/dysaesthesia in spinal cord injury patients: results of a multicentre study. *Spinal Cord* 1997; 35:446–455.

Vecchiet L, Giamberardino MA, Dragani L, Albé-Fessard D. Pain from renal/ureteral calculosis: evaluation of sensory thresholds in the lumbar area. *Pain* 1989; 36:289–295.

Verdugo R, Ochoa JL. Quantitative somatosensory thermotest: a key method for functional evaluation of small calibre afferent channels. *Brain* 1992; 115:1–21.

Warncke T, Stubhaug A, Jørum E. Ketamine, an NMDA receptor antagonist, suppresses spatial and temporal properties of burn-induced secondary hyperalgesia in man: a double-blind, cross-over comparison with morphine and placebo. *Pain* 1997; 72:99–106.

Woolf C, Bennett GJ, Doherty M, et al. Towards a mechanism-based classification of pain. *Pain* 1998; 77:227–229.

Ziegler EA, Magerl W, Meyer RA, Treede RD. Secondary hyperalgesia to punctate mechanical stimuli: central sensitization to A-fibre nociceptor input. *Brain* 1999; 122:2245–2257.

Correspondence to: Ellen Jørum, MD, PhD, The National Hospital, Sognsvannsveien 20, 0027 Oslo, Norway. Tel: 47 23 07 08 32 (office), 47 23 07 35 81 (laboratory); Fax: 47 23 07 35 78; email: ellen.jorum@rikshospitalet.no.

Spinal Cord Injury Pain: Assessment, Mechanisms, Management. Progress in Pain Research and Management, Vol. 23, edited by Robert P. Yezierski and Kim J. Burchiel, IASP Press, Seattle, © 2002.

5

Evaluation of Clinical Characteristics of Pain and Psychosocial Factors after Spinal Cord Injury

Eva G. Widerström-Noga

Miami Project to Cure Paralysis, Department of Neurological Surgery, Lois Pope LIFE Center, University of Miami School of Medicine, and Veterans Affairs Medical Center, Miami, Florida, USA

Chronic pain is one of the most frequently reported reasons for reduced quality of life following spinal cord injury (SCI) (Lundqvist et al. 1991; Stensman 1994; Westgren and Levi 1998). For some it may be a life-long experience that can become progressively worse over time (Pentland et al. 1995; Lal 1998). Results from recent studies support a high incidence of chronic pain following SCI and high pain intensity ratings (Demirel 1998; Rintala et al. 1998; Siddall et al. 1999; Turner and Cardenas 1999; Turner et al. 2001; Finnerup et al. 2001; Widerström-Noga et al. 2001a), and emphasize that for years after injury, pain continues to be a significant problem for large numbers of individuals with SCI. Thus, despite an increased understanding of the mechanisms responsible for the different types of pain observed following SCI (for recent reviews see Vierck et al. 2000; Siddall and Loeser 2001) and the development of new pharmacological therapies, these pain conditions continue to be a challenge for the health care community.

Unfortunately, individuals who suffer from pain associated with SCI rarely experience spontaneous remission of pain. For example, Störmer et al. (1997) reported that only 5.8% of those who suffered from either pain or distressing dysesthesia following SCI completely recovered, either spontaneously or due to treatment. Furthermore, no treatment approaches have been proven to be consistently effective for central neuropathic pain after SCI (see Chapter 20 for a review of pharmacological approaches). Despite the complexity of these pain conditions, it appears that relatively few patients receive appropriate pharmacological intervention (Finnerup et al. 2001) or enroll in multidisciplinary pain programs (Murphy and Reid 2001). Although central pain may also be associated with conditions like multiple sclerosis, stroke, epilepsy, and Parkinson's disease (Bonica 1991), it is unclear whether central pain due to these various conditions responds differently to treatment.

Chronic pain in the SCI population is heterogeneous (Tunks 1986; Fenollosa et al. 1993; Levi et al. 1995; Bowsher 1996; Siddall et al. 1997; Siddall and Loeser 2001), and most persons with SCI experience more than one type of pain simultaneously (Turner and Cardenas 1999; Murphy and Reid 2001; Turner et al. 2001; Widerström-Noga et al. 2001a). The recent taxonomies for SCI proposed by Bryce and Ragnarsson (2000) and Siddall et al. (2000) classify chronic pain in SCI both relative to level of injury and according to putative mechanisms (for details, see Chapter 2 of this volume). Including level of injury in the classification is a positive step because it improves diagnosis and evaluation. Moreover, classification according to mechanism is important as it suggests treatment strategies (Ragnarsson 1997; Eide 1998; Siddall and Loeser 2001).

Although the various types of pain following SCI are caused by partly different mechanisms (Bryce and Ragnarsson 2000; Siddall et al. 2000), the maintenance and aggravation of a painful condition depends on a variety of factors, some of them unrelated to pathophysiology of pain, both in heterogeneous pain populations (Turk and Rudy 1988) and among SCI patients (Summers et al. 1991; Richards 1992; Störmer et al. 1997). Similar to observations with other pain populations, the severity of SCI-associated neuropathic pain conditions is likely to be influenced by psychological factors such as depressed mood (Haythornthwaite and Benrud-Larson 2000). Therefore, in order to understand and optimally treat SCI pain, we must focus not only on the causative factors but also on the factors responsible for sustaining and aggravating these pain conditions.

Furthermore, the refractory nature of the painful conditions related to SCI suggests that personal characteristics related to adaptation and coping skills are crucial for improving quality of life (Haythornthwaite and Benrud-Larson 2000). Indeed, psychological factors such as anxiety, sadness, and a perception of excessive fatigue are commonly acknowledged by those experiencing SCI-related pain (Rose et al. 1988; Summers et al. 1991; Jacob et al. 1995; Kennedy et al. 1997; Widerström-Noga 2001b). These factors significantly affect coping and adjustment to SCI (Scivoletto et al. 1997; King and Kennedy 1999; Kemp and Krause 1999).

ASSESSMENT PRINCIPLES

The biopsychosocial view of pain incorporates a dynamic interaction among physical, psychological, and social factors that evolve over time. This perspective not only includes the pathophysiological mechanisms underlying the cause of pain, but may also include the psychological and psychosocial factors that can be important in maintaining and exacerbating a chronic painful condition (Turk 1996). This model provides a theoretical foundation that takes into account the fact that individuals with pain may differ in regard to important variables that influence coping and adaptation. The evaluation and treatment strategy for people with chronic pain and SCI should rely on an assessment procedure reflecting psychosocial factors and behavioral factors (Richards et al. 1980; Mariano 1992; Richards 1992; Umlauf 1992; Kishi et al. 1994), as well as the pathophysiological mechanisms described in this volume (see Chapters 6, 7, 9, 14).

The assessment of pain following SCI is complicated by the fact that SCI has a number of medical consequences (Levi et al. 1995; Widerström-Noga 1999), some which are directly related to the extent of nervous tissue injury. In contrast, the pathophysiology of chronic SCI pain is not as well known, and few conclusive relationships between injury characteristics and chronic pain have been demonstrated (Siddall and Loeser 2001).

Although several assessment instruments have been developed for chronic pain patients in general (Turk and Melzack 2001), they may not be appropriate for SCI pain because of other consequences of injury that may influence patients' perception of pain and subsequent responses in different ways. Thus, it is inappropriate to assume that measures developed for use with other chronic pain populations can be generalized to individuals with SCI.

Several important factors must be considered in the evaluation of SCI pain. For example, the nature of the pain must be defined because different types of pain may respond differently to treatment (Ragnarsson 1997; Eide 1998). Thus, attempts should be made to determine whether the pain is nociceptive or neuropathic. A classification of pain can be made based on a comprehensive pain history in combination with a neurological examination defining the extent of neurological deficit. The evaluator should obtain information regarding the location and quality of pain, its temporal pattern and intensity, aggravating and pain-relieving factors, effects of medication and treatments, and changes in location and intensity. In addition to changes in intensity, changes in temporal pattern may also provide valuable information concerning the pain-relieving efficacy of a particular therapy.

Effects of a pain therapy can also be continuously evaluated in a "pain diary," which can be recorded on paper or electronically (Jamison et al. 2001). Clinicians can ask patients with SCI to record the intensity, location, and description of pain at regular intervals. The diary can also include ratings of alleviating and aggravating factors, use of medication, mood state, and activities (Feldman et al. 1999). Recording levels of pain and related factors every day in a diary reduces the risk of recall bias related to reports of level of pain and medication use for the previous day or week (Smith and Safer 1993).

In addition to the evaluation of spontaneous pain, a comprehensive pain evaluation can include an assessment of evoked pain and abnormal sensations, given that sensory dysfunction is an integral part of a neuropathic pain condition and can provide insights into its mechanisms (Eide et al. 1996; Defrin et al. 2001). Thus, it may be helpful for choice of therapy as well as for evaluation of treatment efficacy. Assessment may include *quantitative* abnormalities, such as threshold changes like hypo- or hyperesthesia, or *qualitative* abnormalities, such as allodynia, dysesthesia, or paresthesia (Lindblom 1994). Quantitative sensory assessment is dealt with in depth by Jørum (Chapter 4).

Chronic pain, regardless of origin, affects people differently, and a individual's response to chronic pain depends on a variety of psychological and behavioral factors (Turk and Flor 1992; Jensen et al. 1994; Turk 1996). To increase the likelihood of a positive outcome, the assessment procedure and subsequent treatment intervention should be tailored not only to the specific features of pain but also to each person's psychological characteristics and life circumstances (Turk 1990; Summers et al. 1991; Wegener and Elliott 1992; Haythornthwaite and Benrud-Larson 2001).

A patient's overall well-being can be evaluated to determine the impact of pain on his or her life as well as the efficacy of a treatment. Psychosocial and behavioral factors may also have a synergistic effect and may be reflected in quality of life, interference of pain with activities and functioning, or effects of pain on mood. For example, frequent interference with daily activities may result in a patient feeling unable to deal with or control chronic pain. Feelings of low levels of internal control may result in negative affect and excessive dependence on others. Similar relationships among disability, low levels of control, and depression have been observed in studies that included heterogeneous chronic pain samples (Arnstein et al. 1999).

PAIN HISTORY

Because of the subjective nature of pain (Merskey 1979), a comprehensive evaluation of pain must take into account patients' perceptions of their pain (Fields 1987). In addition to a pain drawing (Margolis et al. 1988), adjectives describing quality of pain are always part of a pain history. The most common questionnaire that includes these components is the McGill Pain Questionnaire (Melzack 1975). A short form is available (Melzack 1987) that includes 15 descriptors from the sensory and affective categories of words, which are rated on an intensity scale as 0 = none, 1 = mild, 2 = moderate, or 3 = severe. For the differentiation of pain following SCI, a pain history should be combined with a neurological examination of motor and sensory function, so that pain descriptors are used along with information concerning location of pain relative to neurological deficit. This assessment may also include a quantitative sensory testing (QST) protocol and other examinations involving imaging and electrophysiological techniques (Siddall and Loeser 2001). An example of a structured pain history that can be used for evaluating SCI pain, similar to the assessment tool used in our studies (Widerström-Noga et al. 2001a,b), is included in Appendix A. This version includes a pain drawing, adjective descriptors from the sensory domain, a numerical rating scale for evaluating pain intensity, questions concerning interference with daily life, previous pain, onset of present pain, temporal aspects of pain, changes in pain over time, the patient's identification of his or her most disturbing pain (if there are several types), and pain-relieving and aggravating factors. This pain history is designed to relate different clinical characteristics to a specific pain location if needed. It includes a basic evaluation that can be supplemented with other aspects, such as information about previous treatments. A thorough pain history provides important information and serves many purposes. Although factors like location, quality, and temporal pattern are essential in differentiating the type of pain, other variables such as interference with daily life, chronicity, aggravation and attenuation of pain, previous treatments and outcomes, and changes in pain also give the evaluator useful clinical information on which to base a treatment plan and prognosis.

The descriptor "burning" in an area of sensory deficit is often associated with neuropathic pain (Fenollosa et al. 1993; Ragnarsson 1997; Siddall et al. 1999), "aching" located in an area above the level of injury is often associated with pain in the musculoskeletal system (Tunks 1986; Siddall et al. 1999). In SCI, the verbal description of pain is complicated by the presence of many types of pain simultaneously (Bowsher 1996; Eide 1998; Turner et al. 2001; Widerström-Noga et al. 2001a). For example, neuropathic pain at or below the level of injury is often accompanied by nociceptive pain such as musculoskeletal pain in the neck and shoulder area (Nepomuceno et al. 1979; Eide et al. 1996; Ragnarsson 1997; Siddall et al. 1999). We examined the relationships among clinical characteristics of chronic pain following

SCI in 217 subjects with chronic pain and SCI (Widerström-Noga et al. 2001a). The response rate in our study was 67%, which included subjects from a previous study where 330 persons rated their difficulty to deal with chronic pain (Widerström-Noga et al. 1999). We found that participants had a slightly harder time dealing with their pain compared to those who did not participate. Thus, participants in surveys may have more severe pain. However, Störmer et al. (1997) investigated a large group of people with SCI considered to be representative of the entire population in a multicenter study, and reported that 70% of their patients rated their pain intensity as 6 or above on a visual analogue scale (VAS). In our study 43.6% scored 6 or above on a numerical rating scale (NRS) ranging from 0 to 10. Thus, it appears that the participants may have experienced slightly more pain than the entire group, but when compared to subjects in the study by Störmer et al. (1997), our subjects experienced less intense pain on average. Pain was frequently reported in several areas of the body using multiple descriptors. Our finding that pain was most commonly represented in the back and lower extremities is consistent with others (Turner et al. 2001). Back pain following SCI can be nociceptive in origin, even in complete tetraplegics (Ragnarsson 1997), because some of the back muscles receive their innervation from the upper cervical segments and the cranial nerves. Considering that a sensory stimulus such as bowel impaction or a full bladder can instigate or aggravate pain in SCI, it is reasonable to assume that a nociceptive stimulus such as musculoskeletal pain may exacerbate other types of pain. Therefore, effective treatment of musculoskeletal pain in an SCI patient with several different types of pain may also indirectly decrease the intensity of more therapy-resistant types of pain.

Level of injury affects the area of pain distribution. We compared persons with tetraplegia and paraplegia and found that a similar distribution of pain in all body areas except the shoulder-neck areas and upper extremity areas, in which pain was significantly more common in persons with tetraplegia (51.7% and 48.3%) than in those with paraplegia (24.5% and 11.2%; see Table I). Curtis et al. (1999) also found that the prevalence of shoulder pain was greater in people with tetraplegia (59%) than with paraplegia (42%), and similar observations were made by Turner et al. (2001). The demands on the shoulder region in activities of daily life are high in a person who is wheelchair dependent, thus it seems reasonable that pain would be more common in this region following a cervical injury in which the muscles of the shoulders may be partly denervated (Subbarao et al. 1995; Curtis et al. 1999). In addition, a higher injury involving the cervical segments and impairing sensory and motor function in the arms and hands increases the risk for neuropathic pain in these regions.

Table I
Frequency of different body areas marked in the pain drawing, comparing persons with tetraplegia (n = 118) and paraplegia (n = 98)

	Frequency (%)	
Location of Pain	Tetraplegia	Paraplegia
Head	15 (12.7%)	5 (5.1%) ns
Neck and shoulder	61 (51.7%)	24 (24.5%)***
Arms and hands	57 (48.3%)	11 (11.2%)***
Genitals and frontal aspect of torso	49 (41.5%)	48 (49.0%) ns
Back	71 (60.2%)	62 (63.2%) ns
Buttocks	59 (50.0%)	50 (51.0%) ns
Thighs	58 (49.2%)	61 (62.2%) ns
Legs and feet	59 (50.0%)	53 (54.1%) ns

Note: ns = no significant difference between groups; *** = $P < 0.001$ (Bonferroni adjusted).

Fifty-nine percent of the subjects in our study reported that their pain began within the first 6 months after injury. This finding is consistent with results of a recent longitudinal study in SCI subjects conducted by Siddall et al. (1999), showing that 64% of the participants experienced pain at 6 months following injury. Furthermore, 41.4% of our sample experienced constant pain without breaks or with short periods of remission lasting up to an hour.

In an attempt to elucidate relationships among common clinical characteristics obtained from the pain history, we entered the following variables into a factor analysis: pain in the neck and shoulder region, pain in the lower extremities, number of pain sites, average pain intensity rating (0–10 on an NRS), onset of pain, duration of pain breaks, descriptors "burning" or "aching," and level of injury. An exploratory factor analysis is a way to study the correlation of a large number of variables by grouping them in "factors" so that variables within each factor are more highly associated with variables in that factor than with variables in other factors. This statistical method highlights common patterns among multiple variables. Three groups of clinical characteristics emerged from our analysis (see Table II).

The first factor included: (a) number of painful regions, (b) pain located in the thighs or legs/feet, and (c) the descriptor "burning." This grouping indicates that a common pattern in our group of subjects was pain located in the lower extremities, described as "burning" and associated with a wide distribution. The level of injury did not correlate with this factor, suggesting that this pattern was not dependent on level of injury. The second factor we identified included: (a) pain in the neck/shoulder area; (b) the descriptor "aching"; and (c) cervical level of injury. This grouping shows relationships among pain located in the neck and shoulder region, described as aching

Table II
Exploratory factor analysis including the factor loadings for each of the three subgroups of clinical characteristics

Clinical Characteristic	1	2	3
Number of painful regions	**0.82**	0.30	0.16
Pain located in legs and feet	**0.78**	–0.02	0.11
Pain located in thighs	**0.73**	–0.12	0.23
"Burning" pain	**0.66**	–0.06	–0.23
Pain located in neck/shoulders	0.02	**0.70**	–0.16
"Aching" pain	–0.12	**0.70**	0.35
Level of injury	0.08	**0.67**	–0.16
Duration of pain breaks	0.05	–0.02	**0.77**
Average pain intensity	0.11	0.11	**0.72**
Onset of pain	0.01	–0.30	**0.60**

Source: Data from Widerström-Noga et al. (2001a), with permission.
Note: The factor loadings were sorted in ascending order for each factor and rotated. Boldface type indicates the factor with which a variable is primarily associated.

and common in persons with tetraplegia. The third factor contained: (a) continuous pain or brief periods of relief lasting less than 1 hour; (b) high average pain intensity; and (c) onset of pain within the first 6 months after injury. The relationships between average pain intensity, onset of pain, and duration of breaks suggest that pain starting soon after injury may be related to more intense pain in the chronic stages. Furthermore, pain that is continuous or includes only short pain-free periods is perceived as more intense than pain states associated with longer breaks. The relationship between pain intensity and early onset of pain is interesting because it may suggest a role for preemptive analgesia (Siddall and Cousins 1997). However, because of the possibility of retrospective reporting bias (Raphael and Marbach 1997), such a relationship must be confirmed in a prospective longitudinal study.

LIFE INTERFERENCE DUE TO CHRONIC PAIN

The consequences of SCI impose limitations on a person's ability to perform and participate in daily activities (Dalyan et al. 1999; Ravenscroft et al. 2000; Widerström-Noga et al. 2001b), and the relationship between pain and decreased quality of life (Rintala et al. 1998; Westgren and Levi 1998) suggests that pain-related interference may be an important factor influencing quality of life (Lundqvist et al. 1991). For example, the interference of pain with daily activities may result in decreased independence, ultimately leading to affective distress (Turk and Rudy 1988) and reduced motivation to participate in activities essential for reaching optimal levels of functional independence following SCI (Kishi et al. 1994; Fuhrer 1996). It is important to define factors that influence the extent to which pain interferes in various daily activities because such relationships provide insights for treatment and rehabilitation strategies. In addition, the complexity of interactions among the various consequences of SCI (Widerström-Noga et al. 1999; Ville et al. 2001) indicates that relationships among clinical characteristics of pain as well as psychosocial factors must be further clarified. For example, greater life satisfaction following SCI displays positive relationships with factors including education, income, employment, and social/recreational activities, whereas medical complications are often inversely correlated (Vogel et al. 1998). Moreover, being injured when older is also often associated with a lower level of well-being, poorer health, and a less active lifestyle (Krause 1998).

We examined the extent of pain's interference with common daily activities as well as relationships between interference and pain characteristics, demographic factors, and psychosocial factors in a study including 217 persons with SCI and chronic pain (Widerström-Noga et al. 2001b). Chronic pain frequently interfered with common activities such as sleep, household chores, exercise, work, and other daily activities. Pain interfered "often" to "always" with one or several of these different areas in 77.3% of subjects.

In particular, difficulties with either going to sleep or staying asleep because of pain were reported "often" to "always" by 38.3% and 40.0% of subjects, respectively. The variables that most significantly predicted the extent of interference with falling asleep were pain described with multiple descriptors and high average pain intensity. Similarly, the frequency of interference with staying asleep was significantly predicted by a combination of factors including intense pain, as well as other variables such as male gender, higher age at time of injury, and psychological factors including anxiety. This finding is consistent with a report by Edwards et al. (2000) showing that only in men were there significant relationships among high severity of pain, anxiety, and pain interference in 215 individuals with heterogeneous pain.

We also rated the extent of interference from pain and examined predictors of interference with household chores, exercise, work and other daily activities. Daily household chores were performed by 62.2% of the sample, and frequent interference was more likely to be experienced by men who also reported excessive fatigue, described their pain as intense, and used multiple descriptors, indicating that they had several different types of pain.

Exercise has profoundly beneficial effects on a variety of health issues following SCI (Noreau and Shepherd 1995; Dallmeijer et al. 1999). In our sample, 34.9% reported that pain frequently interfered with exercise; this limitation appeared to depend primarily on pain intensity rather than on any of the other assessed variables. Demographic factors such as gender and age at injury, level of injury, psychological factors, and psychosocial factors such as employment or level of education were less important in this regard.

Work interference is another area of primary importance. Employment opportunities for persons with SCI are more limited than for able-bodied persons, and chronic pain creates an additional burden. Employment is often viewed as an indicator of successful adaptation to injury (Krause and Anson 1996; McColl et al. 1999), and a low level of engagement in work correlates to lower quality of life following SCI (Kreuter 1997). Of the 53.5% who worked or were in educational programs in our study, 33.6% reported that pain frequently interfered with their work. Frequent pain interference was more likely when individuals suffered from several different kinds of pain, were injured when older, had education at or below high school level, and experienced anxiety.

Although it is important to keep in mind that correlation does not provide any indication of causality, one of the most significant factors related to frequent pain interference in our study was high pain intensity. Thus, the more intense pain is perceived to be, the more frequently pain is reported to interfere. Indeed, Jensen et al. (2001) suggested that the relationship between pain intensity and pain interference is nonlinear, i.e., before pain significantly affects a person's function, a pain intensity "threshold level" must be reached. Interestingly, these authors also reported that pain interference was related to type of pain, paralleling our results revealing a relationship between frequent interference and multiple pain types. Thus, even a moderate decrease in intensity of severe pain following an intervention may have significant beneficial effects on overall function and well-being because the level of pain may decrease to below the "threshold." In fact, pain severity was one of the few factors that predicted well-being in a large study in 1668 persons with tetraplegia (Ville et al. 2001). Furthermore, pain was perceived as being very difficult to deal with by a large proportion of individuals with SCI, and this rating was strongly correlated with intensity of pain (Widerström-Noga et al. 2001a).

Although no gender differences were found in areas such as exercise and work, male gender predicted frequent pain interference with chores and other daily activities. This finding may possibly be due to differences in gender roles, given that women may be more active in domestic chores

(Underlid 1996). Another possibility for the association with male gender and frequent interference is the difference in utilization of coping strategies, with women engaging to a greater extent than men in problem solving, using social support, and making positive self-statements (Unruh et al. 1999).

MULTIDIMENSIONAL IMPACT OF PAIN

As with other types of chronic pain, it is important to realize that physical pathology by itself is insufficient to determine how patients will respond to an SCI or its treatment. Although determining the type of pain is important for the choice of medical treatment strategy, evaluation of the relevant psychosocial factors is critical for a comprehensive approach and a successful treatment outcome (Richards 1992; Turk 1993). While level of satisfaction with life usually is lower following SCI, factors like type of injury only appear to be minimally related (Post et al. 1998). Therefore, factors affecting coping and adjustment are important for long-term therapeutic success in SCI where chronic pain may be long-lasting and is likely to respond poorly to treatment (Störmer et al. 1997).

Many aspects related to the psychosocial and behavioral domains are highly relevant to chronic pain in persons with SCI. However, these relationships are often complex and may be specific to the SCI pain population. For example, chronic pain can negatively influence a person's ability to cope with the consequences of SCI (Stensman 1994), and negative coping following SCI is associated with depression (Kemp and Krause 1999), yet several factors may mediate the association between affective distress and chronic pain. For example, Turk and colleagues (Rudy et al. 1988; Turk et al. 1995) reported that perceived interference of pain with ability to function mediated the association between pain and depression. Activities of daily living are affected not only by pain, but also by other consequences resulting from SCI. Thus, affective distress may not only be directly related to chronic pain but rather to how successfully a person is able to cope with the impact of SCI (Scivoletti et al. 1997).

The Multidimensional Pain Inventory (MPI) is a comprehensive instrument designed not only to assess a broad range of behavioral and psychosocial factors associated with chronic pain syndromes but also to evaluate the relationships among these factors (Kerns et al. 1985; Turk and Rudy 1988). It has been used to assess various pain states such as back pain, headache, temporomandibular disorders, fibromyalgia, and cancer (Turk et al. 1996, 1998; Turk and Rudy 1988). Its factor structure has been confirmed for several specific pain populations (Bergström et al. 1998; Lousberg et al.

1999; Riley et al. 1999). The MPI assesses several domains important for coping and adaptation and provides possibilities for differentiating subgroups of subjects by its cluster features (Turk and Rudy 1988). The MPI consists of three sections, of which the first includes items concerning perceived severity of pain; the extent to which pain interferes with activities of daily life; perceived degree of support received from one's significant other; level of affective distress experienced; and perceived level of control over life events, including pain. The second section assesses three different types of responses (negative, solicitous, and distracting) of the significant other to the individual's pain. To improve response rates to this section, "significant other" was defined as the person to whom the respondent feels closest (Okifuji et al. 1999). The third section includes the patient's level of participation in various activities. The four factors or groups of items in this section are household chores, activities away from home, social activities, and outdoor activities.

Although the MPI has previously been used in the SCI population (Summers et al. 1991; Conant 1998), no previous study has evaluated whether it is appropriate for use in this population. Therefore, we decided to test the adequacy of the MPI for use in this population by using confirmatory and secondary exploratory factor analyses to estimate how well the factor structure of the MPI established in other chronic pain populations could be replicated (Widerström-Noga et al. 2002). We were also interested in the extent to which pain decreased activity compared to other aspects of injury and whether there were differences in the psychosocial and behavioral responses between cervical and below-cervical injuries.

A group of 120 persons with SCI and chronic pain filled out the MPI. We then statistically analyzed each of the three sections of the MPI. Because more than half of persons with SCI are unemployed at 1 year after injury (Krause et al. 1999), MPI items concerning work interference and work satisfaction did not appear relevant. Consequently, removal of these and two additional cross-loading items improved the statistical "fit" (goodness-of-fit) for Section I (Appendix B). The subsequent exploratory factor analysis replicated the original factor structure and accounted for over 70% of the total variation. Furthermore, the internal consistency values for each factor were similar to those observed in other pain samples (Bergström et al. 1998). Of the five subscales (factors), life control had the lowest value, and even though internal locus of control and pain severity following SCI are significantly related (Conant 1998), control over one's life following SCI is related to other consequences of injury as well as chronic pain (Macleod and Macleod 1998). Although our data did not perfectly fit the original MPI factor structure, displayed as moderate fit indices (Marsh et al. 1988), we replicated the original factor structure for Section I in the analyses. Thus, the cognitive-behavioral theory on which the five factors making up Section I was based appears to be valid for persons with SCI.

The same procedure was applied to Sections II (perceived responses from significant others) and III (activities) of the MPI. After deleting two items from Section II, the statistical indices indicated a satisfactory goodness-of-fit. The analysis of Section III did not show a satisfactory fit, but a subsequent exploratory factor analysis resulted in an activity scale where all original items were retained but in different factors. For example, car-related work, originally loading on the subscale "Outdoor work," instead loaded on "Social Activities," suggesting that after SCI this type of activity is more of a social activity that is performed together with friends. This finding suggests that the activity scale of the MPI-SCI should be used as a general measure of activity. Bergström et al. (1998) found similar problems in the Swedish version of the MPI, and suggested the same solution.

It is difficult to determine the reason for decreased activity in people with chronic pain and SCI. We attempted to address this issue by including two questions for each activity that asked about the extent to which pain and other consequences of SCI, respectively, reduced participation in a particular activity. The results reveal that activity levels, as measured by the MPI, were judged to be significantly more affected by other consequences of SCI than by pain itself. The strong relationship between decrease in activity due to the various sequelae of SCI and decrease in activity due to pain reflects a person's overall coping and physical ability. Similarly, difficulty in dealing with pain is also related to difficulty in dealing with other consequences of injury, such as abnormal nonpainful sensations, muscle spasms, and sadness (Widerström-Noga et al. 1999).

As would be anticipated and similar to relationships observed in other studies of heterogeneous pain patients (Turk and Rudy 1988; Turk et al. 1996; Jensen et al. 2001) and following SCI (Rintala et al. 1998; Widerström-Noga et al. 2001b), the more severe pain is perceived to be, the greater is the probability that pain will negatively affect level of activity. Because overall activity levels were more affected by the other consequences of SCI than by pain, we explored the relationships between activity levels and level of injury (i.e., tetraplegia or paraplegia). As might be expected, activity levels were significantly higher in persons with paraplegia than in those with tetraplegia. Those with tetraplegia also reported significantly less participation in various activities due to "other consequences" of injury than did those with paraplegia. In contrast, a comparison of persons with tetraplegia and those with paraplegia found no significant difference with regard to decreased activities due to chronic pain.

The analysis of the appropriateness of using the MPI in persons with chronic SCI pain showed that while similarities in the responses of the specific SCI and heterogeneous pain populations were apparent, several aspects were unique to SCI. Even though the factor structure and consequently the theoretical foundation were similar following SCI, it is evident that other consequences of SCI beyond the presence of pain have a significant impact on life.

The revised MPI presented in Appendix B appears to be a reasonable instrument to evaluate the impact of SCI pain and the response of significant others to pain. However, because activity levels are different depending on whether a person has tetraplegia or paraplegia and because other consequences of SCI decrease activity levels more than pain, less participation in a particular activity may not necessarily reflect impairment due to pain itself. Reduction in activity levels due to pain appeared to be independent of injury level, so this measure appears to more directly assess how pain affects activity levels. Future research must address the psychometric properties of the revised MPI and the use of complementary ways to assess psychosocial and behavioral aspects of chronic SCI pain.

We have conducted preliminary cluster analyses of MPI data according to the revised MPI (unpublished observations) and found that the proportion of people falling into the "Adaptive coper/Minimizer" cluster appears to be much larger than in other pain populations. Interestingly, Cohen et al. (1988) used the MPQ and the Minnesota Multiphasic Pain Inventory (MMPI) to assess pain in persons with SCI and found differences in the profiles compared to able-bodied populations with heterogeneous pain as well as differences between incomplete and complete SCI. While persons with incomplete injuries reported pain to be as severe as did a heterogeneous chronic pain population, those with complete injuries reported less severe pain but had a significantly more elevated MMPI profile, indicating more psychological distress. These inconsistencies emphasize that there are important differences among the various subgroups of SCI patients as well as differences between heterogeneous pain populations and the SCI population. Therefore, we must better define the various psychosocial and psychological responses to chronic pain specific to the SCI population with the goal of better understanding and improved treatment of chronic pain following SCI.

CONCLUSIONS

New knowledge concerning the pathophysiological mechanisms of chronic SCI pain may well stimulate exciting new pharmacological treatment approaches, yet it is unrealistic to assume that persons who have suffered pain for many years will completely recover and return to "normal" activities, even with new, more effective treatments. Thus, in order to provide optimal pain relief and enhance quality of life following SCI, clinicians must assess and treat these pain conditions from a multidisciplinary perspective. A comprehensive assessment protocol and a tailored therapeutic approach based on pain type and neurological characteristics as well as psychosocial and behavioral factors should provide a better possibility to significantly relieve chronic SCI pain and decrease its impact on patients' lives.

ACKNOWLEDGMENTS

The research presented in this chapter and the preparation of the manuscript were supported by The Miami Project to Cure Paralysis; The State of Florida; VAMC, Miami; The Hollfelder Foundation; and The Gordon Family Foundation. The author gratefully acknowledges the persons with SCI and chronic pain who volunteered to provide detailed information concerning their pain and my colleagues who contributed with their enthusiasm and expertise in the studies. In addition, I would like to thank Drs. Dennis Turk and Robert Yezierski for helpful comments and suggestions concerning this chapter.

REFERENCES

Arnstein P, Caudill M, Mandle CL, Norris A, Beasley R. Self-efficacy as a mediator between pain intensity, disability, and depression in chronic pain. *Pain* 1999; 80:483–491.

Bergström G, Jensen IB, Bodin L, et al. Reliability and factor structure of the Multidimensional Pain Inventory—Swedish language version (MPI-S). *Pain* 1998; 75:101–110.

Bonica JJ. Introduction: semantic, epidemiologic, and educational issues. In: Casey KL (Ed). *Pain and Central Nervous System Disease: The Central Pain Syndromes.* New York: Raven Press, 1991, pp 13–29.

Bowsher D. Central pain: clinical and physiological characteristics. *J Neurol Neurosurg Psychiatry* 1996; 61:62–69.

Bryce TN, Ragnarsson KT. Pain after spinal cord injury. *Phys Med Rehabil Clin N Am* 2000; 11:157–168.

Cairns DM, Adkins RH, Scott MD. Pain and depression in acute traumatic spinal cord injury: origins of chronic problematic pain? *Arch Phys Med Rehabil* 1996; 77:329–335.

Cohen MJ, McArthur DL, Vulpe M, Schandler SL, Gerber KE. Comparing chronic pain from spinal cord injury to chronic pain of other origins. *Pain* 1988; 35:57–63.

Conant LL. Psychological variables associated with pain perceptions among individuals with chronic spinal cord injury pain. *J Clin Psychol Med Settings* 1998; 5:71–90.

Curtis KA, Drysdale GA, Lanza RD, et al. Shoulder pain in wheelchair users with tetraplegia and paraplegia. *Arch Phys Med Rehabil* 1999; 80:453–457.

Dallmeijer AJ, van der Woude LH, Hollander AP, van As HH. Physical performance during rehabilitation in persons with spinal cord injuries. *Med Sci Sports Exerc* 1999; 31:1330–1335.

Dalyan M, Cardenas DD, Gerard B. Upper extremity pain after spinal cord injury. *Spinal Cord* 1999; 37:191–195.
Defrin R, Ohry A, Blumen N, Urca G. Characterization of chronic pain and somatosensory function in spinal cord injury subjects. *Pain* 2001; 89:253–263.
Demirel G, Yllmaz H, Gencosmanoglu B, Kesiktas N. Pain following spinal cord injury. *Spinal Cord* 1998; 36:25–28.
Edwards R, Augustson EM, Fillingim R. Sex-specific effects of pain-related anxiety on adjustment to chronic pain. *Clin J Pain* 2000; 16:46–53.
Eide PK. Pathophysiological mechanisms of central neuropathic pain after spinal cord injury. *Spinal Cord* 1998; 36:601–612.
Eide PK, Jørum E, Stenehjelm AE. Somatosensory findings in patients with spinal cord injury and central dysesthesia pain. *J Neurol Neurosurg Psychiatry* 1996; 60:411–415.
Feldman SI, Downey G, Schaffer-Neitz R. Pain, negative mood, and perceived support in chronic pain patients: a daily diary study of people with reflex sympathetic dystrophy syndrome. *J Consult Clin Psychol* 1999; 67:776–785.
Fields HL. *Pain.* New York: McGraw-Hill, 1987.
Fenollosa P, Pallares J, Cervera J, et al. Chronic pain in the spinal cord injured: statistical approach and pharmacological treatment. *Paraplegia* 1993; 31:722–729.
Finnerup NB, Johannesen IL, Sindrup SH, Bach FW, Jensen TS. Pain and dysesthesia in patients with spinal cord injury: a postal survey. *Spinal Cord* 2001; 39:256–262.
Fuhrer MJ. The subjective well-being of people with spinal cord injury: relationships to impairment, disability, and handicap. *Top Spinal Cord Injury Rehabil* 1996; 1:56–71.
Haythornthwaite JA, Benrud-Larson LM. Psychological aspects of neuropathic pain. *Clin J Pain* 2000; 16:101–105.
Haythornthwaite JA, Benrud-Larson LM. Psychological assessment and treatment of patients with neuropathic pain. *Curr Pain Headache Rep* 2001; 5:124–129.
Jacob KS, Zachariah K, Bhattacharji S. Depression in individuals with spinal cord injury: methodological issues. *Paraplegia* 1995; 33:377–380.
Jamison RN, Raymond SA, Levine JG, et al. Electronic diaries for monitoring chronic pain: 1-year validation study. *Pain* 2001; 91:277–281.
Jensen MP, Turner JA, Romano JM, Lawler BK. Relationship of pain-specific beliefs to chronic pain adjustment. *Pain* 1994; 57:301–309.
Jensen MP, Smith DG, Ehde DM, Robinson LR. Pain site and the effects of amputation pain: further clarification of the meaning of mild, moderate, and severe pain. *Pain* 2001; 91:317–322.
Kemp BJ, Krause JS. Depression and life satisfaction among people ageing with post-polio and spinal cord injury. *Disabil Rehabil* 1999; 21:241–249.
Kennedy P, Frankel H, Gardner B, Nuseibeh I. Factors associated with acute and chronic pain following traumatic spinal cord injuries. *Spinal Cord* 1997; 35:814–817.
Kerns RD, Turk DC, Rudy TE. The West Haven-Yale multidimensional pain inventory (WHYMPI). *Pain* 1985; 23:345–356.
King C, Kennedy P. Coping effectiveness training for people with spinal cord injury: preliminary results of a controlled trial. *Br J Clin Psychol* 1999; 38:5–14.
Kishi Y, Robinson RG, Forrester AW. Prospective longitudinal study of depression following spinal cord injury. *J Neuropsychiatry Clin Neurosci* 1994; 6:237–244.
Krause JS. Aging and life adjustment after spinal cord injury. *Spinal Cord* 1998; 36:320–328.
Krause JS, Anson CA. Employment after spinal cord injury: relations to related participant characteristics. *Arch Phys Med Rehabil* 1996; 77:737– 743.
Krause JS, Kewman D, DeVivo MJ, et al. Employment after spinal cord injury: an analysis of cases from the Model Spinal Cord Injury Systems. *Arch Phys Med Rehabil* 1999; 80(11):1492–1500.
Kreuter M. Partner relationships, sexuality and quality of life in persons with traumatic spinal cord injury and brain injury. Dissertation, Göteborg University, Sweden, 1997.
Lal S. Premature degenerative shoulder changes in spinal cord injury patients. *Spinal Cord* 1998; 36:186–189.

Levi R, Hulting C, Nash M, Seiger Å. The Stockholm spinal cord injury study. 1. Medical problems in a regional SCI population. *Paraplegia* 1995; 33:308–315.

Lundqvist C, Siösteen A, Sullivan L, Lind B, Sullivan M. Spinal cord injuries: clinical, functional, and emotional status. *Spine* 1991; 16:78–83.

Lindblom U. Analysis of abnormal touch, pain, and temperature sensation in patients. In: Boivie J, Hansson P, Lindblom U (Eds). *Touch, Temperature, and Pain in Health and Disease: Mechanisms and Assessments,* Progress in Pain Research and Management, Vol. 3. Seattle: IASP Press, 1994, pp 63–84.

Lousberg R, Van Breukelen GJ, Groenman NH, et al. Psychometric properties of the Multidimensional Pain Inventory, Dutch language version (MPI-DLV). *Behav Res Ther* 1999; 37:167–182.

Lundqvist C, Siosteen A, Blomstrand C, Lind B, Sullivan M. Spinal cord injuries: clinical, functional, and emotional status. *Spine* 1991; 16:78–83.

Macleod L, Macleod G. Control cognitions and psychological disturbance in people with contrasting physically disabling conditions. *Disabil Rehabil* 1998; 20:448–456.

Margolis RB, Chibnall JT, Tait RC. Test-retest reliability of the pain drawing instrument. *Pain* 1988; 33:49–51.

Mariano AJ. Chronic pain and spinal cord injury. *Clin J Pain* 1992; 8:87–92.

Marsh HW, Balla JR, McDonald RO. Goodness-of-fit indexes in confirmatory factor analysis: the effect of sample size. *Psychol Bull* 1988; 103:391–410.

McColl MA, Stirling P, Walker J, Wilkins R. Expectations of independence and life satisfaction among aging spinal cord injured adults. *Disabil Rehabil* 1999; 21:231–240.

Melzack R. The McGill Pain Questionnaire: major properties and scoring methods. *Pain* 1975; 1:277–299.

Melzack R. The short-form McGill Pain Questionnaire. *Pain* 1987; 30:191–197.

Merskey H. Pain terms: a list with definitions and notes on usage. *Pain* 1979; 6:249–252.

Murphy D, Reid DB. Pain treatment satisfaction in spinal cord injury. *Spinal Cord* 2001; 39:44–46.

Nepomuceno C, Fine PR, Richards JS, et al. Pain in patients with spinal cord injury. *Arch Phys Med Rehabil* 1979; 60:605–609.

Noreau L, Shephard RJ. Spinal cord injury, exercise and quality of life. *Sports Med* 1995; 20:226–250.

Okifuji A, Turk DC, Eveleigh DJ. Improving the rate of classification of patients with the multidimensional pain inventory (MPI): clarifying the meaning of "significant other." *Clin J Pain* 1999; 15:290–296.

Pentland W, McColl MA, Rosenthal C. The effect of aging and duration of disability on long term health outcomes following spinal cord injury. *Paraplegia* 1995; 33:367–373.

Post MW, de Witte LP, van Asbeck FW, van Dijk AJ, Schrijver S. Predictors of health status and life satisfaction in spinal cord injury. *Arch Phys Med Rehabil* 1998; 79(4):395–401.

Ragnarsson KT. Management of pain in persons with spinal cord injury. *J Spinal Cord Med* 1997; 20:186–199.

Raphael KG, Marbach JJ. When did your pain start?: reliability of self-reported age of onset of facial pain. *Clin J Pain* 1997; 13:352–359.

Ravenscroft A, Ahmed YS, Burnside IG. Chronic pain after SCI: a patient survey. *Spinal Cord* 2000; 38:611–614.

Richards JS. Chronic pain and spinal cord injury: review and comment. *Clin J Pain* 1992; 8:119–122.

Richards JS, Meredith RL, Nepomuceno C, Fine PR, Bennett G. Psycho-social aspects of chronic pain in spinal cord injury. *Pain* 1980; 8:355–366.

Riley JL III, Zawacki TM, Robinson ME, Geisser ME. Empirical test of the factor structure of the West Haven-Yale Multidimensional Pain Inventory. *Clin J Pain* 1999; 15:24–30.

Rintala DH, Loubser PG, Castro J, Hart KA, Fuhrer MJ. Chronic pain in a community-based sample of men with spinal cord injury: prevalence, severity, and relationships with impairment, disability, handicap, and subjective well-being. *Arch Phys Med Rehabil* 1998; 79:604–614.

Rose M, Robinson JE, Ells P, Cole JD. Pain following spinal cord injury: results from a postal survey. *Pain* 1988; 34:101–102.

Rudy TE, Kerns RD, Turk DC. Chronic pain and depression: toward a cognitive-behavioral mediation model. *Pain* 1988; 35:129–140.

Scivoletto G, Petrelli A, Di Lucente L, Castellano VI. Psychological investigation of spinal cord injury patients. *Spinal Cord* 1997; 35:516–520.

Siddall PJ, Taylor DA, Cousins MJ. Classification of pain following spinal cord injury. *Spinal Cord* 1997; 35:69–75.

Siddall PJ, Loeser JD. Pain following spinal cord injury. *Spinal Cord* 2001; 39:63–73.

Siddall PJ, Cousins MJ. Spine update: spinal mechanisms. *Spine* 1997; 22:98–104.

Siddall PJ, Taylor DA, McClelland JM, Rutkowski SB, Cousins MJ. Pain report and the relationship of pain to physical factors in the first 6 months following injury. *Pain* 1999; 81:187–197.

Siddall PJ, Yezierski RP, Loeser JD. Pain following spinal cord injury: clinical features, prevalence, and taxonomy. *IASP Newsletter* 2000; 3:3–7.

Smith WB, Safer MA. Effects of present pain level on recall of chronic pain and medication use. *Pain* 1993; 55:355–361.

Stensman R. Adjustment to traumatic spinal cord injury: a longitudinal study of self-reported quality of life. *Paraplegia* 1994; 32:416–422.

Störmer S, Gerner HJ, Gruninger W, et al. Chronic pain/dysesthesiae in spinal cord injury patients: results of a multicentre study. *Spinal Cord* 1997; 35:446–455.

Subbarao JV, Klopfstein J, Turpin R. Prevalence and impact of wrist and shoulder pain in patients with spinal cord injury. *J Spinal Cord Med* 1995; 18:9–13.

Summers JD, Rapoff MA, Varghese G, Porter K, Palmer RE. Psychosocial factors in chronic spinal cord injury pain. *Pain* 1991; 47:183–189.

Tunks E. Pain in spinal cord injured patients. In: Bloch RF, Basbaum M (Eds). *Management of Spinal Cord Injuries.* Baltimore: Williams and Wilkins, 1986, pp 180–211.

Turner JA, Cardenas DD. Chronic pain problems in individuals with spinal cord injuries. *Semin Clin Neuropsychiatry* 1999; 4:186–194.

Turner JA, Cardenas DD, Warms CA, McClellan CB. Chronic pain associated with spinal cord injuries: a community survey. *Arch Phys Med Rehabil* 2001; 82:501–509.

Turk DC. Customizing treatment for chronic pain patients: who, what, and why? *Clin J Pain* 1990; 6:255–270.

Turk DC. Assess the person, not just the pain. *Pain: Clin Updates* 1993; 1:1–4.

Turk DC. Biopsychosocial perspective on chronic pain. In: Gatchel RJ, Turk DC (Eds). *Psychosocial Approaches to Pain Management: A Practitioners Handbook.* New York: Guilford Press, 1996, pp 3–32.

Turk DC, Flor H. Chronic pain: a biobehavioral perspective. In: Gatchel RJ, Turk DC (Eds). *Psychosocial Factors in Pain: Critical Perspectives.* New York: Guilford Press, 1992, pp 481–494.

Turk DC, Melzack R (Eds). *Handbook of Pain Assessment,* 2nd ed. New York: Guilford Press, 2001.

Turk DC, Rudy TE. Toward an empirically derived taxonomy of chronic pain patients: integration of psychological assessment data. *J Consult Clin Psychol* 1988; 56:233–238.

Turk DC, Okifuji A, Scharff L. Chronic pain and depression: role of perceived impact and perceived control in different age cohorts. *Pain* 1995; 61:93–102.

Turk DC, Okifuji A, Sinclair JD, Starz TW. Pain, disability, and physical functioning in subgroups of fibromyalgia patients. *J Rheumatol* 1996; 23:1255–1262.

Turk DC, Sist TC, Okifuji A, et al. Adaptation to metastatic cancer pain, regional/local cancer pain and non-cancer pain: role of psychological and behavioral factors. *Pain* 1998; 74:247–256.

Umlauf RL. Psychological interventions for chronic pain following spinal cord injury. *Clin J Pain* 1992; 8:111–118.

Underlid K. Activity during unemployment and mental health. *Scand J Psychol* 1996; 37:269–281.

Unruh AM, Ritchie J, Merskey H. Does gender affect appraisal of pain and pain coping strategies? *Clin J Pain* 1999; 15:31–40.

Vierck CJ, Siddall P, Yezierski RP. Pain following spinal cord injury: animal models and mechanistic studies. *Pain* 2000; 89:1–5.

Ville I, Ravaud JF. Tetrafigap Group. Subjective well-being and severe motor impairments: the Tetrafigap survey on the long-term outcome of tetraplegic spinal cord injured persons. *Soc Sci Med* 2001; 52:369–384.

Vogel LC, Klaas SJ, Lubicky JP, Anderson CJ. Long-term outcomes and life satisfaction for adults who had pediatric spinal cord injuries. *Arch Phys Med Rehabil* 1998; 79:1496–1503.

Wegener ST, Elliott TR. Pain assessment in spinal cord injury. *Clin J Pain* 1992; 8:93–101.

Westgren N, Levi R. Quality of life and traumatic spinal cord injury. *Arch Phys Med Rehabil* 1998; 79:1433–1439

Widerström-Noga EG, Felipe-Cuervo E, Broton JG, Duncan RC, Yezierski RP. Perceived difficulty in dealing with consequences of spinal cord injury. *Arch Phys Med Rehabil* 1999; 80:580–586.

Widerström-Noga EG, Felipe-Cuervo E, Yezierski RP. Relationships among clinical characteristics of chronic pain following spinal cord injury. *Arch Phys Med Rehabil* 2001a; 82(9):1191–1197.

Widerström-Noga EG, Felipe-Cuervo E, Yezierski RP. Chronic pain following spinal cord injury: interference with sleep and activities. *Arch Phys Med Rehabil* 2001b; 82(11):1571–1577.

Widerström-Noga EG, Duncan R, Felipe-Cuervo E, Turk DC. Assessment of the impact of pain and impairments associated with spinal cord injuries. *Arch Phys Med Rehabil* 2002; 83(3): in press.

Correspondence to: Eva Widerström-Noga, DDS, PhD, Miami Project to Cure Paralysis, Department of Neurological Surgery, Lois Pope LIFE Center, University of Miami School of Medicine, P.O. Box 016960 (R-48), Miami, FL 33101, USA. Tel: 305-243-7125; Fax: 305-243-3921; email: ewiderst@miamiproject.med.miami.edu.

Spinal Cord Injury Pain: Assessment, Mechanisms, Management. Progress in Pain Research and Management, Vol. 23, edited by Robert P. Yezierski and Kim J. Burchiel, IASP Press, Seattle, © 2002.

Appendix A

Pain History (Interview Format, SCI Version)

(1) A person may have pain in one or several places. **Where do you have pain?** Please mark the area(s) in the figures that show the location of your pain.

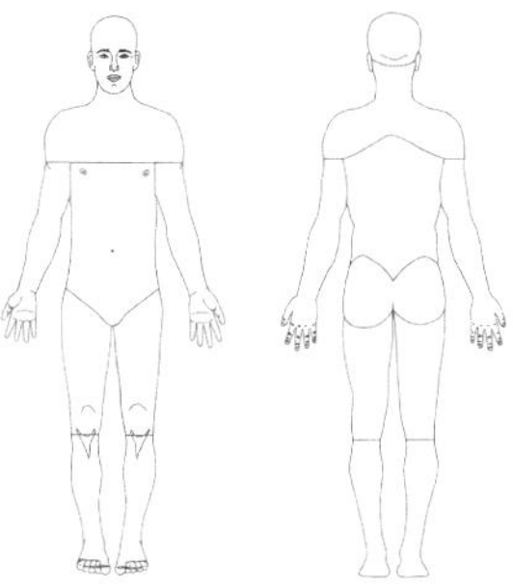

H head
NS neck and shoulder
AH arms and hands
FG front and genitals
BA back
BU buttocks
T thighs
LF legs and feet

(2) Listed below are words used to describe pain. Please write the letters corresponding to the painful area(s)in front of the words that best describe <u>your</u> pain. You can also use your own word(s).

__sharp	__shooting	__stinging	__electric
__stabbing	__flashing	__shocking	__lancinating
__crushing	__pinching	__penetrating	__lacerating
__burning	__pricking	__cramping	__cutting
__aching	__throbbing	__pressing	__pulsating
__radiating	__dull	__cold	__biting

H head
NS neck and shoulder
AH arms and hands
FG front and genitals
BA back
BU buttocks
T thighs
LF legs and feet

______________ ______________ ______________

(3) The following question concern: (a) how intense your pain is on average; and (b) how unpleasant your pain is on average. Please rate your pain(s) by circling the numbers and link each pain rating (if the various areas differ) with the letters corresponding to a particular area.

How <u>intense</u> is the pain on average?

no pain 0 1 2 3 4 5 6 7 8 9 10 most intense pain imaginable

H NS AH FG BA BU T LF

How <u>unpleasant</u> is the pain on average?

no pain 0 1 2 3 4 5 6 7 8 9 10 most unpleasant pain imaginable

H NS AH FG BA BU T LF

(4) How often is it difficult to go to sleep because of pain? Indicate using the letters for each area if different.

_____ never
_____ every night
_____ three to six nights per week
_____ one or two nights per week
_____ one to three nights per month

(5) How often do you wake up because of pain? Indicate using the letters for each area if different.

_____ never
_____ every night
_____ three to six nights per week
_____ one or two nights per week
_____ one to three nights per month

(6) How much does pain interfere with your exercise habits? Indicate using the letters for each area if different.

_____ I do not normally exercise
_____ pain never interferes with my exercise
_____ pain sometimes interferes with my exercise
_____ pain often interferes with my exercise
_____ pain always interferes with my exercise

(7) How much does pain interfere with you doing household chores? Indicate using the letters for each area if different.

_____ I do not normally do household chores
_____ pain never interferes with my household chores
_____ pain sometimes interferes with my household chores
_____ pain often interferes with my household chores
_____ pain always interferes with my household chores

(8) How much does pain interfere with your work? Indicate using the letters for each area if different.

_____ I am not working because of reasons other than pain
_____ pain never interferes with my work
_____ pain sometimes interferes with my work
_____ pain often interferes with my work
_____ pain always interferes with my work

(9) How much does pain interfere with other daily activities?

_____ pain never interferes with other daily activities
_____ pain sometimes interferes with other daily activities
_____ pain often interferes with other daily activities
_____ pain always interferes with other daily activities

(10) Did you have pain that lasted more than 6 months before you got injured?

☐ **No**

☐ **Yes**

If yes, circle the letters corresponding to the area below.

H NS AH FG BA BU T LF

(11) After your SCI, when did you pain(s) start? Indicate using the letters for each area if different.

_____ immediately following injury
_____ within the first month following injury
_____ 1–3 months following injury
_____ 3–6 months following injury
_____ 6 months to a year following injury
_____ 1–2 years after injury
_____ more than two years following injury

(12) Does your pain(s) vary in how much it hurts? Indicate using the letters for each area if different.

____ **No**
____ **Yes. If yes:**

(A) When does it usually hurt the <u>least:</u>

_____ in the morning
_____ around noon
_____ in the afternoon
_____ at night
_____ no predictable pattern

(B) When does it usually hurt the <u>most:</u>

_____ in the morning
_____ around noon
_____ in the afternoon
_____ at night
_____ no predictable pattern

(13) How often do you have pain? Indicate using the letters for each area if different.

_____ every day
_____ 3–6 days per week
_____ 1–2 days per week
_____ 1–3 days per month
_____ no predictable pattern

(14) How long are the breaks from this pain? Indicate using the letters for each area if different.

_____ I have no breaks from the pain
_____ I have short breaks (less than five minutes)
_____ I have breaks of 5 minutes and up to one hour
_____ I have breaks of several hours
_____ I have breaks of one day to several days
_____ I have week-long breaks
_____ no predictable pattern

(15) Do you have "attacks" (less then five minutes) of pain?

_____ **No**
_____ **Yes. If yes, how frequent are these attacks?**
_____ More than 5 times per day
_____ 1–5 times per day
_____ 3–6 times per week
_____ 1–2 times per week
_____ 1–3 times per month
_____ no predictable pattern

(16) Pain can change with time. This change may be related to how it feels and/or where it is located.
Has your pain(s) changed significantly since it started? Indicate using the letters for each area if different. <u>Please note that several alternatives can be selected</u>.

_____ **No**
_____ **Yes**, it is <u>more</u> intense now than at the time it started
_____ **Yes**, it is <u>less</u> intense now than at the time it started
_____ **Yes**, the painful area has become <u>smaller</u>
_____ **Yes**, the painful area has become <u>larger</u>
_____ **Yes**, the pain has moved from one location to another
_____ **Yes,** the pain has changed from a painful sensation to non-painful

(17) If your pain has changed significantly since it started, can you explain why? Indicate using the letters for each area if different.

_____ My pain has not changed a lot
_____ I have received an effective treatment
_____ I don't know
_____ **Other reason** ____

(18) If you have pain in several areas, which one is the most disturbing?

_____ No area is more disturbing than another
_____ I have pain in one area only
_____ **Yes.** If yes, circle the area that is most disturbing

H NS AH FG BA BU T LF

(19) The following list contains factors and situations that may affect your pain. Please mark with the letters corresponding to the area how these factors affect your pain. If there are factors/situations that affect your pain which are not listed, please add these below.

Factor or Situation	Do not know	Makes pain disappear	Makes pain considerably better	Makes pain slightly better	No effect on pain	Makes pain worse	Makes pain considerably worse
lying down							
getting out of bed							
going outside							
sudden movements							
muscle spasms							
coughing or sneezing							
exercise							
sexual activity							
anger							
anxiety							
feeling sad							
fatigue							
touch							
noise							
listening to music							
alcohol							
cigarettes							
caffeine							
recreational drugs							
infections							
hot climate							
cold climate							
wet climate							
full bladder							
constipation							
prolonged sitting							
change of position							

Spinal Cord Injury Pain: Assessment, Mechanisms, Management. Progress in Pain Research and Management, Vol. 23, edited by Robert P. Yezierski and Kim J. Burchiel, IASP Press, Seattle, © 2002.

Appendix B

Multidimensional Pain Inventory (SCI Version)[1]

Today's date: ____________________
ID: ________________________
When did your pain first start? Month: ______ Year: ________

Instructions
An important part of our evaluation includes examination of pain from ***your*** perspective because you know your pain better than anyone else. The following questions are designed to help us learn more about your pain and how it affects your life. The questionnaire has three sections. Under each question is a scale to mark your answer. Read each question carefully and then ***circle a number*** on the scale under that question to indicate how that specific question applies to you. If there is a question that you think does not apply to you, please circle ***the number*** of that question. After you have completed the questionnaire, check your responses to make sure that you have answered each question. Please use the last page to add any additional information or comments that you think would be of help to us in better understanding your pain problem.

Before you begin, please answer the two pre-evaluation questions below:

1. Some of the questions in this questionnaire refer to your "significant other." A significant other is **the *person with whom you feel closest***. This includes ***anyone*** that you relate to on a regular or frequent basis. It is very important that you identify someone as your "significant other." Please indicate below who your significant other is (please check only one):

   __ Spouse __ Partner/companion __ Housemate/roommate
   __ Friend __ Neighbor __ Parent, child or other relative
   __ Other: ____

2. Do you currently live with this person?
   __ Yes
   __ No

When you answer questions on the following pages about "your significant other," always respond in reference to the specific person you just indicated.

---

[1] The original items of the MPI are reprinted with permission from the copyright holders, Robert Kerns, Thomas Rudy, and Dennis Turk. The SCI version of the MPI was previously published by Widerström-Noga et al. (2002); reprinted with permission.

Section I

This part asks questions to help us learn more about your pain and how it affects your life. Under each question is a scale to mark your answer. Read each question carefully and then ***circle a number*** on the scale under that question to indicate how that specific question applies to you. The following example may help you to better understand how you should answer these questions.

Example

How nervous are you when you ride in a car when the traffic is heavy?

Not at all nervous 0 1 2 3 4 5 6 Extremely nervous

If you are not at all nervous when riding in a car in heavy traffic, you would want to ***circle*** the number 0. If you are very nervous when riding in a car in heavy traffic, you would then circle the number 6. Lower numbers would be used for less nervousness, and higher numbers for more nervousness.

1. Rate the level of your pain at the present moment.

No pain 0 1 2 3 4 5 6 Very intense pain

2. How much has your pain changed the amount of satisfaction or enjoyment you get from taking part in social and recreational activities?

No change 0 1 2 3 4 5 6 Extreme change

3. How supportive or helpful is your spouse (significant other) to you in relation to your pain?

Not at all supportive 0 1 2 3 4 5 6 Extremely supportive

4. Rate your overall mood during the past week

Extremely low 0 1 2 3 4 5 6 Extremely high

5. On the average, how severe has your pain been during the last week?

Not at all severe 0 1 2 3 4 5 6 Extremely severe

6. How much has your pain changed your ability to take part in recreational and other social activities?

No change 0 1 2 3 4 5 6 Extreme change

7. How much do you limit your activities in order to keep your pain from getting worse?

Not at all 0 1 2 3 4 5 6 Very much

8. How much has your pain changed the amount of satisfaction or enjoyment you get from family-related activities?

No change 0 1 2 3 4 5 6 Extreme change

9. How worried is your spouse (significant other) about you because of your pain?

Not at all worried 0 1 2 3 4 5 6 Extremely worried

10. During the past week how much control do you feel that you have had over your life?

No control 0 1 2 3 4 5 6 Extreme control

11. How much suffering do you experience because of your pain?
No suffering 0 1 2 3 4 5 6 Extreme suffering

12. How much has your pain changed your relationship with your spouse, family, or significant other?
No change 0 1 2 3 4 5 6 Extreme change

13. How attentive is your spouse (significant other) to you because of your pain?
Not at all attentive 0 1 2 3 4 5 6 Extremely attentive

14. During the <u>past week</u> how much do you feel that you've been able to deal with your problems?
Not at all 0 1 2 3 4 5 6 Extremely well

15. How much control do you feel that you have over your pain?
No control at all 0 1 2 3 4 5 6 A great deal of control

16. How much has your pain changed your ability to do household chores?
No change 0 1 2 3 4 5 6 Extreme change

17. How much has your pain interfered with your ability to plan activities?
No interference 0 1 2 3 4 5 6 Extreme interference

18. During the <u>past week</u> how irritable have you been?
Not at all irritable 0 1 2 3 4 5 6 Extremely irritable

19. How much has your pain changed or interfered with your friendships with people other than your family?
No change 0 1 2 3 4 5 6 Extreme change

20. During the <u>past week</u> how tense or anxious have you been?
Not at all tense or anxious 0 1 2 3 4 5 6 Extremely tense and anxious

Section II

In this section, we are interested in knowing how your spouse (or significant other) responds to you when he or she knows that you are in pain. On the scale listed below each question, **circle a number** to indicate **how often** your spouse (or significant other) responds to you in that particular way when you are in pain. ***(All questions below are answered on the following response scale)***

Never 0 1 2 3 4 5 6 Very often

21. Asks me what he/she can do to help.
22. Reads to me.
23. Gets irritated with me.
24. Takes over my jobs or duties.
25. Talks to me about something else to take my mind off the pain.
26. Gets frustrated with me.
27. Tries to get me to rest.

28. Tries to involve me in some activity.
29. Gets angry with me.
30. Gets me pain medication.
31. Encourages me to work on a hobby.
32. Gets me something to eat or drink.

Section III

Listed below are 18 daily activities. Please indicate:
How often you do each of these by ***circling a number*** on the scale listed below ***(All questions below are answered on the following response scale)***

Never 0 1 2 3 4 5 6 Very often

For each item please also circle the number indicating how ***pain*** has affected how often you participate in these activities on the following response scale ***(All questions below are answered on the following response scale)***

Pain has reduced my participation in this activity:

Not at all 0 1 2 3 4 5 6 Extremely

33. How often do you wash dishes?
34. How often do you mow the lawn?
(___ Check here, if you do not have a lawn to mow).
35. How often do you go out to eat?
36. How often do you play cards or other games?
37. How often do you go grocery shopping?
38. How often do you work in the garden?
(___ Check here, if you do not have a garden)
39. How often do you go to a movie?
40. How often do you visit friends?
41. How often do you help with the house cleaning?
42. How often do you work on the car?
(__ Check here, if you do not have a car)
43. How often do you take a ride in a car or bus?
44. How often do you visit relatives?
(__ Check here, if you do not have relatives within 100 miles)
45. How often do you prepare a meal?
14. How often do you wash the car?
(__ Check here, if you do not have a car)
46. How often do you take a trip?
16. How often do you go to a park or beach?
47. How often do you do the laundry?
48. How often do you work on a needed household repair?

Part II

Experimental Studies

Spinal Cord Injury Pain: Assessment, Mechanisms, Management. Progress in Pain Research and Management, Vol. 23, edited by Robert P. Yezierski and Kim J. Burchiel, IASP Press, Seattle, © 2002.

6

Possible Mechanisms of Central Neuropathic Pain

William D. Willis

Department of Anatomy and Neurosciences, University of Texas Medical Branch, Galveston, Texas, USA

Injury or disease in the central nervous system (CNS) can result in chronic pain (Cassinari and Pagni 1969; Tasker 1990; Casey 1991; Boivie 1994; Pagni 1998). The definition of central neuropathic pain as "pain initiated or caused by a primary lesion or dysfunction in the central nervous system" by the International Association for the Study of Pain (Merskey and Bogduk 1994) excludes pain due to peripheral nerve damage with resultant CNS changes (Boivie 1994). However, some of the mechanisms that underlie neuropathic pain most likely are common to both peripheral and central neuropathic pain states. For example, damage to neurons at lower levels of the pain transmission system can result in transsynaptic alterations in neurons at higher levels of the system. Primary afferent neurons directly affected by injuries may result in peripheral neuropathic pain, but such injuries lead to secondary changes in dorsal horn neurons. Therefore, it is reasonable to expect that injury to the spinal cord might cause alterations of neurons at the thalamic and cerebral cortical levels secondary to injury of spinothalamic neurons or of the dorsal column.

ETIOLOGY OF CENTRAL PAIN

Lesions that cause central neuropathic pain are most frequently located in the spinal cord (Davidoff et al. 1987; Beric et al. 1988), the lower brainstem, especially the lateral medulla (Tasker 1990), or the thalamus (Dejerine and Roussy 1906; see review by Boivie 1994). When a lesion that causes central pain is located in the thalamus, the region affected seems always to include the ventral posterior nuclei (Bogousslavsky et al. 1988; Mauguière and

Desmedt 1988; Leijon et al. 1989; see Pagni 1998). Central neuropathic pain can also follow lesions of cortical and subcortical regions (Biemond 1956; Fields and Adams 1974; Leijon et al. 1989; Schmahmann and Leifer 1992; see Pagni 1998). When damage to the cerebral cortex is the source of central pain, there may be associated painful epileptic seizures (see Albé-Fessard et al. 1985; Boivie 1994; Pagni 1998). Iatrogenic lesions that may lead to central pain include several neurosurgical procedures meant to relieve pain: thalamotomies that impinge on the ventral posterior lateral (VPL) and ventral posterior medial (VPM) nuclei, lateral mesencephalotomies, bulbar trigeminal tractotomies, and anterolateral cordotomies (Fig. 1; Pagni 1998). Central pain may also result from Lissauer's tractotomies, dorsal root entry zone lesions (Chapter 25), and commissural myelotomies (Tasker 1990).

Disorders that can be associated with central neuropathic pain are diverse and include neurotrauma, multiple sclerosis, syringomyelia, and

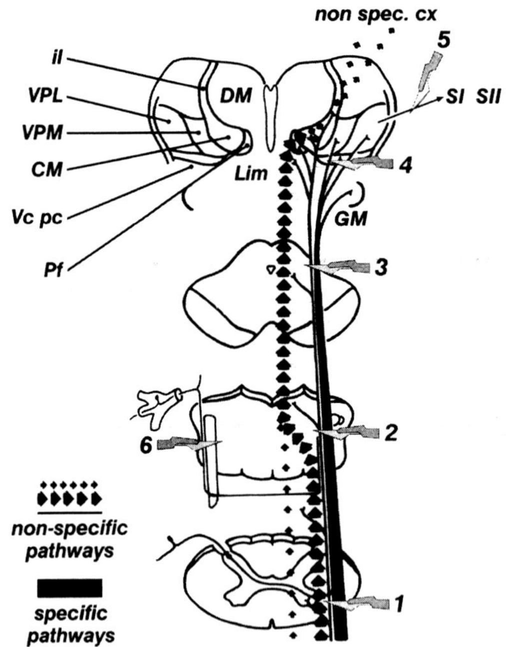

Fig. 1. Neurosurgical procedures that can result in central neuropathic pain. Lesions can be in the (1) spinal cord, (2) medulla, (3) midbrain, (4) ventral posterior thalamus, (5) thalamocortical projections, or (6) spinal tract of the trigeminal nerve. CM = center median nucleus; DM = dorsal medial nucleus; GM = medial geniculate nucleus; il = intralaminar nuclei; Lim = nucleus limitans; nonspec. cx = nonspecific areas of cortex; Pf = parafascicular nucleus; Vc pc = ventrocaudal parvocellular nucleus; VPL, VPM = ventral posterior lateral and medial nuclei. (From Pagni 1998.)

cerebrovascular disease (Table I; see also Moulin et al. 1988; Boivie 1994; Madsen et al. 1994). Central pain occurs in 10–30% of cases of spinal cord injury (SCI), follows 1–8% of strokes, and is seen in 19% of patients with multiple sclerosis (Pagni 1998). SCI also results in other types of pain, and the incidence of pain following traumatic SCI may be as high as 80–94% (according to literature cited by Richardson et al. 1980).

Pagni (1998) states that "any kind of spontaneous or surgical lesion can trigger central pain, provided the spinothalamic tract is damaged, whatever is the involved neuron (first, second, third)." Thus, central pain appears to be a consequence of interruption of the spinothalamocortical pathway.

CHARACTERISTICS OF CENTRAL PAIN

Explanations of central neuropathic pain should account for several clinical features of these disorders:

1) The time of onset of central neuropathic pain varies in different patients from immediately to years after the lesion occurs (Pagni 1998). A rapid onset of central pain suggests that damage to the CNS interrupts or alters maintained functional activity, such as tonic inhibition of pain transmission neurons. A delayed onset allows time for processes to occur that require changes in gene expression.

2) There is a strong relationship between the presence of central neuropathic pain and abnormalities of somatic sensation. For example, there is

Table I
Etiology of central pain

Vascular lesions of the brain or spinal cord
Infarct
Hemorrhage
Vascular malformation
Multiple sclerosis
Traumatic spinal cord injury; cordotomy
Traumatic brain injury
Syringomyelia and syringobulbia
Tumors
Abscesses
Inflammatory diseases other than multiple sclerosis; myelitis caused by viruses, syphilis
Epilepsy
Parkinson's disease

Source: Boivie (1994).

often a partial or complete deficit in pain and temperature sensations (Tasker 1990; Boivie 1994; Pagni 1998), and where an overt deficit cannot be demonstrated, a subclinical deficit is possible (Tasker 1990). Such minor deficits can be detected by quantitative sensory testing (Lindblom and Ochoa 1986; Boivie et al. 1989). Sensory evoked potentials in response to electrical stimulation of peripheral nerves can demonstrate deficits in touch and vibratory sense (Mauguière and Desmedt 1988; Holmgren et al. 1990), and laser activation of cutaneous thermal nociceptors can detect abnormalities in pain and thermal sensation (Bromm and Treede 1987; Pertovaara et al. 1988). A thalamic lesion will often diminish not only spinothalamic but also dorsal column–medial lemniscus sensory modalities, and sometimes SCI may abolish all sensation. However, a dissociated sensory loss of spinothalamic modalities with intact dorsal column and medial lemniscus modalities is seen in the central neuropathic pain that occurs after cordotomy and in the Wallenberg syndrome (Boivie 1994). The common finding of a reduction in evocable pain and temperature sensation suggests that central neuropathic pain depends on lesions that affect the spinothalamic tract (STT) and associated pathways (Beric et al. 1988; Boivie et al. 1989; see Boivie 1994; Pagni 1998). There is no correlation between the presence of central neuropathic pain and neurological deficits that do not involve sensation, such as motor system signs (Riddoch 1938; Beric et al. 1988; Leijon et al. 1989; see Tasker 1990; Boivie 1994; Pagni 1998).

3) Central neuropathic pain may be projected to a large area of the body, such as one side or the lower body, but it can also be projected to a smaller area, such as part of a hand or one side of the face. Therefore, it is not appropriate to consider the pain as diffuse (Boivie 1994). The distribution of the pain corresponds somatotopically to the site of the lesion. For example, in the Wallenberg syndrome, the pain is projected to the ipsilateral face and contralateral body, in keeping with damage to the spinal nucleus and tract of the trigeminal nerve and the crossed STT (Riddoch 1938; Leijon et al. 1989; Holmgren et al. 1990). After cordotomy, the pain is felt on the side contralateral to the lesion (Boivie 1994). Thus, apparently central pain cannot be explained by enhanced activity of nociceptive neurons that have very large, non-somatotopically organized receptive fields, as is the case with many spinoreticular neurons (Fields et al. 1977; Haber et al. 1982) and spinothalamic neurons that project to the medial but not to the lateral thalamus (Giesler et al. 1981).

4) The pain in central neuropathic pain syndromes can have any quality (Boivie 1994), and in a given case, there may be pains of different qualities (see, e.g., Davidoff et al. 1987). The most common quality of central pain seems to be burning pain (Cassinari and Pagni 1969; Beric et al. 1988; Leijon et al. 1989; Tasker 1990). However, burning pain is less common in

patients with thalamic than with supratentorial lesions (Leijon et al. 1989). Central pain has also been described as "intermittent, shooting, lancinating," and there may be "hyperesthesia, hyperalgesia, allodynia, hyperpathia" (Pagni 1998). There does not seem to be any strong correlation between pain quality and the location of the causal lesion (Boivie 1994).

5) Central neuropathic pain sometimes stops after some months, but it is often permanent (Boivie 1994; Pagni 1998).

6) Central neuropathic pain can be influenced by stimulation of the skin, movement, visceral stimuli, and psychological state, including emotional responses (Boivie 1994; Pagni 1998).

7) Only a fraction of individuals who develop a lesion in a location that is sometimes associated with central neuropathic pain go on to develop such a pain state (Tasker 1990; Boivie 1994).

MECHANISMS PROPOSED TO UNDERLIE CENTRAL NEUROPATHIC PAIN

Several mechanisms have been proposed to explain central neuropathic pain. These include (1) enhanced excitability of neurons in the pain transmission system, (2) disinhibition of pain transmission, (3) substitution of alternative pain pathways, and (4) reorganization of neural circuits.

ENHANCED EXCITABILITY

Irritable focus. Damage to the CNS may lead to the development of an "irritable focus" (Dejerine and Roussy 1906; Livingston 1943; see Pagni 1998). An irritable focus is a region of nervous tissue in which neural circuits become hyperexcitable. It is easier than normal for these neurons to be activated, and activity of the irritable focus evokes central pain.

One version of this theory is the idea that ascending sensory projection cells, such as STT neurons, might be "irritated" following a spinal cord lesion, and consequently their increased activity might evoke pain (Riddoch 1938). A parallel mechanism in peripheral neuropathic pain is the upregulation of sodium channels in primary afferent neurons after nerve damage and the development of ectopic discharges from the region of the neuroma or from dorsal root ganglion cells (Devor et al. 1993; Matzner and Devor 1994; Lyu et al. 2000).

A recent observation is that exposure of a lesioned lateral funiculus to blood in rats can result in enhanced nociceptive responses on the side ipsilateral to the lesion, although nociceptive responses are reduced on the contralateral side for at least 20 weeks postoperatively (Fig. 2; Vierck and

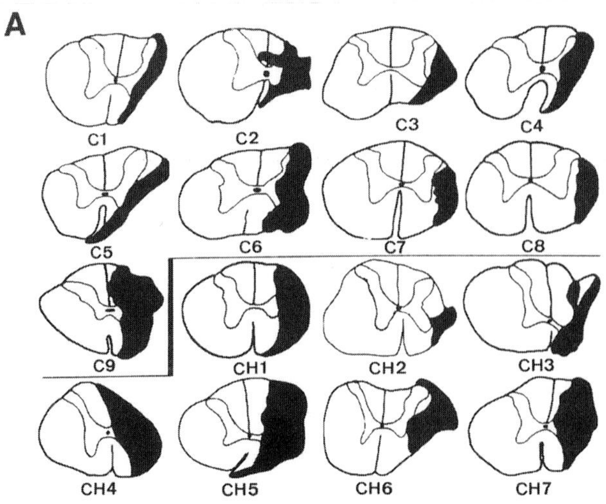
A
C1
C2
C3
C4
C5
C6
C7
C8
C9
CH1
CH2
CH3
CH4
CH5
CH6
CH7

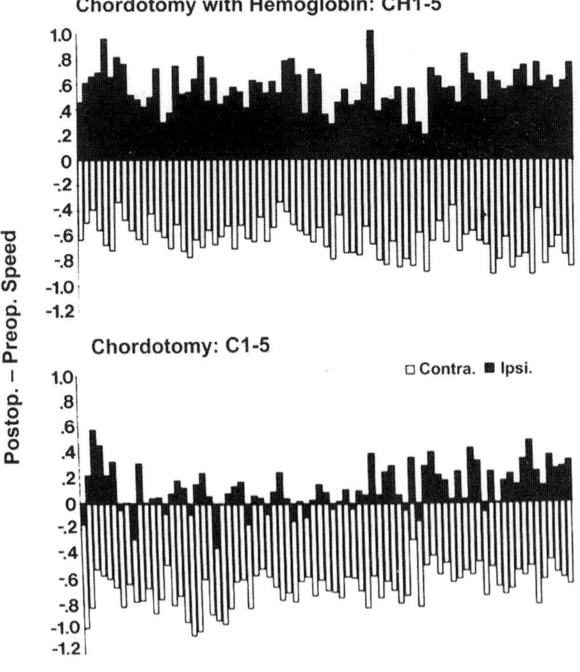
B
Chordotomy with Hemoglobin: CH1-5
Postop. – Preop. Speed
Chordotomy: C1-5
□ Contra. ■ Ipsi.
1.0
.8
.6
.4
.2
0
-.2
-.4
-.6
-.8
-1.0
-1.2

Light 1999). Presumably, substances in the blood cause increased excitability of neurons in the gray matter whose axons ascend in the ipsilateral lateral funiculus. The cytokine tumor necrosis factor α can produce ectopic discharges of axons in a peripheral nerve (Sorkin et al. 1997), and so involvement of the gray matter may not be necessary for an irritable focus to develop under some conditions.

The usual presentation of central neuropathic pain involves loss of somatic sensation, especially of spinothalamic modalities, and surgical interruption of the spinothalamic system does not relieve central neuropathic pain (Tasker 1990). These observations argue against the idea that irritated spinothalamic neurons are responsible for central neuropathic pain after a spinal cord lesion. On the other hand, an irritable focus could well develop in spinal neurons that give rise to ascending nociceptive pathways other than the STT.

Central sensitization. The development of central sensitization of neurons in the pain transmission system could explain increases in spontaneous activity and in evoked responses and central pain (Willis 2001a). Central sensitization has been studied extensively at the spinal cord level in models of acute inflammation. For example, intradermal injection of capsaicin results in enhanced responses of primate STT neurons to stimulation of mechanoreceptors in a region of skin surrounding the injection site. Sensory receptors in this region are unaffected by the capsaicin (Baumann et al. 1991), and so the enhanced responses of STT neurons can help explain secondary mechanical allodynia (Simone et al. 1991; Dougherty and Willis 1992).

Central sensitization of STT neurons following intradermal capsaicin injection has been found to depend on the activation of both ionotropic and metabotropic glutamate receptors and neuropeptide receptors such as NK1 receptors (Dougherty and Willis 1991, 1992; Dougherty et al. 1992, 1994; Neugebauer et al. 1999, 2000). These neurotransmitter events lead to activation of intracellular signal transduction pathways involving a number of protein kinases, including calcium/calmodulin-dependent protein kinase II (CaMKII), protein kinase C (PKC), nitric oxide/protein kinase G (NO/PKG), and protein kinase A (PKA) (Lin et al. 1996a, 1997, 1999; Wu et al. 1998; Zou et al. 2000).

← **Fig. 2.** (A) Lesions of the right side of the rat spinal cord placed at a lower thoracic level. For nine animals in group C (cordotomy, animals C1–C9), no blood was placed in the lesion cavity, whereas for seven animals in group CH (cordotomy with hemoglobin, animals CH1–CH7), blood-soaked Gelfoam was put into the lesion cavity. (B) Differences in speed of escape from electrical stimulation of the skin before and after the spinal cord lesion. Five animals in groups C and CH were tested during 76 postoperative sessions. Contralateral escape speed was comparable for the two groups, indicating slowed responses. However, ipsilateral escape speeds were increased in CH animals. (From Vierck and Light 1999.)

Consequences of the activation of protein kinases include phosphorylation of *N*-methyl-D-aspartate (NMDA) receptors (Zou et al. 2000) and of α-amino-3-hydroxy-5-methyl-4-isoxazole propionate (AMPA) receptors (Fang et al. 2000). Phosphorylation of excitatory amino acid receptors can enhance their responsiveness (Chen and Huang 1991, 1992). These mechanisms are similar to those involved in long-term potentiation (LTP) in brain structures such as the hippocampus, and so it is reasonable to consider central sensitization in the spinal cord to be a form of LTP (Willis 1997, 2001b). Long-lasting central sensitization, like long-term LTP, presumably requires changes in gene expression. These changes may be initiated in response to activation of immediate early genes, such as *c-fos*. *Fos* expression is increased when central sensitization is produced by intradermal injection of capsaicin and also when nitric oxide is released in the dorsal horn of the spinal cord (Wu et al. 2000). Changes in gene expression presumably underlie the transsynaptic induction of substances such as RL-29, in dorsal horn neurons in the chronic constriction injury model of neuropathic pain (Cameron et al. 1993), and presumably similar changes could occur in neurons that are upstream in the pain system after lesions that interrupt the spinothalamocortical pathway.

Central sensitization may play an important role in peripheral neuropathic pain (Yoon et al. 1996), and evidence supports a role of NMDA receptors and of nitric oxide release in peripheral neuropathic pain (Yoon et al. 1998; Burton et al. 1999; Isaev et al. 2000). The Chung spinal nerve ligation (SNL) model of neuropathic pain (Kim and Chung 1992) results in severe mechanical allodynia when applied in monkeys (Palecek et al. 1992; Carlton et al. 1994). Recordings from STT neurons in neuropathic monkeys revealed increased background activity and increased responses to innocuous mechanical and thermal stimuli in the segment rostral to the level of SNL (Fig. 3). However, the responses of cells at the level of SNL were reduced. Presumably, in the intact animal, there would be a sensory deficit for stimuli applied to the L7 dermatome but allodynia following stimulation

---

Fig. 3. Responses of four different wide-dynamic-range (WDR) spinothalamic tract (STT) neurons in a neuropathic monkey (L7 spinal nerve ligation) to mechanical and thermal stimulation of the cutaneous receptive fields. (A, B) Peristimulus time histograms show the enhanced responses of two STT cells located rostral to the L6/L7 border (EPN R) to mechanical stimuli. E and F show the enhanced responses of the same neurons to graded heat stimuli, and I and J show those to cooling stimuli. C, G, and K show reduced responses of a WDR STT neuron located within L7 to mechanical and thermal stimuli. D, H, and L show the presumed normal responses of an STT neuron on the contralateral side to the same stimuli. The drawings at the bottom show the most responsive sites in the receptive fields of the neurons (marked by arrows). EPN = experiment peripheral neuropathy (From Palecek et al. 1992.) ⟶

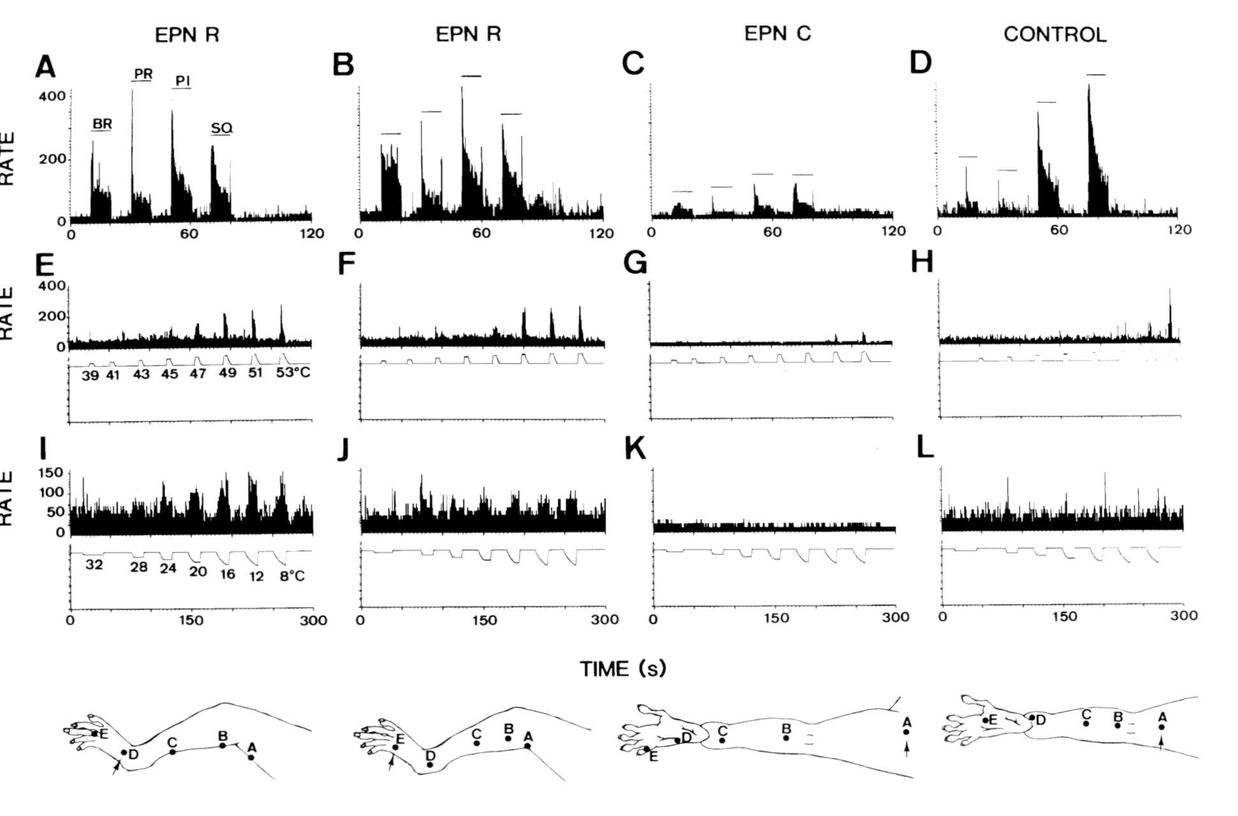

EPN R
EPN R
EPN C
CONTROL
A
B
C
D
BR
PR
PI
SQ
RATE
400
200
0
60
120
E
F
G
H
39 41 43 45 47 49 51 53°C
I
J
K
L
150
100
50
32 28 24 20 16 12 8°C
150
300
TIME (s)

in the L6 dermatome. No evidence was obtained to determine whether the hyperexcitable responses were due to peripheral input from ectopic spike generators, to central sensitization, or to both mechanisms. However, the increased evoked responses were apparently produced by activation of intact axons following sensory stimulation of the skin.

The arguments that there is a reduction in sensations mediated by the spinothalamic system and that lesions of the STT do not eliminate central neuropathic pain after spinal cord lesions are inconsistent with a major role of central sensitization of STT neurons in central pain originating from a spinal cord lesion that interrupts the STT. However, central sensitization could presumably be produced in other types of nociceptive neurons in the spinal cord, such as spinoreticular neurons, or of nociceptive neurons at any of several different levels of the pain transmission system, including not only the spinal cord, but also structures at levels rostral to the lesion, such as the thalamus or cerebral cortex (Fig. 4; cf. Guilbaud et al. 1990, 1992; Boivie 1992; Jones 1992; Lenz 1992; Salt 1992). Changes in excitability have been described for neurons in the ventrobasal thalamus that depend on the activation of NMDA and metabotropic glutamate receptors and second messenger systems, similar to the processes that underlie central sensitization of spinal cord neurons (Eaton and Salt 1991; Shaw and Salt 1997; Shaw et al. 1999; Salt and Binns 2000). Interruption of the STT in cats resulted in increased spontaneous and evoked activity in neurons of the VPL nucleus (Koyama et al. 1993). This enhanced activity was reduced by administration of MK801, an NMDA glutamate receptor antagonist, whereas MK801 had no effect on neurons recorded in sham-operated controls. These experiments suggest that VPL neurons become hyperactive following interruption of the STT and that NMDA receptors may play an important role in this change.

REDUCED INHIBITION

Disinhibition. Thalamic pain has been suggested to result from disinhibition. Interruption of the dorsal column–medial lemniscus pathway could lead to disinhibition of transmission through the STT and associated nociceptive pathways (Foerster 1927). This idea would be consistent with the fact that stimulation of the dorsal column can be used to relieve pain (Shealy et al. 1967), possibly by inhibiting nociceptive transmission at a supraspinal level (see discussion in Gybels and Sweet 1989; Meyerson 1990). However, good evidence shows that central neuropathic pain can occur with no deficit in dorsal column–medial lemniscus sensory modalities, including touch, vibratory sense, and proprioception (Biemond 1956; Beric et al. 1988; Mauguière and Desmedt 1988; Boivie et al. 1989; Holmgren et al. 1990).

Even though there can be a deficit in these modalities in some individuals, interruption of the dorsal column–medial lemniscus pathway is clearly not a requirement for central neuropathic pain because central pain does not appear to develop following lesions of the posterior column in patients (see review by Pagni 1998).

On the other hand, central sensitization may well involve disinhibition due to loss of effectiveness of inhibitory mechanisms within the spinothalamocortical pathway. Transsynaptic loss of dorsal horn inhibitory interneurons after peripheral nerve injury may contribute to peripheral neuropathic pain (see Sugimoto et al. 1990). The loss of dorsal horn interneurons may relate to excitotoxicity produced by release of an excessive amount of glutamate from Aβ fibers that sprout and then grow into the superficial dorsal horn (Woolf et al. 1992; Coggeshall et al. 2001). The central sensitization that follows intradermal injection of capsaicin is associated not only with increased responsiveness of *excitatory* amino acid receptors, but also with decreased responsiveness of *inhibitory* amino acid receptors (Fig. 5; see Lin et al. 1996b). In addition, inhibition in response to stimulation of the periaqueductal gray is reduced (Lin et al. 1997). Gamma-aminobutyric acid-A ($GABA_A$) receptors were diminished in the VPL nucleus of monkeys that had a chronic pain syndrome following extensive dorsal rhizotomies at the cervical level (Fig. 6; Rausell et al. 1992). The chronic dorsal rhizotomies did not significantly reduce the population of GABAergic interneurons in the VPL nucleus (Rausell et al. 1992). However, a lesion of the dorsal column in monkeys reduced the number of GABAergic contacts onto thalamocortical relay neurons (Ralston et al. 1996). The loss of inhibitory amino acid receptors and/or a reduction in GABAergic synaptic contacts would presumably lead to enhanced excitability of thalamic neurons.

Another suggestion is that disinhibition is produced by interruption of corticothalamic inhibitory projections that end in the lateral thalamus, resulting in increased responsiveness within the thalamus (Head and Holmes 1911). Alternatively, interruption of projections from the reticular nucleus of the thalamus could lead to disinhibition of thalamic neurons (Mauguière and Desmedt 1988; Cesaro et al. 1991) following a lesion that impinges on the thalamus. Disinhibition could also contribute to central neuropathic pain that originates from other parts of the CNS. For example, injury to the spinal cord could interrupt inhibitory pathways that descend from the brain to the spinal cord, known as the endogenous analgesia system (Fields and Besson 1988). However, Pagni (1998) states: "No central pain ever followed damage of descending pain-suppressing fibers or of the endogenous opiate system."

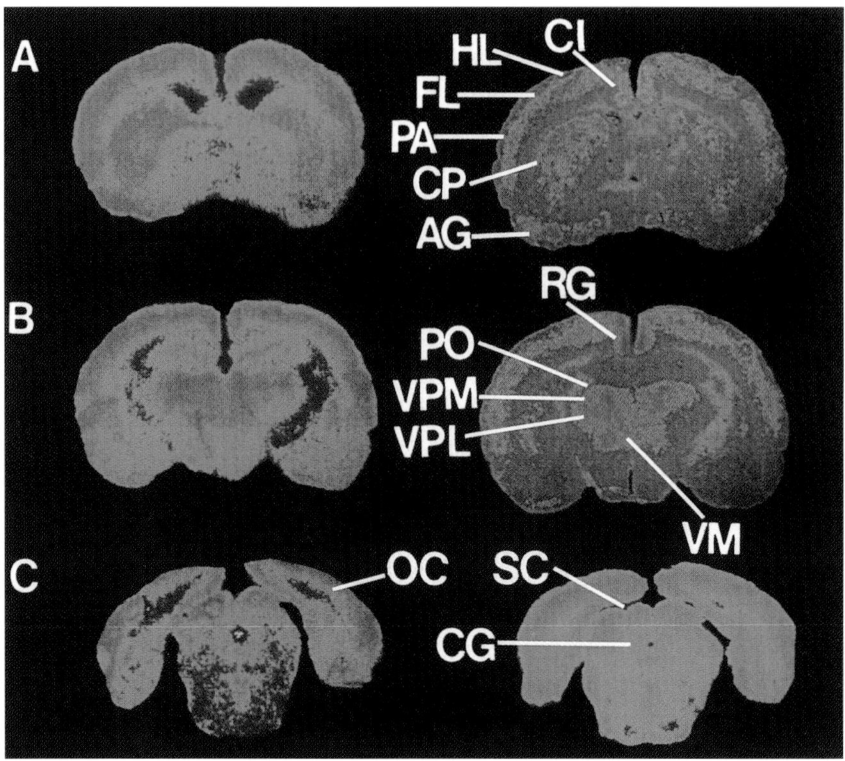

Fig. 4. Increases in metabolic activity in the thalamus and other brain structures in a rat with peripheral neuropathic pain. The colored areas indicate the levels of ^{14}C-2-deoxyglucose in neurons at several levels of the brains of a sham-operated control animal and an animal with a chronic constriction injury of the sciatic nerve (A–C). The sections on the left were from the control animal, whereas the sections on the right were from the neuropathic animal. AG = amygdala; CG = central gray; Cl = cingulate gyrus; CP = caudate putamen; FL = forelimb area; HL = hindlimb area; OC = occipital cortex; PA = parietal area; PO = posterior thalamic nucleus; RG = retrosplenial granular cortex; SC = superior colliculus; VM = ventral medial nucleus; VPL, VPM = ventral posterior lateral and medial nuclei. (From Mao et al. 1993.)

SUBSTITUTION OF ALTERNATIVE NOCICEPTIVE PATHWAYS

Interruption of the spinothalamic tract. Central neuropathic pain may occur only after lesions that interrupt the spinothalamic pathways, whether or not the dorsal column–medial lemniscus system is also affected (Boivie et al. 1989; Pagni 1998).

Nuclei in the ventroposterior thalamus that receive nociceptive spinothalamic and trigeminothalamic projections include the ventral posterior lateral

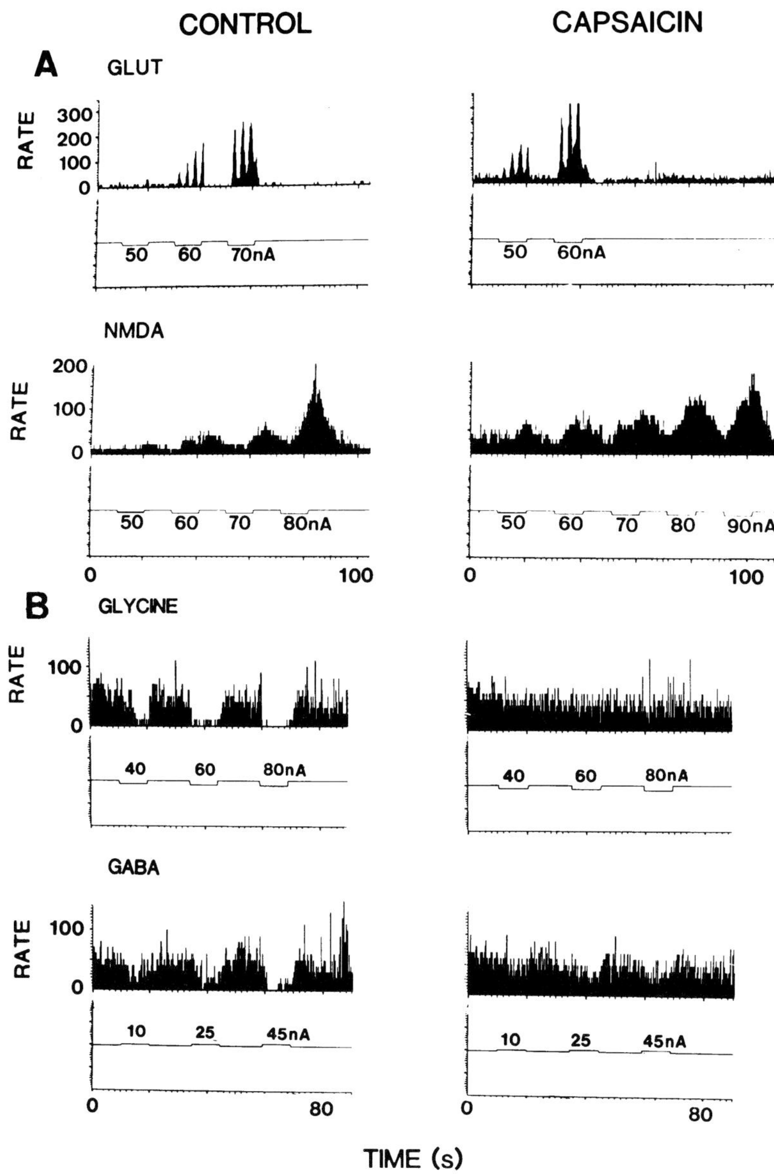

Fig. 5. (A) Enhancement of responses of spinothalamic tract (STT) cells to excitatory amino acids; and (B) reduction of responses of STT cells to inhibitory amino acids during central sensitization evoked by intradermal capsaicin injection. Rate is spikes/bin; one bin = 100 ms. (From Dougherty and Willis 1992 and Lin et al. 1996b).

(VPL) nucleus, its trigeminal equivalent, the ventral posterior medial (VPM) nucleus, and the ventral posterior inferior nucleus (VPI), as well as parts of

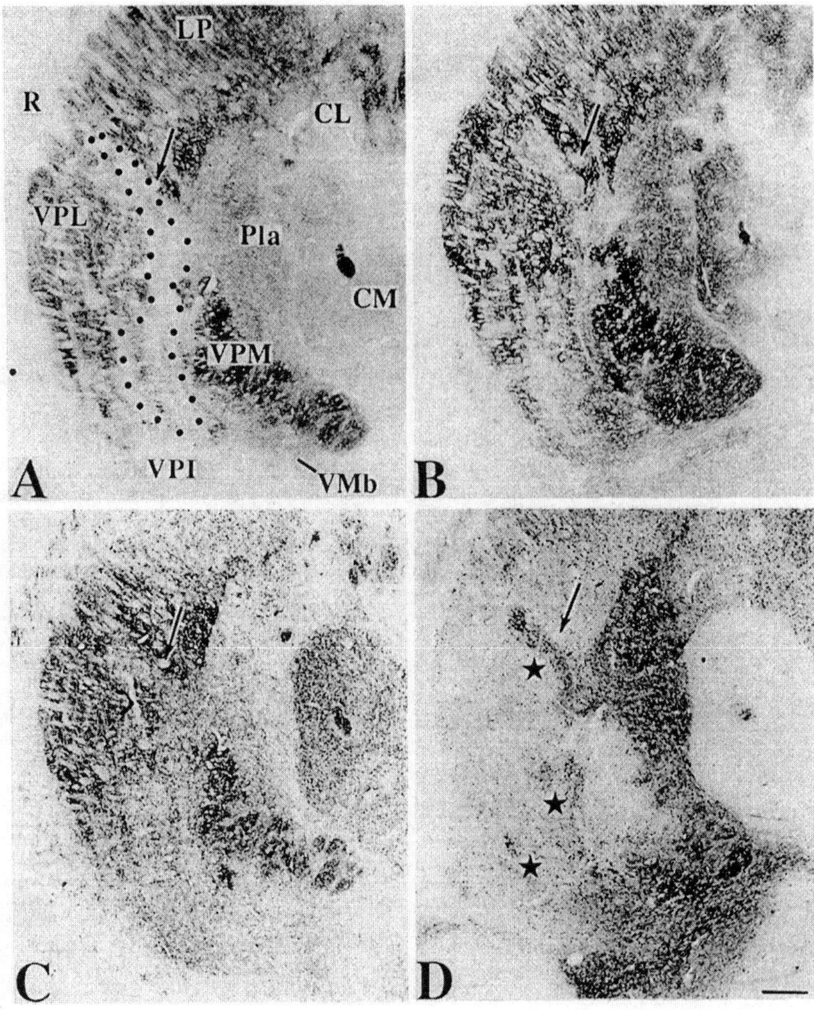

Fig. 6. Immunocytochemical changes in the ventral posterior and adjacent nuclei contralateral to chronic dorsal rhizotomies in the segments of the cervical enlargement in a monkey. The section in panel A is stained for cytochrome oxidase, which is reduced in the area that corresponds to the representation of the upper extremity (area enclosed by dotted line). The section in panel B is stained for $GABA_A$ receptors, that in C for parvalbumin, and that in D for calbindin. The affected area shows a loss of $GABA_A$ and parvalbumin staining and an increase in calbindin staining. CL = central lateral nucleus; CM = center median nucleus; LP = lateral posterior; Pla = anterior pulvinar nucleus; R = reticular nucleus; VPL, VPM, VPI = ventral posterior lateral, medial, and inferior nuclei; VMb = basal part of ventral medial nucleus. (From Rausell et al. 1992.)

the posterior complex (Mehler et al. 1960; Mehler 1962; Applebaum et al. 1979; Boivie 1979; Berkley 1980; Apkarian and Hodge 1989; Zhang et al. 2000; Willis et al. 2001). Nociceptive responses have been recorded from neurons in all of these nuclei (Pollin and Albé-Fessard 1979; Kenshalo et al. 1980; Casey and Morrow 1983; Chung et al. 1986; Bushnell et al. 1993; Duncan et al. 1993; Apkarian and Shi 1994; Craig et al. 1994; Lenz et al. 1994).

Why interruption of input to this region of the thalamus over the spinothalamic system should result in chronic pain is not immediately obvious, but a possibility is that upstream neurons in the pain transmission system develop spontaneous activity and perhaps heightened responsiveness to inputs over other pathways (see Levitt and Levitt 1981). Evidence in support of this suggestion is the observation of burst discharges in thalamic neurons in human patients and the development of novel receptive fields following SCI (Lenz et al. 1987; Lenz 1989; see, however, Radhakrishnan et al. 1999). In experimental animals with peripheral neuropathic pain, metabolism is increased dramatically in neurons of the VPL and VPM nuclei and other brain structures (Fig. 4; Mao et al. 1993), as is nerve impulse activity (Guilbaud et al. 1990). Such changes could occur if the altered responses were in neurons that have undergone central sensitization. Central sensitization results from strong and prolonged activation of nociceptive pathways, and so central sensitization of upstream neurons in the pain system could be due to strong activation of STT neurons at the time of SCI or a stroke affecting the lateral medulla, or there could be a more prolonged activation of STT neurons by a slowly progressing pathological process such as syringomyelia or multiple sclerosis. Another way in which upstream neurons could be affected by the loss of a major input would be through upregulation of neurotransmitter receptors, a form of denervation supersensitivity. Another change could be transneuronal degeneration and subsequent reorganization of the remaining postsynaptic neurons. Such changes could also explain why stimulation in the ventroposterior thalamus can often evoke pain after deafferentation following a spinal cord or peripheral lesion, although stimulation in a similar region in patients who do not have chronic pain fails to elicit pain (Tasker et al. 1980; Gorecki et al. 1989; Lenz et al. 1998). However, thalamic lesions would prevent thalamic activity if the neurons in the damaged area died. In this case, changes leading to central neuropathic pain might involve cortical neurons (see Guilbaud et al. 1992).

Alternative nociceptive pathways. Another theory of central neuropathic pain is that when nociceptive transmission is completely interrupted in the spinothalamic system on one side, nociceptive transmission may occur through alternative nociceptive pathways (Craig 1991), such as the ipsilateral STT, the postsynaptic dorsal column pathway (including the newly described visceral

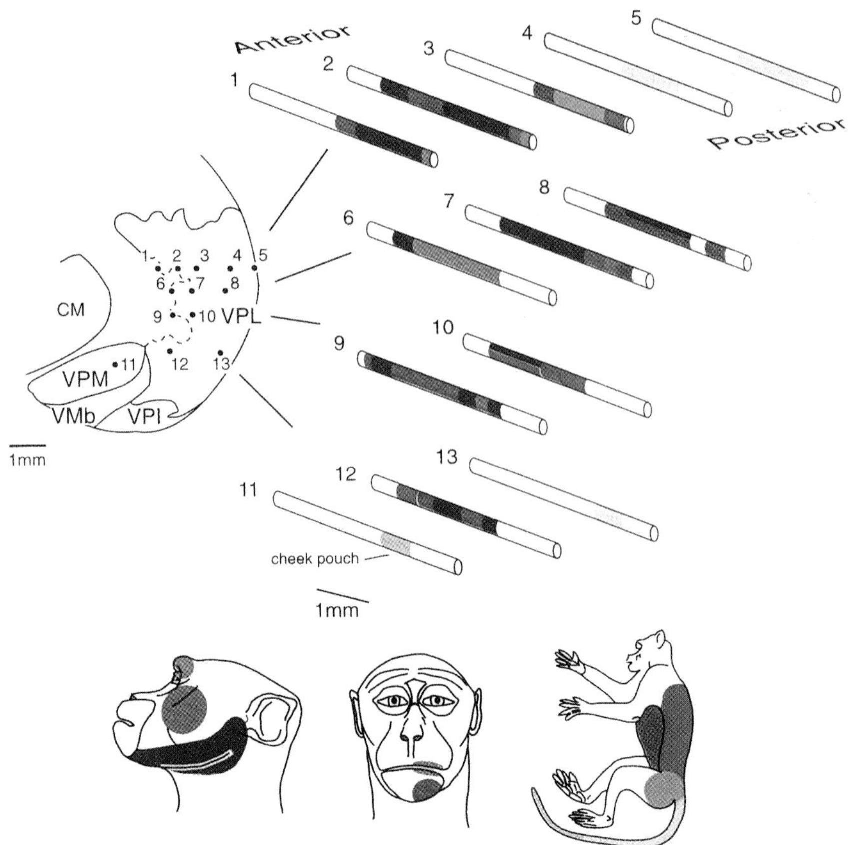

Fig. 7. Thalamic mapping in a monkey following chronic dorsal rhizotomy of the cervical enlargement. Tracks were made horizontally through the thalamus. The locations of tracks 1–13 are shown in the drawing of a coronal section through the posterior thalamus. The receptive fields of thalamic units found in these tracks are shown on the drawings of the monkey at the bottom. The cylinders represent the 13 tracks and show the zones that correspond to cells having receptive fields on the face, trunk, or tail. No receptive fields were found on the forelimb. Abbreviations are as in Fig. 6. (From Jones and Pons 1998.)

pain pathway that ascends in the dorsal column), the spinocervical tract, the spinoparabrachial tract, the spinohypothalamic tract, spinolimbic tracts, and the spinoreticular tract (e.g., Cervero et al. 1977; Willis et al. 1979; Haber et al. 1982; Burstein et al. 1987; Downie et al. 1988; Ferrington et al. 1988; Noble and Riddell 1988; Bernard and Besson 1990; Cliffer et al. 1992; Al-Chaer et al. 1996a,b; Hirshberg et al. 1996; see review by Willis and Coggeshall 1991). Thus, nociceptive transmission could occur in ascending tracts that are often regarded as tactile pathways, but that do include a nociceptive component. It is conceivable that upstream neurons in the pain system could undergo central sensitization because of activity in such alternative nociceptive pathways. However, in monkeys with an anterolateral cordotomy, contralateral nociceptive responses are least likely to return when the lesion of the white matter of the lateral funiculus is relatively superficial, despite maximal sparing of alternative nociceptive pathways (Vierck et al. 1990).

REORGANIZATION OF NEURAL CIRCUITS

Rewiring. Damage to the CNS can result in sprouting of axons and rewiring of circuits, even in the adult. This process has been proposed as a mechanism for allodynia in peripheral neuropathic pain because large, presumably tactile primary afferents sprout collaterals that terminate in lamina II following sciatic nerve injury (Woolf et al. 1992, 1995). After chronic SCI in the hemisection model, there is massive sprouting of primary afferent neurons that contain calcitonin gene-related peptide (CGRP: Christensen and Hulsebosch 1997a,b). These afferents may be involved in maintaining the central pain state because the mechanical and thermal allodynia seen in these animals can be relieved by an antagonist of CGRP receptors, $CGRP_{8-37}$ (Bennett et al. 2000).

Reorganization within the thalamus following injury to the nervous system has been observed. For example, systematic mapping of the principal sensory nucleus (presumably the VPL and VPI nuclei) using intrathalamic microstimulation was conducted in patients with neuropathic pain, and the results were compared with those in patients with motor disorders but no pain (Lenz et al. 1998). Pain responses to intrathalamic microstimulation were found much more frequently and warm and cool responses much less frequently in the neuropathic pain patients. The mechanism of this modality reorganization was uncertain, but it might relate to the morphological reorganization that has been reported in monkeys following dorsal rhizotomies or interruption of the dorsal column (Figs. 6 and 7; Rausell et al. 1992; Ralston et al. 1996; Jones and Pons 1998). In monkeys that had dorsal rhizotomies of the cervical enlargement on one side 12–20 years earlier, several transneuronal morphological changes were noted. There was marked reduction in the size of the cuneate fasciculus and nucleus on the rhizotomized side (Jones and Pons 1998) and a loss of cytochrome oxidase and parvalbumin staining (Fig. 6A and C) in the region of the contralateral VPL nucleus to which the cuneate nucleus had originally projected (Rausell et al. 1992), as well as a loss in $GABA_A$ receptors (Fig. 6B). By contrast, there was an increased staining for calbindin (Fig. 6D) in the forelimb representation of the VPL nucleus. Recordings from the VPL nucleus in these animals demonstrated a reorganization of receptive fields (Jones and Pons 1998). Forelimb receptive fields were not observed in what had been the forelimb representation. Instead, receptive fields in this region were on the face or on the trunk (Fig. 7). Factors that might contribute to this reorganization include transneuronal degeneration in the cuneate and VPL nuclei, followed by expression of the activity of previously ineffective synapses (Jones and Pons 1998). For example, collaterals of trigeminothalamic afferents to the face region that synapse in the forelimb region but that are normally ineffective might now become effective in exciting residual forelimb VPL neurons, converting these to neurons that respond to stimulation of the face. Presumably, sprouting could also contribute, although there was no evidence for this possibility. The VPL neurons of the former forelimb representation would then convert the projection to the cerebral cortical forelimb area to a face projection, thus altering the cortical somatotopic map. The enhanced staining for calbindin in the forelimb part of the VPL nucleus could result from increased activity in this region, presumably in response to the intact spinothalamic input (Rausell et al. 1992). Increased activity in VPL neurons would be facilitated by the observed downregulation in $GABA_A$ receptors, as well as by a reduction of GABAergic synaptic connections to thalamocortical relay neurons (Ralston et al. 1996). Such changes might contribute to a central pain state. However, if so, it is unclear why dorsal column lesions in human patients do not seem to lead to central pain.

Release of activity in medial thalamus. A lesion of the ventroposterior thalamus might lessen corticofugal suppression of medial thalamic nuclei, such as the nucleus submedius (Craig 1991) or an area in the posterior thalamus adjacent to the basal part of the ventral medial nucleus (VMb) (Craig et al. 1994). The nucleus submedius projects to the lateral orbital cortex (Craig et al. 1982), and the area near the VMb is thought to project to the insula (Craig et al. 1994). However, bilateral lesions of the nucleus submedius in rats result in hyperalgesia, and stimulation in the nucleus submedius produces an antinociceptive action, suggesting that the nucleus submedius is part of the endogenous analgesia system (Roberts and Dong 1994; Zhang et al. 1995, 1998). The role of the posterior region near the VMb is unclear, although Craig et al. (1994) proposed that this region is concerned with thermal and pain sensations.

GENETIC SUSCEPTIBILITY

Genetic variations. Similar lesions result in central neuropathic pain in only a fraction of cases (Tasker 1990). The liability for developing a chronic pain state following peripheral nerve injury has a genetic component (Inbal et al. 1980; Mogil et al. 1999a,b), and it would not be surprising if a similar genetic dependence applies to central pain. Evidence for a genetic component of SCI pain was reported by Levitt and Levitt (1981), who observed that stumptail macaques were much more likely than other species of monkey to develop a pain syndrome after experimental lesions of the spinal cord.

INVOLVEMENT OF THE SYMPATHETIC NERVOUS SYSTEM

There may be changes in sympathetic function in central neuropathic pain (Riddoch 1938; Tasker 1990), and sympathetic blocks can provide pain relief in this pain state, as well as in peripheral neuropathic pain (Loh et al. 1981). However, little is known about the possible role of the sympathetic nervous system in central pain states.

EXPERIMENTAL MODELS OF CENTRAL NEUROPATHIC PAIN

Few experimental models have been developed to study the mechanisms of central neuropathic pain, and most pertain to the pain associated with SCI and other disorders of the spinal cord, such as cordotomy and syringomyelia. Models are needed for the pain of the Wallenberg syndrome, thalamic pain, and central pain following cortical and subcortical damage. This section discusses experimental models of pain resulting from damage to the spinal cord and briefly reviews reports of central pain following experimental alterations at the thalamic or cortical level.

MODELS OF SCI PAIN

Cordotomy model. In this model, a unilateral cordotomy is performed to interrupt the STT and accompanying ascending pathways, and changes in nociceptive responses are examined over time (Levitt and Levitt 1981; Vierck et al. 1990; Ovelmen-Levitt et al. 1995; Vierck and Light 1999). The objective is to mimic the changes in nociception following anterolateral cordotomy to treat pain in patients. Clinically, these changes include a reduction in nociception contralaterally below the lesion, but in some cases the later development of a central pain state contralaterally (White and Sweet 1969), ipsilaterally (Bowsher 1988) or bilaterally (Graf 1960). The return of pain after a cordotomy may be associated with abnormal discharges of neurons in the ventroposterior thalamus that no longer receive spinothalamic input (Lenz et al. 1987; see Koyama et al. 1993).

In experimental studies in monkeys, a lesion of the lateral funiculus that extended medially to near the gray matter initially resulted in reduced speeds of escape responses to electrical stimulation of the skin, but the response speeds gradually recovered in half of the monkeys and even became faster than normal, indicating hyperalgesia (Vierck et al. 1990). Recovery was most likely to occur in animals that had the most medially extensive lesions and did not occur when invasion of the gray matter was minimal. This finding led to the hypothesis that postcordotomy pain may depend on the extent of bleeding at the lesion site and may result from a hemotoxic effect on the spinal cord gray matter that enhances nociceptive responses. This hypothesis was tested in rats (Fig. 2; Vierck and Light 1999). A lesion was made of the lateral funiculus at a thoracic level, and in some animals blood-soaked Gelfoam was placed within the lesion site to investigate hemotoxic effects on the gray matter. Nociceptive behavioral tests included the speed of escape responses following noxious electrical stimulation of the skin, as well as flexion reflexes and vocalization in response to the same stimuli. The speed of nociceptive escape responses to electrical stimuli was reduced on the contralateral side below the lesion. However, the speed of escape responses to similar stimuli applied ipsilaterally was increased if blood had been applied to the lesion site. Interestingly, flexion reflexes were not increased on the ipsilateral side, despite the development of hyperalgesia. This dissociation serves as a reminder that flexion reflexes do not necessarily parallel sensory changes. Vocalizations to contralateral stimulation were greatly reduced, but those to ipsilateral stimulation were essentially unchanged; again, vocalizations and sensory changes do not necessarily change in parallel. The findings were interpreted to mean that hemotoxic injury to the gray matter near a cordotomy can lead to increased nociceptive transmission.

Weng et al. (2000) made recordings in the VPL nucleus of the thalamus in monkeys following a lesion of the STT at a thoracic level. No wide-dynamic-range (WDR) neurons were found in the sample of neurons from the VPL nucleus on the side of the lesion (compared to 4% of the neurons on the side with an intact STT). Low-threshold cells had similar properties whether or not the STT was lesioned. However, there were distinct changes in multireceptive VPL neurons that received approximately equal input from mechanoreceptors and mechanical nociceptors. The recordings revealed increased spontaneous activity, enhanced responses to cutaneous stimulation, and larger receptive fields in these neurons. These thalamic neurons also showed an increase in spike-bursts, similar to those seen in human thalamic neurons recorded in patients with central pain (Lenz et al. 1987, 1989). Such abnormally discharging VPL neurons might contribute to spontaneous pain (see, however, Radhakrishnan et al. 1999), and the enhanced responses of these cells to lemniscal inputs might contribute to an increase in evoked pain.

Spinal cord contusion injury model. A model used in several experimental studies produces contusion injury by dropping a weight on the dorsal aspect of the spinal cord (Beattie et al. 1997). This model has the advantage of mimicking the most common type of SCI, that produced by trauma. The purpose of most such studies has been to produce a controlled injury to define the natural history of the associated motor deficits, to investigate attempts by the spinal cord to repair itself, and to examine the effects of various forms of therapy on repair processes. Recent researchers have attempted to determine whether central pain occurs secondary to contusion injury and have begun to study the time course of pain development, the relationship of the pain state to the volume of the injury, and the effects of therapeutic interventions (Siddall et al. 1995; Hulsebosch et al. 2000). One of the problems with this model is variability in the extent of the damage. However, carefully controlled conditions (dropping a defined weight a defined distance onto a defined area of the exposed spinal cord) can minimize variability. Impact injury to the spinal cord elevates the concentration of excitatory amino acids in the extracellular space (Liu et al. 1991; Xu et al. 1998; Liu et al. 1999; McAdoo et al. 2000); such increases in the spinal cord dorsal horn are associated with hyperalgesia and allodynia (Sluka and Westlund 1993a,b).

Spinal cord hemisection model. Another SCI model involves hemisection of the spinal cord at a midthoracic level (Christensen et al. 1996; Christensen and Hulsebosch 1997a). The clinical condition that this model most closely resembles is the Brown-Sequard syndrome, which occurs only rarely. However, the model has the advantage that it is quite reproducible. Over a period of weeks, the animals develop severe allodynia over the trunk and, perhaps surprisingly, can develop mechanical allodynia and thermal hyperalgesia of both hindlimbs and forelimbs. An important finding is a substantial increase in the number of axons that immunostain for calcitonin gene-related peptide (CGRP) in the dorsal horn several segments above and below the lesion (Christensen and Hulsebosch 1997b). Since CGRP occurs only in primary afferent fibers in the dorsal horn (Chung et al. 1988), these axons must represent sprouting axons of peptidergic primary afferent fibers.

Quisqualate model. In this model, an injection of quisqualic acid is made into the spinal cord gray matter (Yezierski et al. 1993, 1998). The neurotoxic action of this glutamate receptor agonist results in the development of a cavity that resembles to some extent the cavity resulting from damage from a contusion injury or, perhaps, a syrinx (Yezierski et al. 1993;

Madsen et al. 1994). The most striking behavioral consequence of the lesion is the development of a unique overgrooming behavior in which the animal scratches its coat in an area somatotopically related to the lesion. This area also develops mechanical allodynia. Dorsal horn neurons in this model of central pain show increased background activity and increased sensitivity to mechanical stimulation of the skin, as well as prolonged afterdischarges (Yezierski and Park 1993).

Ischemia model. In this model, a lesion is made of the spinal cord gray matter by focusing a laser beam at a region of spinal cord through which blood that contains a photosensitive dye is circulating. The reaction between the laser beam and the photopigment results in an ischemic lesion by occluding blood vessels. Following such a lesion, the animals typically develop truncal mechanical allodynia (Hao et al. 1991a; Xu et al. 1992), as shown by vocalization when the animals are touched during handling and by agitation when the flanks are brushed. The extent of the lesion can be controlled by altering the time of exposure to the laser beam. With longer exposure times, the allodynia can persist for months. Interestingly, responses to noxious heat are unchanged in this model (Hao et al. 1992a). Hao et al. (1991b, 1992b) made recordings of the responses of WDR neurons in the dorsal horn of decerebrate, spinalized rats before and after an ischemic lesion was made. The sensitivity of WDR cells was increased 4 days after the lesion, suggesting that the lesion increased the responsiveness of these neurons. The authors proposed that such changes could underlie the allodynia and that the lesion might have caused the loss of GABAergic inhibitory interneurons, which might have increased the excitability of nociceptive dorsal horn neurons. The number of neurons that could be immunostained for GABA was reduced after transient spinal cord ischemia (Zhang et al. 1994).

MODELS OF POST-STROKE PAIN

Thalamic lesions. To produce a model of thalamic pain, lesions have been made in the thalamus in rats (Saadé et al. 1999; LaBuda et al. 2000). In the first study, the thalamic lesions were electrolytic and were placed in the lateral or medial thalamus. Behavioral tests included the paw pressure, hot-plate, and tail-flick tests and the formalin test (Saadé et al. 1999). After a subtotal thalamic lesion, there was an initial period in which motor signs were present, but the rats recovered from the procedure within a week. At this time, the latencies for withdrawal in the paw pressure (bilaterally), hot–plate, and tail-flick tests were reduced, and pain scores increased in both phases of the formalin test. Similar effects followed a lesion restricted to the lateral thalamus, although in this case the latency in the tail-flick test was unchanged, and the responses in the formalin test were increased mostly during the tonic phase. After a lesion of the medial thalamus, the withdrawal latencies in the paw pressure test were greater contralateral to the lesion. Latencies in the hot-plate and tail-flick tests were also reduced, and pain scores in the formalin test were increased between the acute and tonic phases.

In the other study, a lesion was made in the VPL nucleus of rats by an injection of kainic acid (LaBuda et al. 2000). Kainic acid is thought to cause loss of neuronal cell bodies but is not believed to interrupt axons of passage. Paw withdrawals to mechanical stimuli (von Frey filaments) and to thermal stimuli (radiant heat) were used to demonstrate mechanical and thermal allodynia. When the VPL nucleus was damaged by the kainate lesion, there was a leftward shift in the stimulus-response function for the mechanical stimuli, indicating an increase in the frequency of responses. This change was significant 24 hours after the lesion and maximal at 48 hours. The latency of withdrawal from a heat stimulus was also reduced at 48 hours. When the VPL nucleus was missed by the lesion, no such change occurred.

Cortical injection of picrotoxin. The injection of picrotoxin, an antagonist of $GABA_A$ receptors, into the hindpaw region of the rat sensorimotor cerebral cortex results in electrophysiological evidence of seizure activity (Oliveras and Montagne-Clavel 1996). Accompanying this damage is pain-like behavior resembling that seen after injection of formalin into the hindpaw. This model may be a good model of central pain.

FUTURE STUDIES

Additional work is required to define further the mechanisms of central neuropathic pain. It seems likely, as with peripheral neuropathic pain, that multiple mechanisms are involved. A starting point will be the use of currently available models of central neuropathic pain. However, new models are desirable, especially for central pain syndromes that result from strokes that affect brain structures such as the lateral medulla, ventroposterior thalamus, and cerebral cortex. If research continues to suggest that central sensitization plays an important role in central neuropathic pain, the possibility should be pursued that central sensitization occurs in neurons of the pain system that are upstream from the site of damage. Many studies have already begun to evaluate therapeutic interventions that alleviate pain in the currently available models. Positive evidence from such studies will be valuable both to provide clues about possible therapies and to offer new insight into the mechanisms of this pain state.

ACKNOWLEDGMENTS

The author thanks Griselda Gonzales for her assistance with the illustrations. The work in the author's laboratory was supported by NIH grants NS 09743 and NS 11255.

REFERENCES

Al-Chaer ED, Lawand NB, Westlund KN, Willis WD. Visceral nociceptive input into the ventral posterolateral nucleus of the thalamus: a new function for the dorsal column pathway. *J Neurophysiol* 1996a; 76:2661–2674.

Al-Chaer ED, Lawand NB, Westlund KN, Willis WD. Pelvic visceral input into the nucleus gracilis is largely mediated by the postsynaptic dorsal column pathway. *J Neurophysiol* 1996b; 76:2675–2690.

Albé-Fessard D, Berkley KJ, Kruger L, Ralston HJ, Willis WD. Diencephalic mechanisms of pain sensation. *Brain Res Rev* 1985; 9:217–296.

Apkarian AV, Hodge CJ. Primate spinothalamic pathways: III. Thalamic terminations of the dorsolateral and ventral spinothalamic pathways. *J Comp Neurol* 1989; 288:493–511.

Apkarian AV, Shi T. Squirrel monkey lateral thalamus. I. Somatic nociresponsive neurons and their relation to spinothalamic terminals. *J Neurosci* 1994; 14:6779–6795.

Applebaum AE, Leonard RB, Kenshalo DR, Martin RF, Willis WD. Nuclei in which functionally identified spinothalamic tract neurons terminate. *J Comp Neurol* 1979; 188:575–586.

Baumann TK, Simone DA, Shain CN, LaMotte RH. Neurogenic hyperalgesia: the search for the primary cutaneous afferent fibers that contribute to capsaicin-induced pain and hyperalgesia. *J Neurophysiol* 1991; 66:212–227.

Beattie MS, Bresnahan JC, Komon J, et al. Endogenous repair after spinal cord contusion injuries in the rat. *Exp Neurol* 1997; 148:453–463.

Bennett AD, Chastain KM, Hulsebosch CE. Alleviation of mechanical and thermal allodynia by $\mathrm{CGRP}_{8\text{-}37}$ in a rodent model of chronic central pain. *Pain* 2000; 86:163–175.

Beric A, Dimitrijevic MR, Lindblom U. Central dysesthesia syndrome in spinal cord injury patients. *Pain* 1988; 34:109–116.

Berkley KJ. Spatial relationships between the terminations of somatic sensory and motor pathways in the rostral brainstem of cats and monkeys. I. Ascending somatic sensory inputs to lateral diencephalon. *J Comp Neurol* 1980; 193:283–317.

Bernard JF, Besson JM. The spino(trigemino)pontoamygdaloid pathway: electrophysiological evidence for an involvement in pain processes. *J Neurophysiol* 1990; 63:473–490.

Biemond A. The conduction of pain above the level of the thalamus opticus. *Arch Neurol Psychiatry* 1956; 75:231–244.

Bogousslavsky J, Regli F, Uske A. Thalamic infarcts: clinical syndromes, etiology, and prognosis. *Neurology* 1988; 38:837–848.

Boivie J. An anatomical reinvestigation of the termination of the spinothalamic tract in the monkey. *J Comp Neurol* 1979; 186:343–370.

Boivie J. Thalamic mechanisms of central pain as viewed from a clinical perspective. *Am Pain Soc J* 1992; 1:55–57.

Boivie J. Central pain. In: Wall PD, Melzack R (Eds). *Textbook of Pain*, 3rd ed. London: Churchill Livingstone, 1994, pp 871–902.

Boivie J, Leijon G, Johansson I. Central post-stroke pain—a study of the mechanisms through analyses of the sensory abnormalities. *Pain* 1989; 37:173–185.

Bowsher D. The anatomy of thalamic pain. *J Neurol Neurosurg Psychiatry* 1959; 22:81–82.

Bowsher D. Contralateral mirror-image pain following anterolateral chordotomy. *Pain* 1988; 33:63–65.

Bromm B, Treede RD. Human cerebral potentials evoked by CO_2 laser stimuli causing pain. *Exp Brain Res* 1987; 67:153–162.

Burstein R, Cliffer KD, Giesler GJ. Direct somatosensory projections from the spinal cord to the hypothalamus and telencephalon. *J Neurosci* 1987; 7:4159–4164.

Burton AW, Lee DH, Saab C, Chung JM. Preemptive intrathecal ketamine injection produces a long-lasting decrease in neuropathic pain behaviors in a rat model. *Reg Anesth Pain Med* 1999; 24:208–213.

Bushnell MC, Duncan GH, Tremblay N. Thalamic VPM nucleus in the behaving monkey. I. Multimodal and discriminative properties of thermosensitive neurons. *J Neurophysiol* 1993; 69:739–752.

Cameron AA, Dougherty PM, Garrison CJ, Willis WD, Carlton SM. The endogenous lectin RL-29 is transsynaptically induced in dorsal horn neurons following peripheral neuropathy in the rat. *Brain Res* 1993; 620:64–71.

Carlton SM, Lekan HS, Kim SH, Chung JM. Behavioral manifestations of an experimental model for peripheral neuropathy produced by spinal nerve ligation in the primate. *Pain* 1994; 56:155–166.

Casey KL (Ed). *Pain and Central Nervous System Disease: The Central Pain Syndromes.* New York: Raven Press, 1991.

Casey KL, Morrow TJ. Ventral posterior thalamic neurons differentially responsive to noxious stimulation of the awake monkey. *Science* 1983; 221:675–677.

Cassinari V, Pagni CA. *Central Pain: A Neurosurgical Survey.* Cambridge: Harvard University Press, 1969.

Cervero F, Iggo A, Molony V. Responses of spinocervical tract neurones to noxious stimulation of the skin. *J Physiol* 1977; 267:537–558.

Cesaro P, Mann MW, Moretti JL, et al. Central pain and thalamic hyperactivity: a single photon emission computerized tomographic study. *Pain* 1991; 47:329–336.

Chen L, Huang LYM. Sustained potentiation of NMDA receptor-mediated glutamate responses through activation of protein kinase C by a μ opioid. *Neuron* 1991; 7:319–326.

Chen L, Huang LYM. Protein kinase C reduces Mg^{2+} block of NMDA-receptor channels as a mechanism of modulation. *Nature* 1992; 356:521–523.

Christensen MD, Hulsebosch CE. Chronic central pain after spinal cord injury. *J Neurotrauma* 1997a; 14:517–537.

Christensen MD, Hulsebosch CE. Spinal cord injury and anti-NGF treatment results in changes in CGRP density and distribution in the dorsal horn in the rat. *Exp Neurol* 1997b; 147:463–475.

Christensen MD, Everhart AW, Pickelman JT, Hulsebosch CE. Mechanical and thermal allodynia in chronic central pain following spinal cord injury. *Pain* 1996; 68:97–107.

Chung JM, Lee KH, Surmeier DJ, et al. Response characteristics of neurons in the ventral posterior lateral nucleus of the monkey thalamus. *J Neurophysiol* 1986; 56:370–390.

Chung K, Lee WT, Carlton SM. The effects of dorsal rhizotomy and spinal cord isolation on calcitonin gene-related peptide-labeled terminals in the rat lumbar dorsal horn. *Neurosci Lett* 1988; 90:27–32.

Cliffer KD, Hasegawa T, Willis WD. Responses of neurons in the gracile nucleus of cats to innocuous and noxious stimuli: basic characterization and antidromic activation from the thalamus. *J Neurophysiol* 1992; 68:818–832.

Coggeshall RE, Lekan HA, Doubell TP, Allchorne A, Woolf CJ. Central changes in primary afferent fibers following peripheral nerve lesions. *Neuroscience* 1997; 77:1115–1122.

Coggeshall RE, Lekan HA, White FA, Woolf CJ. A-fiber sensory input induces neuronal cell death in the dorsal horn of the adult rat spinal cord. *J Comp Neurol* 2001; 435:276–282.

Craig AD. Supraspinal pathways and mechanisms relevant to central pain. In: Casey KL (Ed). *Pain and Central Nervous System Disease: The Central Pain Syndromes.* New York: Raven Press, 1991, pp 157–170.

Craig AD, Wiegand SJ, Price JL. The thalamo-cortical projection of the nucleus submedius in the cat. *J Comp Neurol* 1982; 206:28–48.

Craig AD, Bushnell MC, Zhang ET, Blomqvist A. A thalamic nucleus specific for pain and temperature sensation. *Nature* 1994; 372:770–773.

Davidoff G, Roth E, Guarracini M, Sliwa J, Yarkony G. Function-limiting dysesthetic pain syndrome among traumatic spinal cord injury patients: a cross-sectional study. *Pain* 1987; 29:39–48.

Dejerine, J, Roussy G. Le syndrome thalamique. *Rev Neurol (Paris)* 1906; 14:521–532.

Devor M, Govrin-Lippmann R, Angelides K. Na^+ channel immunolocalization in peripheral mammalian axons and changes following nerve injury and neuroma formation. *J Neurosci* 1993; 13:1976–1992.

Dougherty PM, Willis WD. Enhancement of spinothalamic neuron responses to chemical and mechanical stimuli following combined micro-iontophoretic application of N-methyl-D-aspartic acid and substance P. *Pain* 1991; 47:85–93.

Dougherty PM, Willis WD. Enhanced responses of spinothalamic tract neurons to excitatory amino acids accompany capsaicin-induced sensitization in the monkey. *J Neurosci* 1992; 12:883–894.

Dougherty PM, Palecek J, Paleckova V, Sorkin LS, Willis WD. The role of NMDA and non-NMDA excitatory amino acid receptors in the excitation of primate spinothalamic tract neurons by mechanical, chemical, thermal and electrical stimuli. *J Neurosci* 1992; 12:3025–3041.

Dougherty PM, Palecek J, Paleckova V, Willis WD. Neurokinin 1 and 2 antagonists attenuate the responses and NK1 antagonists prevent the sensitization of primate spinothalamic tract neurons after intradermal capsaicin. *J Neurophysiol* 1994; 72:1464–1475.

Downie JW, Ferrington DG, Sorkin LS, Willis WD. The primate spinocervicothalamic pathway: responses of cells of the lateral cervical nucleus and spinocervical tract to innocuous and noxious stimuli. *J Neurophysiol* 1988; 59:861–885.

Duncan GH, Bushnell MC, Oliveras JL, Bastrash N, Tremblay N. Thalamic VPM nucleus in the behaving monkey. III. Effects of reversible inactivation by lidocaine on thermal and mechanical discrimination. *J Neurophysiol* 1993; 70:2086–2096.

Eaton SA, Salt TE. Membrane and action potential responses evoked by excitatory amino acids acting at N-methyl-D-aspartate receptors and non-N-methyl-D-aspartate receptors in the rat thalamus in vivo. *Neuroscience* 1991; 44:277–286.

Fang L, Wu J, Willis WD. Enhanced phosphorylation of AMPA receptor (Glu-R1) contributes to central sensitization in rats following intradermal injection of capsaicin. *J Pain* 2001; 2:20.

Ferrington DG, Downie JW, Willis WD. Primate nucleus gracilis neurons: responses to innocuous and noxious stimuli. *J Neurophysiol* 1988; 59:886–907.

Fields HL, Adams JE. Pain after cortical injury relieved by electrical stimulation of the internal capsule. *Brain* 1974; 97:169–178.

Fields HL, Besson JM. (Eds). *Pain Modulation.* Progress in Brain Research, Vol. 77. Amsterdam: Elsevier, 1988.

Fields HL, Clanton CH, Anderson SD. Somatosensory properties of spinoreticular neurons in the cat. *Brain Res* 1977; 120:49–66.

Foerster O. Die Leitungsbahnen des Schmerzgefühls und die chirurgische Behandlung der Schmerzzustände. Berlin: Urban & Schwarzenberg, 1927, pp 77–80.

Giesler GJ, Yezierski RP, Gerhart KD, Willis WD. Spinothalamic tract neurons that project to medial and/or lateral thalamic nuclei: evidence for a physiologically novel population of spinal cord neurons. *J Neurophysiol* 1981; 46:1285–1308.

Gorecki J, Hirayama T, Dostrovsky JO, Tasker RR, Lenz FA. Thalamic stimulation and recording in patients with deafferentation and central pain. *Stereotact Funct Neurosurg* 1989; 52:219–226.

Graf CJ. Consideration in loss of sensory level after bilateral cervical cordotomy. *Arch Neurol* 1960; 3:410–415.

Guilbaud G, Benoist JM, Jazat F, Gautron M. Neuronal responsiveness in the ventrobasal thalamic complex of rats with an experimental peripheral mononeuropathy. *J Neurophysiol* 1990; 64:1537–1554.

Guilbaud G, Benoist JM, Levante A, Gautron M, Willer JC. Primary somatosensory cortex in rats with pain-related behaviours due to a peripheral mononeuropathy after moderate ligation of one sciatic nerve: neuronal responsivity to somatic stimulation. *Exp Brain Res* 1992; 92:227–245.

Gybels JM, Sweet WH. *Neurosurgical Treatment of Persistent Pain.* Basel: Karger, 1989.

Haber LH, Moore BD, Willis WD. Electrophysiological response properties of spinoreticular neurons in the monkey. *J Comp Neurol* 1982; 207:75–84.

Hao JX, Xu XJ, Aldskogius H, Seiger Å, Wiesenfeld-Hallin Z. Allodynia-like effects in rat after ischaemic spinal cord injury photochemically induced by laser irradiation. *Pain* 1991a; 45:175–185.

Hao JX, Xu XJ, Yu YX, Seiger Å, Wiesenfeld-Hallin Z. Hypersensitivity of dorsal horn wide dynamic range neurons to cutaneous mechanical stimuli after transient spinal cord ischemia in the rat. *Neurosci Lett* 1991b; 128:105–108.

Hao JX, Xu XJ, Aldskogius H, Seiger Å, Wiesenfeld-Hallin Z. Photochemically induced transient spinal ischemia induces behavioral hypersensitivity to mechanical and cold stimuli, but not to noxious-heat stimuli, in the rat. *Exp Neurol* 1992a; 118:187–194.

Hao JX, Xu XJ, Yu YX, Seiger Å, Wiesenfeld-Hallin Z. Transient spinal cord ischemia induces temporary hypersensitivity of dorsal horn wide dynamic range neurons to myelinated, but not unmyelinated, fiber input. *J Neurophysiol* 1992b; 68:384–391.

Head H, Holmes G. Sensory disturbances from cerebral lesions. *Brain* 1911; 34:102–254.

Hirshberg RM, Al-Chaer ED, Lawand NB, Westlund KN, Willis WD. Is there a pathway in the posterior funiculus that signals visceral pain? *Pain* 1996; 67:291–305.

Holmgren H, Leijon G, Boivie J, Johansson I, Ilievska L. Central post-stroke pain- somatosensory evoked potentials in relation to location of the lesion and sensory signs. *Pain* 1990; 40:43–52.

Hulsebosch CE, Xu GY, Perez-Polo JR, et al. Rodent model of chronic central pain after spinal cord contusion injury and effects of gabapentin. *J Neurotrauma* 2000; 17:1205–1217.

Inbal R, Devor M, Tuchendler O, Lieblich I. Autotomy following nerve injury: genetic factors in the development of chronic pain. *Pain* 1980; 9:327–337.

Isaev D, Gerber G, Park SK, Chung JM, Randic M. Facilitation of NMDA-induced currents and Ca^{2+} transients in the rat substantia gelatinosa neurons after ligation of L5–L6 spinal nerves. *Neuroreport* 2000; 11:4055–4061.

Jones EG. Thalamus and pain. *Am Pain Soc J* 1992; 1:58–61.

Jones EG, Pons TP. Thalamic and brainstem contributions to large-scale plasticity of primate somatosensory cortex. *Science* 1998; 282:1121–1125.

Kenshalo DR, Giesler GJ, Leonard RB, Willis WD. Responses of neurons in the primate ventral posterior lateral nucleus to noxious stimuli. *J Neurophysiol* 1980; 43:1594–1614.

Kim SH, Chung JM. An experimental model for peripheral neuropathy produced by segmental spinal nerve ligation in the rat. *Pain* 1992; 50:355–363.

Koyama S, Katayama Y, Maejima S, et al. Thalamic neuronal hyperactivity following transection of the spinothalamic tract in the cat: involvement of N-methyl-D-aspartate receptor. *Brain Res* 1993; 61:345–350.

LaBuda CJ, Cutler TD, Dougherty PM, Fuchs PN. Mechanical and thermal hypersensitivity develops following kainate lesion of the ventral posterior lateral thalamus in rats. *Neurosci Lett* 2000; 290:79–83.

Leijon G, Boivie J, Johansson I. Central post-stroke pain- neurological symptoms and pain characteristics. *Pain* 1989; 36:13–25.

Lenz FA. The ventral posterior nucleus of thalamus is involved in the generation of central pain syndromes. *Am Pain Soc J* 1992; 1:42–51.

Lenz FA, Tasker RR, Dostrovsky JO, et al. Abnormal single-unit activity recorded in the somatosensory thalamus of a quadriplegic patient with central pain. *Pain* 1987; 31:225–236.

Lenz FA, Kwan HC, Dostrovsky JO, Tasker RR. Characteristics of the bursting pattern of action potentials that occurs in the thalamus of patients with central pain. *Brain Res* 1989; 496:357–360.

Lenz FA, Gracely RH, Rowland LH, Dougherty PM. A population of cells in the human thalamic principal sensory nucleus respond to painful mechanical stimuli. *Neurosci Lett* 1994; 180:46–50.

Lenz FA, Gracely RH, Baker FH, Richardson RT, Dougherty PM. Reorganization of sensory modalities evoked by microstimulation in region of the thalamic principal sensory nucleus in patients with pain due to nervous system injury. *J Comp Neurol* 1998; 399:125–138.

Levitt M, Levitt JH. The deafferentation syndrome in monkeys: dysesthesias of spinal origin. *Pain* 1981; 10:129–147.

Lin Q, Peng YB, Willis WD. Possible role of protein kinase C in the sensitization of primate spinothalamic tract neurons. *J Neurosci* 1996a; 16:3026–3034.

Lin Q, Peng YB, Willis WD. Inhibition of primate spinothalamic tract neurons by spinal glycine and GABA is reduced during central sensitization. *J Neurophysiol* 1996b; 76:1005–1014.

Lin Q, Peng YB, Wu J, Willis WD. Involvement of cGMP in nociceptive processing by and sensitization of spinothalamic neurons in primates. *J Neurosci* 1997; 17:3293–3302.

Lin Q, Palecek J, Paleckova V, et al. Nitric oxide mediates the central sensitization of primate spinothalamic tract neurons. *J Neurophysiol* 1999; 81:1075–1085.

Lindblom U, Ochoa J. Somatosensory function and dysfunction. In: Asbury AK, McKhann GM, McDonald WI (Eds). *Diseases of the Nervous System: Clinical Neurobiology*, Vol. 1, Philadelphia: W.B. Saunders, 1986, pp 283–298.

Liu D, Thangnipon W, McAdoo DJ. Excitatory amino acids rise to toxic levels upon impact injury to the rat spinal cord. *Brain Res* 1991; 547:344–348.

Liu D, Xu GY, Pan E, McAdoo DJ. Neurotoxicity of glutamate at the concentration released upon spinal cord injury. *Neuroscience* 1999; 93:1383–1389.

Livingston WK. *Pain Mechanisms: A Physiologic Interpretation of Causalgia and its Related States*. New York: Macmillan, 1943.

Loh L, Nathan PW, Schott GD. Pain due to lesions of central nervous system removed by sympathetic block. *Brit Med J* 1981; 282:1026–1028.

Lyu YS, Park SK, Chung K, Chung JM. Low dose of tetrodotoxin reduces neuropathic pain behaviors in an animal model. *Brain Res* 2000; 871:98–103.

Madsen PW, Yezierski RP, Holets VR. Syringomyelia: clinical observations and experimental studies. *J Neurotrauma* 1994; 11:241–254.

Mao J, Mayer DJ, Price DD. Patterns of increased brain activity indicative of pain in a rat model of peripheral mononeuropathy. *J Neuroscience* 1993; 13:2689–2702.

Matzner O, Devor M. Hyperexcitability at sites of nerve injury depends on voltage-sensitive Na^+ channels. *J Neurophysiol* 1994; 72:349–359.

Mauguière F, Desmedt JE. Thalamic pain syndrome of Dejèrine-Roussy. Differentiation of four subtypes assisted by somatosensory evoked potentials data. *Arch Neurol* 1988; 45:1312–1320.

McAdoo DJ, Xu GY, Robak G, Hughes MG, Price EM. Evidence that reversed glutamate uptake contributes significantly to glutamate release following experimental injury to the rat spinal cord. *Brain Res* 2000; 865:283–285.

Mehler WR. The anatomy of the so-called "pain tract" in man: an analysis of the course and distribution of the ascending fibers of the fasciculus anterolateralis. In: French JD, Porter RW (Eds). *Basic Research in Paraplegia*. Springfield: Charles C. Thomas, 1962, pp 26–55.

Mehler WR, Feferman ME, Nauta WJH. Ascending axon degeneration following anterolateral cordotomy. An experimental study in the monkey. *Brain* 1960; 83:718–751.

Merskey H, Bogduk N. (Eds). *Classification of Chronic Pain: Descriptions of Chronic Pain Syndromes and Definitions of Pain Terms*, 2nd ed. Seattle: IASP Press, 1994.

Meyerson BA. Electric stimulation of the spinal cord and brain. In: Bonica JJ (Ed). *The Management of Pain*, Vol. II, Philadelphia: Lea & Febiger, 1990, pp 1862–1877.

Mogil JS, Wilson SG, Bon K, et al. Heritability of nociception I: responses of 11 inbred mouse strains on 12 measures of nociception. *Pain* 1999a; 80:67–82.

Mogil JS, Wilson SG, Bon K, et al. Heritability of nociception II. 'Types' of nociception revealed by genetic correlation analysis. *Pain* 1999b; 80:83–93.

Moulin DE, Foley KM, Ebers GC. Pain syndromes in multiple sclerosis. *Neurology* 1988; 38:1830–1834.

Neugebauer V, Chen PS, Willis WD. Role of metabotropic glutamate receptor subtype mGluR1 in brief nociception and central sensitization of primate STT cells. *J Neurophysiol* 1999; 82:272–282.

Neugebauer V, Chen PS, Willis WD. Groups II and III metabotropic glutamate receptors differentially modulate brief and prolonged nociception in primate STT cells. *J. Neurophysiol* 2000; 84:2998–3009.

Noble R, Riddell JS. Cutaneous excitatory and inhibitory input to neurones of the postsynaptic dorsal column system in the cat. *J Physiol* 1988; 396:497–513.

Oliveras JL, Montagne-Clavel J. Picrotoxin produces a "central" pain-like syndrome when microinjected into the somato-motor cortex of the rat. *Physiol Behav* 1996; 60:1425–1434.

Ovelmen-Levitt J, Gorecki J, Nguyen K, Iskandar B, Nashold BS. Spontaneous and evoked dysesthesias observed in the rat after spinal cordotomies. *Stereotact Funct Neurosurg* 1995; 65:157–160.

Pagni CA. *Central Pain. A Neurosurgical Challenge.* Torino: Edizioni Minerva Medica, 1998.

Palecek J, Dougherty PM, Kim SH, et al. Responses of spinothalamic tract neurons to mechanical and thermal stimuli in an experimental model of peripheral neuropathy in primates. *J Neurophysiol* 1992; 68:1951–1966.

Pertovaara A, Morrow TJ, Casey KL. Cutaneous pain and detection thresholds to short CO_2 laser pulses in humans: evidence on afferent mechanisms and the influence of varying stimulus conditions. *Pain* 1988; 34:261–269.

Pollin B, Albé-Fessard D. Organization of somatic thalamus in monkeys with and without section of dorsal spinal tracts. *Brain Res* 1979; 173:431–449.

Radhakrishnan V, Tsoukatos J, Davis KD, et al. A comparison of the burst activity of lateral thalamic neurons in chronic pain and non-pain patients. *Pain* 1999; 80:567–575.

Ralston HJ, Ohara PT, Meng XW, Wells J, Ralston DD. Transneuronal changes of the inhibitory circuitry in the macaque somatosensory thalamus following lesions of the dorsal column nuclei. *J Comp Neurol* 1996; 371:325–335.

Rausell E, Cusick CG, Taub E, Jones EG. Chronic deafferentation in monkeys differentially affects nociceptive and nonnociceptive pathways distinguished by specific calcium-binding proteins and down-regulates γ-aminobutyric acid type A receptors at thalamic levels. *Proc Natl Acad Sci USA* 1992; 89:2571–2575.

Richardson RR, Meyer PR, Cerullo LJ. Neurostimulation in the modulation of intractable paraplegic and traumatic neuroma pains. *Pain* 1980; 8:75–84.

Riddoch G. The clinical features of central pain. *Lancet* 1938; 234:1093-1098, 1150–1156, 1205–1209.

Roberts VJ, Dong WK. The effect of thalamic nucleus submedius lesions on nociceptive responding in rats. *Pain* 1994; 57:341–349.

Saadé NE, Kafrouni AI, Saab CY, Atweh SF, Jabbur SJ. Chronic thalamotomy increases pain-related behavior in rats. *Pain* 1999; 83:401–409.

Salt TE. The possible involvement of excitatory amino acids and NMDA receptors in thalamic pain mechanisms and central pain syndromes. *Am Pain Soc J* 1992; 1:52–54.

Salt TE, Binns KE. Contributions of mGlu1 and mGlu5 receptors to interactions with N-methyl-D-aspartate receptor-mediated responses and nociceptive sensory responses of rat thalamic neurons. *Neuroscience* 2000; 100:375–380.

Schmahmann JD, Leifer D. Parietal pseudothalamic pain syndrome. Clinical features and anatomic correlates. *Arch Neurol* 1992; 49:1032–1037.

Shaw PJ, Salt TE. Modulation of sensory and excitatory amino acid responses by nitric oxide donors and glutathione in the ventrobasal thalamus of the rat. *Eur J Neurosci* 1997; 9:1507–1513.

Shaw PJ, Charles SL, Salt TE. Actions of 8-bromo-cyclic-GMP on neurones in the rat thalamus in vivo and in vitro. *Brain Res* 1999; 833:272–277.

Shealy CN, Mortimer JT, Reswick J. Electrical inhibition of pain by stimulation of the dorsal columns: preliminary clinical report. *Anesth Analg* 1967; 46:489–491.

Siddall P, Xu CL, Cousins M. Allodynia following traumatic spinal cord injury in the rat. *Neuroreport* 1995; 6:1241–1244.

Simone DA, Sorkin LS, Oh U, et al. Neurogenic hyperalgesia: central neural correlates in responses of spinothalamic tract neurons. *J Neurophysiol* 1991; 66:228–246.

Sluka KA, Westlund KN. An experimental arthritis model in rats: the effects of NMDA and non-NMDA antagonists on aspartate and glutamate release in the dorsal horn. *Neurosci Lett* 1993a; 149:99–102.

Sluka KA, Westlund KN. Behavioral and immunohistochemical changes in an experimental arthritis model in rats. *Pain* 1993b; 55:367–377.

Sorkin LS, Xiao WH, Wagner R, Myers RR. Tumour necrosis factor-alpha induces ectopic activity in nociceptive primary afferent fibres. *Neuroscience* 1997; 81:255–262.

Sugimoto T, Bennett GJ, Kajander KC. Transsynaptic degeneration in the superficial dorsal horn after sciatic nerve injury: effects of a chronic constriction injury, transection, and strychnine. *Pain* 1990; 42:205–213.

Tasker R. Pain resulting from nervous system pathology (central pain). In: Bonica JJ (Ed). *The Management of Pain*, 2nd ed., Vol. 1. Philadelphia: Lea & Febiger, 1990, pp 264–280.

Tasker RR, Organ LW, Hawrylyshyn P. Deafferentation and causalgia. In: Bonica JJ (Ed). *Pain*. New York: Raven Press, 1980, pp 305–329.

Vierck CJ, Light AR. Effects of combined hemotoxic and anterolateral spinal lesions on nociceptive sensitivity. *Pain* 1999; 83:447–457.

Vierck CJ, Greenspan JD, Ritz LA. Long-term changes in purposive and reflexive responses to nociceptive stimulation in monkeys following anterolateral chordotomy. *J Neurosci* 1990; 10:2077–2095.

Weng H, Lee JI, Lenz FA, et al. Functional plasticity in primate somatosensory thalamus following chronic lesion of the ventral lateral spinal cord. *Neuroscience* 2000; 101:393–401.

White JC, Sweet WH. *Pain and the Neurosurgeon: A Forty-year Experience*. Springfield: CC Thomas, 1969.

Willis WD. Is central sensitization of nociceptive transmission in the spinal cord a variety of long-term potentiation? A commentary on the paper by Svendsen, Tjølsen and Hole. *Neuroreport* 1997; 8:iii.

Willis WD. Mechanisms of central sensitization of nociceptive dorsal horn neurons. In: Patterson MM, Grau JW (Eds). *Spinal Cord Plasticity*. New York: Kluwer, 2001a, pp 127–161.

Willis WD. The role of neurotransmitters in sensitization of pain responses. In: Sorg BA, Bell JR (Eds). Role of Neural Plasticity in Chemical Intolerance. *Ann NY Acad Sci* 2001b; 933:142–174.

Willis WD, Coggeshall RE. *Sensory Mechanisms of the Spinal Cord*, 2nd ed. New York: Plenum Press, 1991.

Willis WD, Kenshalo DR, Leonard RB. The cells of origin of the primate spinothalamic tract. *J Comp Neurol* 1979; 188:543–574.

Willis WD, Zhang X, Honda CN, Giesler GJ. Projections from the marginal zone and deep dorsal horn to the ventrobasal nuclei of the primate thalamus. *Pain* 2001; 92:267–276.

Woolf CJ, Shortland P, Coggeshall RE. Peripheral nerve injury triggers central sprouting of myelinated afferents. *Nature* 1992; 355:75–78.

Woolf CJ, Shortland P, Reynolds M, et al. Reorganization of central terminals of myelinated primary afferents in the rat dorsal horn following peripheral axotomy. *J Comp Neurol* 1995; 360:121–134.

Wu J, Lin Q, McAdoo DJ, Willis WD. Nitric oxide contributes to central sensitization following intradermal injection of capsaicin. *Neuroreport* 1998; 9:589–592.

Wu J, Fang L, Lin Q, Willis WD. Fos expression is induced by increased nitric oxide release in rat spinal cord dorsal horn. *Neuroscience* 2000; 96:351–357.

Xu GY, McAdoo DJ, Hughes MG, Robak G, De Castro R. Considerations in the determination by microdialysis of resting extracellular amino acid concentrations and release upon spinal cord injury. *Neuroscience* 1998; 86:1011–1021.

Xu XJ, Hao JX, Aldskogius H, Seiger Å, Wiesenfeld-Hallin Z. Chronic pain-related syndrome in rats after ischemic spinal cord lesion: a possible animal model for pain in patients with spinal cord injury. *Pain* 1992; 48:279–290.

Yezierski RP, Park SH. The mechanosensitivity of spinal sensory neurons following intraspinal injections of quisqualic acid in the rat. *Neurosci Lett* 1993; 157:115–119.

Yezierski RP, Santana M, Park SH, Madsen PW. Neuronal degeneration and spinal cavitation following intraspinal injections of quisqualic acid in the rat. *J Neurotrauma* 1993; 10:445–456.

Yezierski RP, Liu S, Ruenes GL, Kajander KJ, Brewer KL. Excitotoxic spinal cord injury: behavioral and morphological characteristics of a central pain model. *Pain* 1998; 75:141–155.

Yoon YW, Na HS, Chung JM. Contributions of injured and intact afferents to neuropathic pain in an experimental rat model. *Pain* 1996; 64:27–36.

Yoon YW, Sung B, Chung JM. Nitric oxide mediates behavioral signs of neuropathic pain in an experimental rat model. *Neuroreport* 1998; 9:367–372.

Zhang AL, Hao JX, Seiger Å, et al. Decreased GABA immunoreactivity in spinal cord dorsal horn neurons after transient spinal cord ischemia in the rat. *Brain Res* 1994; 656:187–190.

Zhang S, Tang JS, Yuan B, Jia H. Inhibitory effects of glutamate-induced activation of thalamic nucleus submedius are mediated by ventrolateral orbital cortex and periaqueductal gray in rats. *Eur J Pain* 1998; 2:153–163.

Zhang X, Wenk HN, Honda CN, Giesler GJ. Locations of spinothalamic tract axons in cervical and thoracic spinal cord white matter in monkeys. *J Neurophysiol* 2000; 83:2869–2880.

Zhang YQ, Tang JS, Yuan B, Jia H. Effects of thalamic nucleus submedius lesions on the tail flick reflex inhibition evoked by hindlimb electrical stimulation in the rat. *Neuroreport* 1995; 6:1237–1240.

Zou X, Lin Q, Willis WD. Enhanced phosphorylation of NMDA receptor 1 subunits in spinal cord dorsal horn and spinothalamic neurons following intradermal injection of capsaicin in rats. *J Neurosci* 2000; 20:6989–6997.

Correspondence to: William D. Willis, Jr., MD, PhD, Department of Anatomy and Neurosciences, University of Texas Medical Branch, Galveston, TX 77550-1069, USA. Tel: 409-772-2103; Fax: 409-772-4687; email: wdwillis@utmb.edu.

Spinal Cord Injury Pain: Assessment, Mechanisms, Management. Progress in Pain Research and Management, Vol. 23, edited by Robert P. Yezierski and Kim J. Burchiel, IASP Press, Seattle, © 2002.

7

Pathophysiology and Animal Models of Spinal Cord Injury Pain

Robert P. Yezierski

Departments of Orthodontics and Neuroscience, College of Dentistry, and the McKnight Brain Institute, University of Florida, Gainesville, Florida, USA

When discussing the condition of pain following spinal cord injury (SCI) it is important to consider the underlying mechanism responsible for the wide variety of pathological changes associated with ischemic or traumatic insult to the cord. Pain associated with spinal injury is after all a consequence of injury, and thus if we are to understand the end result we must first appreciate the scope of potential causal events contributing to this condition. Obviously, significant structural damage is associated with SCI, leading to a reorganization of spinal and supraspinal circuits responsible for the integration and processing of sensory information. Ischemic or traumatic insult also brings about changes in the expression of intrinsic chemical systems that maintain the homeostatic balance between inhibitory and excitatory circuits. Equally important are the effects on cellular events involved in signaling, transduction, and survival pathways of spinal neurons. Collectively, the complex sequence of primary and secondary injury-induced effects have a profound impact on the survivability and excitability of spinal sensory neurons, ultimately affecting both evoked and resting sensibilities.

Many of the pathophysiological changes associated with spinal injury parallel those thought to be responsible for the development of pain after peripheral nerve and tissue injury (Dubner 1991). This observation led to the proposal of a *central injury cascade* believed to be involved in the initiation of pain-related behaviors following central or peripheral injury (Yezierski et al. 1996). In spite of recent progress directed toward understanding the mechanism(s) of SCI pain, many unanswered questions remain for both basic scientists and health professionals (Bonica 1991; Yezierski

1996, 2000). Different experimental models have provided valuable insights related to the mechanism(s) responsible for the onset of pain following injury (see Chapters 6, 9–12). Continued use of these models should lead to the identification of novel therapeutic targets and the development of more effective treatment strategies.

PATHOPHYSIOLOGY OF SPINAL CORD INJURY

SCI is characterized by pathological changes resulting from mechanical trauma and vascular compromise of the cord parenchyma (Kakulas et al. 1990; Tator and Fehlings 1991). Pain following SCI is believed to be related to the nature of the lesion, the neurological structures damaged, and secondary pathophysiological changes of surviving tissue (Bonica 1991; Yezierski 2000). The most clinically relevant methods used to produce experimental injury are those resulting in morphological changes similar to those associated with the human condition. An initial consequence of SCI, similar to that associated with stroke, hypoxia-ischemia, and traumatic brain injury, is the well-known effects of excitatory amino acids (EAAs) (Regan and Choi 1994). The involvement of glutamate in the secondary pathology of ischemic and traumatic spinal injury is well documented (Faden and Simon 1988; Nag and Riopelle 1990; Hao et al. 1991; Tator and Fehlings 1991; Yezierski et al. 1993; Wrathall et al. 1994). Although the elevation of EAAs occurs for only a brief period, this dramatic change is thought to trigger an injury cascade that includes the production of inflammatory cytokines and prostanoids, as well as the up- and downregulation of cellular messengers and transcription factors that can severely compromise the anatomical and functional integrity of spinal neurons (Young 1987; Tator and Fehlings 1991; Hayashi et al. 2000).

The major components of the central injury cascade include anatomical, neurochemical, excitotoxic, and inflammatory events that collectively interact to influence the functional state of spinal sensory neurons, leading to the onset of various evoked and spontaneous pain states (allodynia, hyperalgesia, and pain). Fig. 1 summarizes some of the different mediators and functional outcomes that have been documented as part of the cascade of secondary events that can follow SCI. In addition to the injury-induced elevation of EAAs and the subsequent neurochemical events characterizing excitotoxicity, one must not ignore parallel events associated with secondary injury, including astrocytic and microglial responses and the initiation of inflammatory and immune processes. Achieving an understanding of the basic biology of these secondary events is pivotal to understanding the

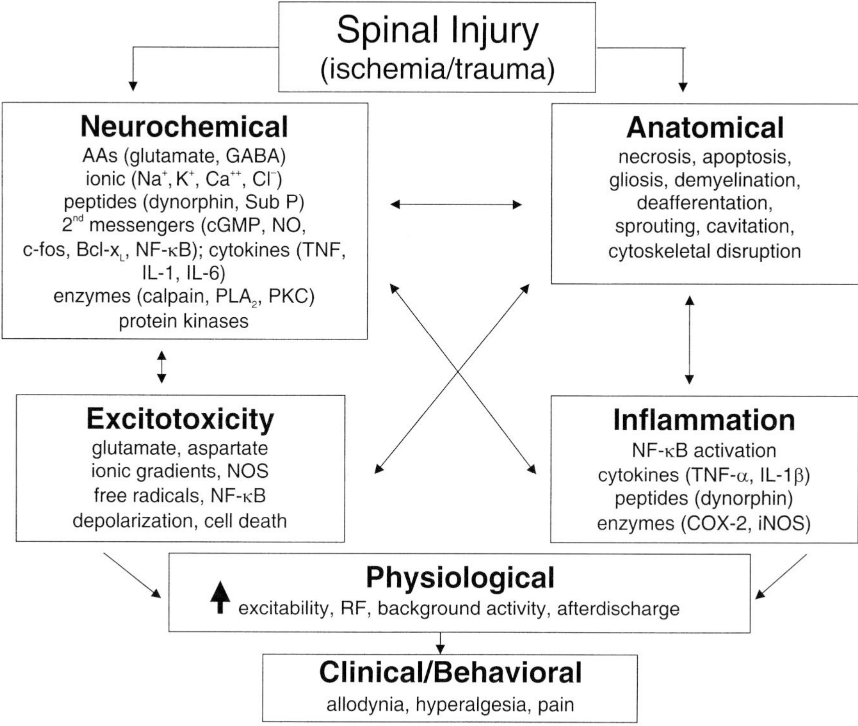

Fig. 1. Summary of the major components of the spinal central injury cascade believed to be responsible for the onset and progression of at-level and below-level pain following ischemic or traumatic spinal injury. Evidence supporting the basic concept of this cascade comes from results of clinical studies as well as those obtained from the use of ischemic, lesion, contusion, and excitotoxic models of SCI. The four major components of the cascade (neurochemical, excitotoxic, anatomical, and inflammatory) are represented as being interactive and collectively lead to changes in the physiological state of spinal and supraspinal neurons. The end result of this cascade is the onset of clinical symptoms, e.g., allodynia, hyperalgesia, and pain. Abbreviations: AAs = amino acids; GABA = γ-aminobutyric acid; Sub P = substance P; cGMP = cyclic guanidine monophosphate; NO = nitric oxide; NF-κB = nuclear factor kappa B; TNF = tumor necrosis factor; IL-1β = interleukin-1β; PLA_2 = phospholipase A2; PKC = protein kinase C; NOS = nitric oxide synthase; COX-2 = cyclooxygenase-2; iNOS = inducible nitric oxide synthase; RF = receptive field. Reprinted from Yezierski (2000), with permission.

mechanisms of pain onset and in designing effective treatments. The pathological sequelae of SCI are by no means simple, nor are they restricted to the site of insult. While most of the focus in the study of spinal injury has been devoted to the spinal cord, we also must consider the often neglected remote effects of SCI, including deafferentation of supraspinal sensory relay nuclei (Lenz 1991; Chapter 13, this volume), chemical and metabolic changes in thalamic nuclei (Chapter 17), elevations in forebrain blood flow (Morrow et al. 2000; Chapter 15, this volume), upregulation of gene expression in the mesencephalon (Brewer et al. 1999), and the increased expression of opioid transmitters in selected supraspinal sites (Abraham et al. 2000, 2001).

The initial elevation in EAAs following SCI is accompanied by the increased production of a number of potentially toxic mediators: (a) endogenous opioids (dynorphin, enkephalin), (b) prostaglandins, (c) cytokines, (d) nitric oxide, and (e) reactive oxygen species (Young 1987; Tator and Fehlings 1991). Upregulation of messenger RNA for *c-fos* and tumor necrosis factor α (TNF-α) and activation of transcription factors have also been reported following SCI (Yakovlev and Faden 1994; Bethea et al. 1998; Abraham and Brewer 2001). Activation of the nuclear factor kappa B (NF-κB) family of transcription factors is a critical step in the inducible regulation of over 150 genes involved in inflammatory, proliferative, and cell death responses (Pahl 1998). Importantly, several of the cellular messengers that are upregulated in response to spinal injury also play a pivotal role in defining the functional state of spinal sensory neurons (Willis 1993).

Traumatic or ischemic insult to the spinal cord initiates immediate changes in ionic gradients that affect survival cascades, leading to programmed cell death (apoptosis) and necrosis. A recent report of SCI-associated changes in the expression of the anti-apoptotic protein Bcl-x_L further supports the influence of SCI on cell survival pathways (Qui et al. 2001). Damage to ascending and descending pathways also results in the deafferentation of supraspinal structures and the loss of transmitter systems, such as serotonergic and noradrenergic terminals, in the spinal cord. The disruption of intracellular and extracellular potassium, sodium, and calcium concentrations affects the functional state of the spinal cord, leading to an increase in excitability secondary to widespread neuronal depolarization. While the full extent of biochemical and molecular changes initiated by SCI has not been defined, those documented provide new insights that could lead to the development of novel strategies targeting cellular events that might restore functional homeostasis.

A critical factor in the onset of pain-like behaviors after SCI is believed to be a loss of inhibitory tone within the injured spinal cord (Wiesenfeld-Hallin 1994; Chapter 10, this volume). The loss of spinal inhibitory control allows for the recruitment of surrounding neurons and the intensification and spread of abnormal sensations, including pain. Existing evidence supports the decreased inhibitory influence of GABAergic neurotransmission in altering the functional properties of neurons in the injured cord. Not to be overlooked is a decreased influence of supraspinal and propriospinal inhibitory pathways that may be compromised after injury. Furthermore, given the well-documented involvement of NMDA receptors in altering the excitability of spinal neurons (Haley and Wilcox 1992; Woolf 1992), it is reasonable to propose that, along with a failed GABAergic inhibitory system, increased NMDA-receptor activation (secondary to injury-induced release of glutamate) could play a role in elevating the excitability of spinal neurons and thus contribute to the cascade of physiological and behavioral changes after spinal injury (Yezierski et al. 1998). Blockade of acute allodynia by the competitive NMDA-receptor antagonist MK-801 supports this hypothesis (Hao et al. 1991), as does the clinical report of Eide and colleagues (1995) showing that central dysesthesia pain after traumatic SCI is dependent on NMDA-receptor activation.

Another component of the pathophysiological sequelae of SCI is the emergence of a "pattern-generating mechanism" (spinal and supraspinal). Melzack and Loeser (1978) concluded that not all post-injury pains are due to noxious input; some may be due to deafferentation or to loss of inhibitory control and subsequent changes in the firing patterns, including burst activity and long afterdischarges of neuronal pools lying adjacent to the site of injury. Consistent with this excitability hypothesis are reports of changes in the functional state of spinal and supraspinal sensory neurons after experimental SCI (Yezierski and Park 1993; Wiesenfeld-Hallin et al. 1994; Hulsebosch et al. 2000; Chapter 12, this volume) and clinical reports of abnormal focal hyperactivity within the superficial laminae of the injured cord (Edgar et al. 1993) and subcortical structures (Lenz 1991; Chapter 13, this volume).

A final consideration related to the pathological consequences of SCI is the initiation of synaptic plasticity. The various categories of plastic changes that alter the functional state of spinal neurons can be broken down into *initiating events*, *maintaining events*, *perpetuating forces*, and *terminal results*. The contribution of these events to the onset and progression of chronic pain is an important focus of research aimed at understanding the central mechanisms of SCI pain and in identifying critical therapeutic targets. Biochemical events that contribute to the initiation of injury-induced plasticity after SCI include membrane lipid peroxidation, perturbed intracellular calcium signaling, neurotransmitter accumulation, cytokine release, activation of protein kinases, and calcium activation of the arachidonic acid cascade. The latter event leads to the synthesis of eicosanoids, which regulate ion channels and the formation of superoxide free radicals (Piomelli 1993; Smith and Dewitt 1995). The production of arachidonic acid exacerbates the injury process by inhibiting sodium-dependent uptake of aspartate and glutamate, thus increasing extracellular levels of these EAAs, and by stimulating exocytosis of glutamate in synergy with protein kinase C (PKC) activation. In parallel with the above sequence of events, which ultimately can influence the normal physiology of spinal neurons, is the initiation of a local inflammatory response that includes increases in the expression of cytokines, chemokines, and adhesion molecules (Hsu et al. 1994). Wilcox and colleagues recently described the role of the inflammatory cytokine interleukin (IL)-1β along with protein synthesis, and activation of NF-κB in synaptic plasticity and chronic pain behaviors in the dynorphin model of SCI pain (Laughlin et al. 2000).

A prime candidate for influencing the functional plasticity of spinal neurons is membrane lipid peroxidation, a free-radical-mediated biochemical reaction leading to the formation of lipid peroxides. This process is one of the first measurable biochemical events after SCI; it is thought to lead to membrane disruption followed by the loss of membrane-bound ionic pumps and transporters that compromise ionic gradients and cell-signaling pathways. Although disruption of the sodium-potassium ion equilibrium threatens the functional state of spinal neurons after injury, perhaps the most significant biochemical event is the derangement of calcium compartmentalization. Elevation in intracellular calcium is one of the most significant pathophysiological events after SCI, influencing signaling pathways, destructive enzymes, production of reactive oxygen radicals, activation of nitric oxide synthase, and disruption of mitochondrial function and thus energy metabolism within cells. Furthermore, the release of the fatty acid oleate directly stimulates PKC. Palecek et al. (1999) recently found that PKC stimulation evokes mechanical allodynia and thermal hyperalgesia, providing further evidence, along with Malmberg et al. (1997), that PKC is involved in modulating nociceptive information in the spinal cord and in producing neuropathic pain. All the above biochemical events potentially influence the excitability and survivability of spinal sensory neurons and thus may contribute to the onset of injury-induced pain states.

Not to be overlooked in the aftermath of SCI are the activation of intrinsic immune cells (microglia), the recruitment of extrinsic immune cells (monocytes, lymphocytes, and natural killer cells), and the activation of astrocytes. Immune cells and astrocytes secrete cytokines such as IL-1 and IL-6 and other potentially neurotoxic substances including TNF-α, quinolinic acid, proteases, and eicosanoids. Considering the potential importance of the inflammatory immune response (DeLeo and Yezierski 2000) and the glial contribution (Watkins et al. 2001) to chronic pain states, these injury-induced responses may be important to the central mechanism responsible for the onset of SCI-induced pain.

ANIMAL MODELS OF SCI PAIN

Several experimental models have been used to study SCI, each with distinctive characteristics related to specific aspects of the human condition (see Chapters 8–12). An important feature of these models is that each is based on a critical component of the primary injury, such as trauma or ischemia. The primary objective in modeling the human condition is to produce the same or similar pathological and behavioral conditions that are described following human SCI. Examples of the pathological condition of specimens from four different models of SCI are shown in Fig. 2. There are many similarities among these models, each of which has provided insight into the mechanism of tissue damage and onset of pain behaviors after injury. Evidence for dysesthesia and pain and for the enhancement of nocifensive responses at the level of spinal lesions comes from models employing excitotoxicity (Yezierski et al. 1998), ischemia (Chapter 10), and contusion injury (Siddall et al. 1995; Chapters 11, 12). For example, lesions

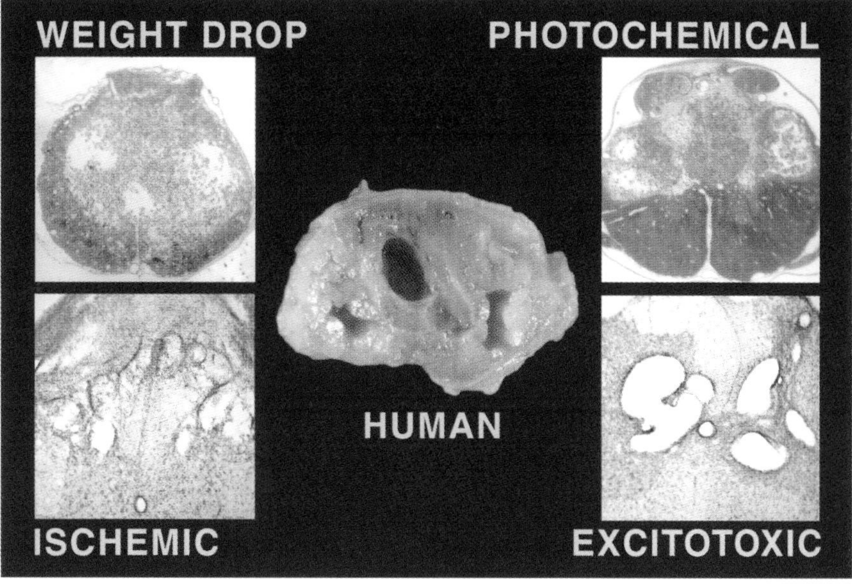

Fig. 2. Examples of histological sections from spinal cords that underwent contusion (WEIGHT DROP), vasoconstriction (ISCHEMIC), ischemic (PHOTOCHEMICAL), and chemical (EXCITOTOXIC) injuries. The objective of each of these experimental models is to simulate different components of the human condition using features (trauma, vascular, chemical) known to be involved in producing primary and/or secondary tissue damage. Sections from the rat spinal cords were taken 3–6 weeks after injury while the human sample was obtained 15 years after a contusion injury.

produced by the intraspinal injection of quisqualic acid result in overgrooming of ipsilateral dermatomes representing segments at the lesion epicenter (Yezierski et al. 1998), and ischemic lesions enhance nocifensive responses to stimuli delivered to dermatomes near the level of injury (Chapter 10). Another approach to the study of altered sensation following SCI involves the use of selected spinal lesions, either alone or in combination with other manipulations (Levitt 1989; Vierck 1991; Vierck and Light 2000; Chapters 9, 11, this volume). All these experimental strategies share the distinction of producing pathological and/or behavioral changes associated with human SCI, and each provides an opportunity to study different aspects of the spinal and supraspinal mechanisms responsible for SCI pain. When discussing different models of SCI pain it is important to point out the parallels between the behavioral consequences of experimental SCI and specific pain conditions known to occur clinically (Chapter 2). In recent years the primary focus of experimental studies has been directed toward at-level and below-level pain (Vierck et al. 2000).

ANIMAL MODELS OF AT-LEVEL PAIN

Animal models of at-level SCI pain have been used to characterize its anatomical, biochemical, molecular, physiological, and pharmacological characteristics. The results implicate a central cascade that exerts a profound influence on the functional state of spinal sensory neurons (Yezierski 2000). The importance of destructive secondary cellular reactions in the development of at-level pain is underscored by the results of studies using neuroprotective or rescuing strategies that reduce the spread of injury-induced tissue damage and limit changes in neuronal excitability. For example, administration of NMDA antagonists can attenuate ischemic damage, prevent the development of segmental hypersensitivity, and reduce chronic SCI pain in humans. Repeated doses of the antiepileptic agent gabapentin alleviates chronic hypersensitivity in spinally injured rats (Chapter 11, this volume; Hao et al., in press). Adrenal chromaffin cells, which produce a "therapeutic cocktail" of neuroprotective and potentially analgesic agents, also have been used to alleviate injury-induced pain behaviors (Brewer and Yezierski 1998; Yu et al. 1998; Hains et al. 2000). Use of the endogenous anti-inflammatory agent IL-10 also has significant neuroprotective properties and beneficial effects on the onset and progression of injury-induced pain behaviors (Brewer et al. 1999; Plunkett et al. 2001).

Consistent with changes in the inhibitory tone brought about by injury are the results reported by Wiesenfeld and colleagues (Chapter 10). The ischemic (photochemical) model of SCI creates two distinct periods of hypersensitivity to mechanical stimuli delivered to dermatomes near the site of injury. The first period lasts 1–5 days, is associated with reduced γ-aminobutyric acid (GABA) immunoreactivity, and is attenuated by GABA-B-receptor agonists. The acute hypersensitivity is insensitive to intrathecal morphine at a time when μ-opioid-receptor immunoreactivity is reduced. By contrast, the chronic enhancement of nocifensive behaviors in this model does not depend on GABAergic mechanisms, but is reduced by intrathecal application of morphine and the α_2 noradrenergic agonist clonidine. Additional studies related to the pharmacology of chronic pain behaviors associated with experimental SCI are described by Hulsebosch (Chapter 11).

Out of consideration for the well-documented elevation of EAAs following SCI, an excitotoxic model was developed to model this chemical change and to evaluate the involvement of non-NMDA receptors in the pathological sequelae of SCI (Yezierski et al. 1993). Results obtained using this model have provided insight into the pathophysiological, molecular, and behavioral consequences initiated by a transient increase in spinal levels of EAAs (Yezierski et al. 1993, 1998; Brewer et al. 1997; Brewer and Yezierski 1998; Morrow et al. 2000; Abraham et al. 2001; Abraham and Brewer 2001; Gorman et al. 2001). One of the behavioral consequences of the excitotoxic model is excessive grooming, a spontaneous at-level pain behavior that has been proposed as a rodent model of central pain following SCI (Yezierski et al. 1998; Yezierski 2000; Gorman et al. 2001). To characterize the events contributing to the onset and progression of this behavior, Gorman et al. (2001) evaluated the relationship between onset and severity and the rostrocaudal spread of injury-induced neuronal loss in three different strains of male rats.

Spinal injections of quisqualic acid were made in Sprague Dawley (SDM), Long Evans (LEM), and Wistar Furth (WFM) male rats. Differences in grooming characteristics between male and female rats and the modulatory effects of female gonadal hormones were also evaluated in Sprague Dawley females (SDF), bilaterally ovariectomized Sprague Dawley females (OVX), and SDMs treated with either 17-β-estradiol (SDM-Est) or progesterone (SDM-Pro). The results showed that the development of excessive grooming behavior in males and ovariectomized females is related to the rostrocaudal spread of a specific pattern of neuronal loss. Excessive grooming behavior in SDFs was similar to that found in SDMs; however, SDFs did not show a dependence on the extent of injury for the onset of this behavior (Fig. 3). The onset, severity, and progression of excessive grooming in OVX rats were similar to the pattern found in SDMs. Furthermore, estradiol-treated SDMs developed severe grooming characterized by early onset, while progesterone treatment delayed the onset of grooming and attenuated its severity

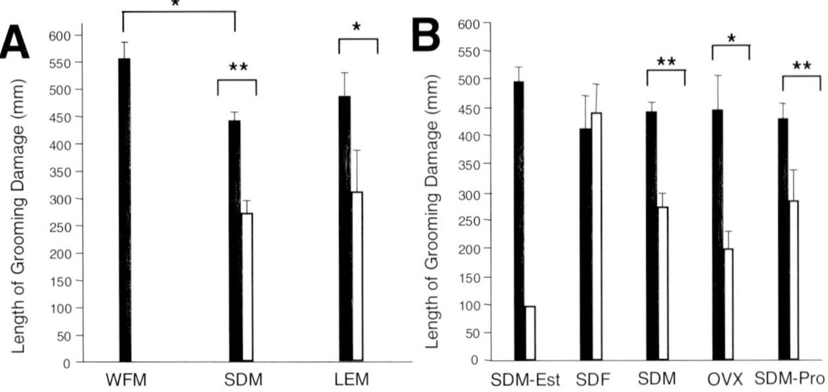

Fig. 3. Total length of grooming-type neuronal loss ipsilateral to the site of injection for both grooming (closed bars) and nongrooming animals (open bars). (A) Grooming-type neuronal loss in different strains of male rats: WFM (n = 11 groomers, 0 nongroomers); SDM (n = 10 groomers, 6 nongroomers); LEM (n = 12 groomers, 5 nongroomers). Significant effects of strain were observed when comparing WFM versus SDM grooming animals ($P < 0.05$). Within each strain significant differences in the extent of grooming-type neuronal loss were observed between grooming and nongrooming animals for SDM ($P < 0.01$) and LEM rats ($P < 0.05$). (B) No significant effects of gender, OVX, or hormone treatment were observed on grooming-type neuronal loss for grooming animals in the different groups that included SDM-Est (n = 7 groomers, 1 nongroomer), SDF (n = 7 groomers, 8 nongroomers), SDM (n = 10 groomers, 6 nongroomers), OVX (n = 5 groomers, 4 nongroomers), and SDM-Pro rats (n = 5 groomers, 5 nongroomers). Significant differences in grooming-type neuronal loss between grooming and nongrooming animals in each subgroup were observed for SDM ($P < 0.01$), OVX ($P < 0.05$), and SDM-Pro rats ($P < 0.01$). Data are represented as mean ± SEM. $^*P < 0.05$; $^{**}P < 0.01$. Reprinted from Gorman et al. (2001), with permission.

and progression (Fig. 4). Strain-related differences were also observed, with WFMs exhibiting more aggressive grooming than SDMs or LEMs. The results of this study suggest that the evolution of pain-like behaviors following SCI is a complex process with gender, strain, and gonadal hormones all potentially influencing the onset and progression of these injury-induced behaviors (Gorman et al. 2001).

An important histological correlate of excessive grooming behavior is a pattern of neuronal loss that includes the neck of the dorsal horn with sparing of the superficial laminae (Fig. 5). Previously, we had speculated that lamina I projection neurons might be part of the substrate for the onset of injury-induced excessive grooming behavior (Yezierski et al. 1998). A conjugate of substance P to saporin, a ribosome-inactivating protein from *Saponaria officinalis,* effectively destroys neurons expressing the neurokinin-1 (NK-1) receptor in the striatum and lamina I of the spinal dorsal horn (Mantyh et al. 1997). This conjugate selectively binds to the NK-1 receptor

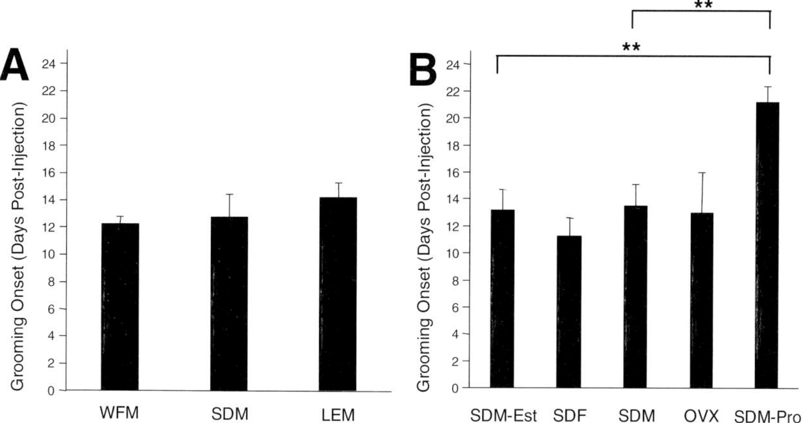

Fig. 4. Onset time for excessive grooming behavior in different strains (A) and groups of Sprague Dawley rats (B). Although Long Evans males had the longest onset-time of the three strains evaluated, no significant effect of strain was observed when comparing Wistar Furth males (WFM, $n = 11$), Sprague Dawley males (SDM, $n = 10$), and Long Evans males (LEM, $n = 12$). (B) The comparison of different Sprague Dawley subgroups showed a significant effect of hormone treatment for the groups examined (SDM-Est, $n = 8$; SDF, $n = 7$; SDM, $n = 10$; OVX, $n = 5$; SDM-Pro, $n = 5$). Significant differences were observed when comparing SDM vs. SDM-Pro ($P < 0.01$), and when comparing SDM-Est vs. SDM-Pro ($P < 0.01$). Data are represented as mean ± SEM for the onset of excessive grooming. $^{**}P < 0.01$. Reprinted from Gorman et al. (2001), with permission.

on the cell surface. Once internalized, the saporin component catalytically inactivates ribosomes, producing irreversible inhibition of protein synthesis and cell death. The effects of the neurotoxin [Sar^9 $Met(O_2)^{11}$] substance P-saporin (SSP-SAP) delivered directly to the dorsal surface of the cord was evaluated in "prevention" and "treatment" protocols against the onset and progression of excessive grooming behavior (Yezierski et al. 2000). The results suggest that selective elimination of neurons with the NK-1 receptor in the superficial dorsal horn plays a significant role in the onset and progression of this behavior (Fig. 6). Of special interest regarding the future treatment of SCI pain was the fact that "treatment" of the pain-like behavior after onset significantly reduced and in many cases eliminated it (Fig. 6). These results support a role of a superficial dorsal horn "pattern generator" in the expression of excessive grooming behavior and suggest the use of this approach, recently referred to as "molecular surgery," as a therapeutic intervention for spontaneous at-level SCI pain.

Although the pathophysiological changes associated with excitotoxic SCI are believed to be in part a consequence of an excitotoxic cascade, one cannot ignore the potential contributions from other components of the secondary injury cascade. Recent evidence supports an inflammatory contribution

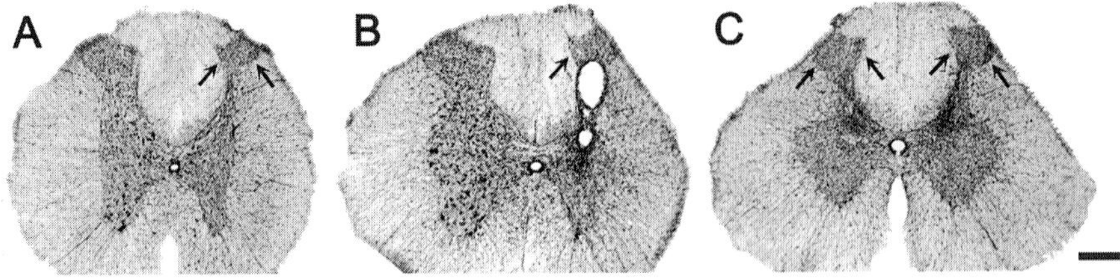

Fig. 5. Photomicrographs of "grooming-type" neuronal loss found in histological sections from animals with unilateral (A,B) or bilateral (C) excessive grooming behavior. In all animals injections of quisqualic acid were made unilaterally on the right side of the cord. Note the pattern of neuronal loss in the neck of the dorsal horn with partial or complete sparing of the superficial laminae (arrows). Scale bar in C equals 380 μm. Reprinted from Gorman et al. (2001), with permission.

to the quisqualic acid injury model. Intraspinal injections of quisqualic acid upregulate mRNAs for IL1-β, cyclooxygenase-2 (COX-2), inducible nitric oxide synthase (iNOS), death-inducing ligand CD-95, and TNF-related apoptosis-inducing ligand (TRAIL) (Plunkett et al. 2001). IL-10, a potent anti-inflammatory cytokine, reduced mRNA levels of IL-1β and iNOS. The behavioral correlate of this decrease was a significant delay in the onset of excessive grooming behavior, a reduction in grooming severity, and a reduction in the longitudinal extent of neuronal loss within the spinal cord (Fig. 7). These results suggest that targeting of injury-induced inflammation is another potentially effective strategy for limiting the extent of neuronal damage following excitotoxic SCI and thus reducing the onset and progression of injury-induced pain behaviors.

Potential mechanisms underlying the onset of excessive grooming behavior were further studied by evaluating the effects of two drugs that target different components of the secondary injury cascade, agmatine and cyclosporin A (Fairbanks et al. 2000; Yu et al. 2000). Use of the NOS inhibitor and NMDA antagonist agmatine or the immunosuppressant cyclosporin A delayed the onset of excessive grooming, reduced the area and severity of grooming, and reduced neuronal loss in the spinal cord compared to saline-treated animals. "Treatment" of excessive grooming behavior with the same drugs also significantly reduced grooming area, grooming severity, and neuronal loss in the spinal cord compared to saline treatment. The conclusion from this study was that systemic administration of agmatine or cyclosporin A can have a significant effect on the onset and progression of a spontaneous pain-related behavior. The effective "treatment" of this behavior suggests that both drugs are capable of modulating events responsible for its progression. These results point to the possibility that using neuroprotective

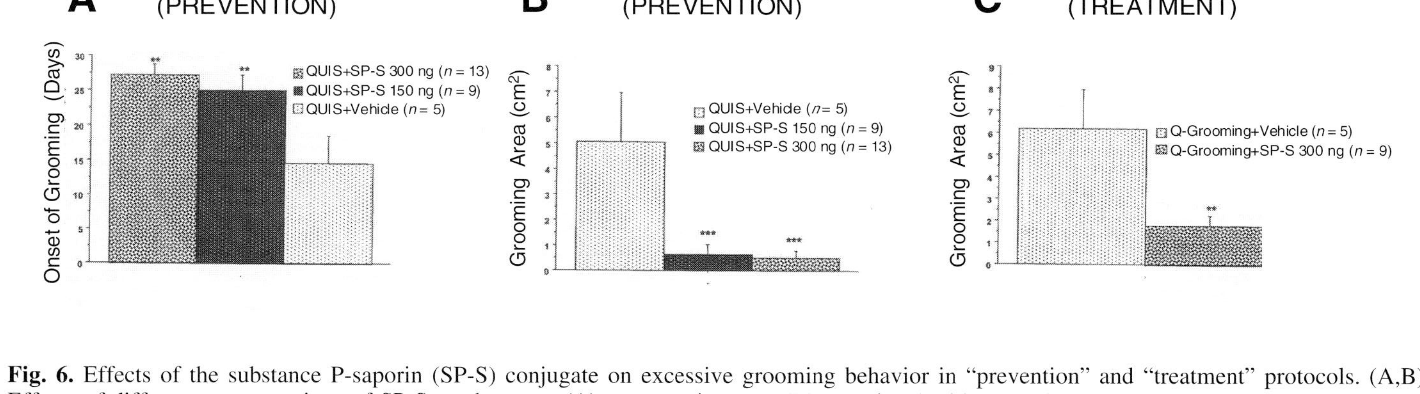

Fig. 6. Effects of the substance P-saporin (SP-S) conjugate on excessive grooming behavior in "prevention" and "treatment" protocols. (A,B) Effects of different concentrations of SP-S on the onset (A) or grooming area (B) associated with excessive grooming behavior in a prevention protocol where SP-S was delivered to the surface of the cord for a period of 10 minutes immediately after the completion of quisqualic acid (QUIS) injections. (C) Effects of SP-S on the area of skin targeted for grooming behavior in a "treatment" protocol where SP-S was delivered to the cord after the onset of excessive grooming behavior. Note the decrease in grooming area relative to animals receiving control (vehicle) injections. Data are represented as means ± SEM. $^{**}P < 0.01$; $^{***}P < 0.001$.

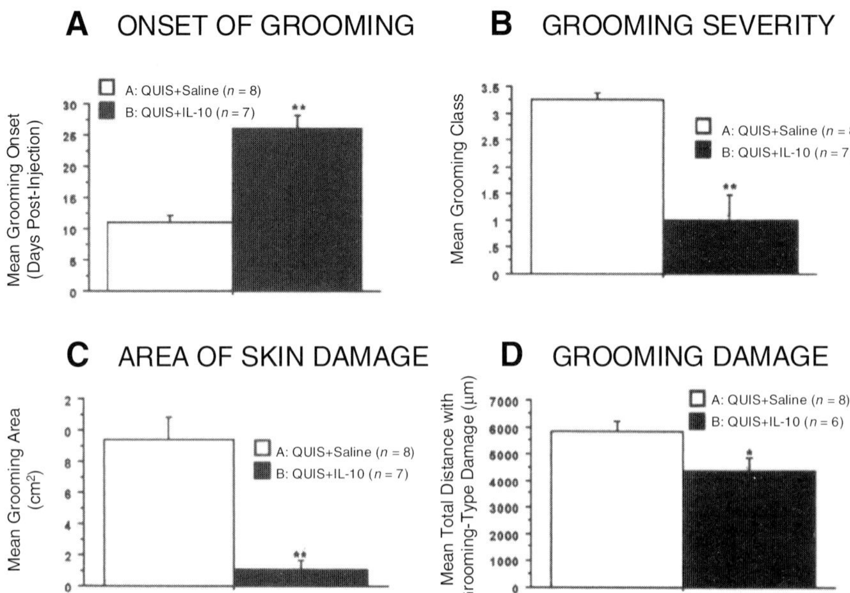

Fig. 7. Assessment of excessive grooming behavior following intraspinal injection of the AMPA/metabotropic agonist quisqualic acid (QUIS). (A) Onset of grooming behavior: saline treatment 30 minutes post-QUIS injury resulted in an average onset time of 11.1 + 0.9 days (bar A), and treatment with IL-10 30 minutes post-QUIS injury resulted in a significant delay in onset of grooming behavior of 26.1 ± 1.9 days ($P < 0.01$) (bar B). (B) Grooming severity: treatment with IL-10 significantly reduced grooming severity (bar B) ($P < 0.01$) versus saline treatment (bar A). (C) Final area of skin damage: treatment with IL-10 significantly reduced the skin area targeted for grooming (bar B) ($P < 0.01$) versus saline treatment (bar A). (D) Grooming-type damage in the dorsal horn: treatment with IL-10 resulted in a significant reduction in the longitudinal extent of grooming-type neuronal loss (bar B) ($P < 0.05$) versus saline treatment (bar A). Error bars represent (mean ± SEM) (*$P < 0.05$, **$P < 0.01$). Reprinted from Plunkett et al. (2001), with permission.

strategies that target selective components of the spinal injury cascade and interfere with death-inducing events of spinal neurons may be useful in the prevention or treatment of pain conditions associated with SCI.

ANIMAL MODELS OF BELOW-LEVEL PAIN

Interruption of the spinothalamic tract has been implicated in the clinical literature as an important condition in the production of chronic central pain (Pagni 1998). Consistent with this conclusion, recent studies have implicated below-level SCI pain as depending upon the partial deafferentation of projection targets associated with the spinothalamic and associated pathways (Vierck 1991; Chapters 8 and 9, this volume). A possible explanation for this conclusion is that below-level pain may be expressed when supraspinal targets lose their input from classic pain pathway(s) and are activated instead by other sources of spontaneous or evoked activity from the spinal cord. This type of pain behavior (including caudally directed overgrooming and autotomy) can be produced by mechanical lesions of the anterolateral spinal column in monkeys and rats (Levitt and Levitt 1981). Similarly, allodynia and hyperalgesia are a variable sequel to "recovery" from contralateral hypoalgesia after anterolateral cordotomy in humans (Lahuerta et al. 1994), monkeys (Vierck 1991), and rats (Chapter 8). Interruption of one anterolateral quadrant of the spinal cord reliably results in contralateral hypoalgesia, but in some cases subjects eventually develop a contralateral or ipsilateral dysesthesia/pain or allodynia/hyperalgesia (Vierck 1991).

In an effort to better simulate the human condition of SCI, ischemic damage of the gray matter was combined with spinothalamic tractotomy. Vierck and Light (2000) introduced blood into anterolateral lesion cavities of rats. Animals with this combination of lesions were consistently hypersensitive to stimulation delivered ipsilateral to and below the level of the lesion. Contralateral sensitivity was variable over time for all animals. Additional studies using restricted lesions of selected cord regions have shown that a lateral hemisection at T13 results in the bilateral enhancement of nocifensive behaviors for both forelimbs (above-level) and both hindlimbs (below-level) of rats (Christensen et al. 1996). Thus, the below-level effects of spinal lesions on nociception do not appear to be limited to a contralateral distribution. The behavioral effects of hemisection are accompanied by evidence for bilateral spinal reorganization, including sprouting (Christensen and Hulsebosch 1997).

Interruption of other spinal pathways and abnormal activity in rostrally conducting systems are also likely to participate in the establishment of below-level pain (Hubscher and Johnson 1999). Below-level SCI pain may, for example, involve the dorsal columns. The involvement of dorsal pathways is exemplified by pain associated with syringomyelia, which is more prevalent when a central cavity expands to include dorsal pathways (Milhorat et al. 1996). Similarly, animal models of injury-evoked dysesthesia or pain have shown that interruption of the dorsal or dorsolateral columns increases the incidence and onset of caudal overgrooming and autotomy after peripheral nerve injury (Saade et al. 1992). Allodynia and hyperalgesia are observed in response to stimulation caudal and ipsilateral to dorsolateral column lesions in monkeys (Vierck et al. 1986). These results suggest that dorsal spinal pathways are likely to be involved in the production of below-level neuropathic pain.

Although there is support for the involvement of white and gray matter damage in both at-level and below-level pain, in the discussion of different experimental models and the clinical condition it is important to distinguish between these regionally distinct pain categories. After SCI the emergence of abnormal pain states tends to follow a progressive sequence from at-level to below-level pain, suggesting a common or interactive mechanism of these two types of pain. For this reason, abnormal spinal or supraspinal neural activity associated with at-level pain may predispose an individual to develop below-level pain. Interestingly, below-level pain along with allodynia and hyperalgesia in persons with SCI are described as episodic (Eide et al. 1995). Similarly, grooming and autotomy by monkeys after anterolateral cordotomy also follow an episodic pattern (Levitt and Levitt 1981). In addition to the potential influence of abnormal activity from gray matter damage, below-level pain may develop only when a specific pattern or amount of white matter damage occurs. After loss of input to supraspinal targets of the spinothalamic tract, abnormal patterns of resting or evoked activity are observed in rostral projection targets, especially in the ventrobasal thalamus (Pollock et al. 1951; Lenz 1991; Chapter 13, this volume). Whether these patterns or distributions are related to or responsible for below-level pain is controversial.

CONCLUSIONS

The cellular, molecular, biochemical, anatomical, and ultimately, functional changes initiated by traumatic or ischemic injury to the spinal cord are believed to be important components of an injury cascade responsible for the onset and progression of SCI-related pain states. Achieving a better understanding of the different secondary injury cascades associated with SCI will provide valuable insights into the underlying mechanisms responsible for different pain syndromes. Animal models suggest that at-level SCI pain results from excitotoxic and/or ischemic damage to the spinal gray and white matter. Experimental models have identified putative mechanisms for the generation of at-level pain and have suggested a number of potential therapeutic approaches, including pharmacological strategies targeting inhibitory systems or spinal mediators of cellular survival. Of special importance is control over secondary signaling and survival pathways along with injury-induced chemical and molecular changes that modulate neuronal excitability. Additionally, current evidence suggests that restricting the extent of excitotoxic or ischemic damage after traumatic SCI might prevent at-level and below-level neuropathic pain by reducing excitatory influences and by limiting white matter damage. Below-level neuropathic pain may result not only from interruption of spinothalamic projections, but also from interruption or activation of other pathways, including propriospinal systems. Continued use of available animal models of at-level and below-level pain should help researchers to provide an increasingly precise definition of the mechanisms of SCI pain and to identify potential therapeutic targets.

ACKNOWLEDGMENTS

The author would like to thank the collaborative assistance of Drs. Shanliang Liu, Kori Brewer, Chen-Guang Yu, Jeffery Plunkett, and Laurel Gorman. Expert technical assistance was provided by Gladys Ruenes and Dimarys Sanchez. The work of the author was supported by NS40096.

REFERENCES

Abraham KE, Brewer KL. Expression of c-fos mRNA is increased and related to dynorphin mRNA expression following excitotoxic spinal cord injury in the rat. *Neurosci Lett* 2001; 307:187–191.

Abraham KE, Brewer KL, McGinty JF. Opioid peptide messenger RNA expression is increased at spinal and supraspinal levels following excitotoxic spinal cord injury. *Neuroscience* 2000; 99:189–197.

Abraham KE, McGinty JF, Brewer KL. Spinal and supraspinal changes in opioid mRNA expression are related to the onset of pain behaviors following excitotoxic spinal cord injury. *Pain* 2001; 90:181–190.

Bethea JR, Castro MC, Lee TT, Dietrich WD, Yezierski RP. Traumatic spinal cord injury induces nuclear factor kappa-B activation. *J Neurosci* 1998; 18:3251–3260.

Bonica JJ. Semantic, epidemiologic and educational issues of central pain. In: Casey KL (Ed). *Pain and Central Nervous System Disease: The Central Pain Syndromes.* New York: Raven Press, 1990, pp 13–29.

Brewer KL, Yezierski RP. Effects of adrenal medullary transplants on pain-related behaviors following excitotoxic spinal cord injury. *Brain Res* 1998; 798:83–92.

Brewer K, Yezierski RP, Bethea JR. Excitotoxic spinal cord injury induces diencephalic changes in gene expression. *Soc Neurosci Abstracts* 1997; 23:438.

Brewer KL, Bethea JR, Yezierski RP. Neuroprotective effects of interleukin-10 following excitotoxic spinal cord injury. *Exp Neurol* 1999; 159:484–493.

Christensen MD, Hulsebosch CE. Chronic pain after spinal cord injury. *J Neurotrauma* 1997; 14:517–537.

Christensen MD, Everhart AW, Pickeman J, Hulsebosch CE. Mechanical and thermal allodynia in chronic central pain following spinal cord injury. *Pain* 1996; 68:97–107.

DeLeo JA, Yezierski RP. The role of neuroinflammation in persistent pain. *Pain* 2001; 90:1–6.

Dubner R. Neuronal plasticity and pain following peripheral tissue inflammation or nerve injury. In: *Proceedings of the VIth World Congress on Pain.* New York: Elsevier, 1991, pp 263–276.

Edgar RE, Best LG, Quail PA, Obert AD. Computer-assisted DREZ microcoagulation: post-traumatic spinal deafferentation pain. *J Spinal Disord* 1993; 6:48–56.

Eide PK, Stubhaug A, Stenehjem AE. Central dysesthesia pain after traumatic spinal cord injury is dependent on *N*-methyl-D-aspartate receptor activation. *Neurosurgery* 1995; 37:1080–1087.

Faden AI, Simon RP. A potential role for excitotoxins in the pathophysiology of spinal cord injury. *Ann Neurol* 1988; 24:623–626.

Fairbanks CA, Schreiber KM, Brewer KL, et al. Agmatine reverses pain induced by inflammation, neuropathy and spinal cord injury. *Proc Natl Acad Sci USA* 2000; 97:10584–10589.

Gorman AL, Yu C-G, Ruenes GR, Daniels L, Yezierski RP. Conditions affecting the onset, severity and progression of a spontaneous pain-like behavior following excitotoxic spinal cord injury. *J Pain* 2001; 2:229–240.

Hains BC, Chastain KM, Evberhart AW, McAdoo DJ, Hulsebosch CE. Transplants of adrenal medullary chromaffin cells reduce forelimb and hindlimb allodynia in a rodent model of chronic central pain after spinal cord hemisection injury. *Exp Neurol* 2000; 164:426–437.

Hao J-X, Xu X-J, Aldskogius H, Seiger Å, Wiesenfeld-Hallin Z. The excitatory amino acid receptor antagonist MK-801 prevents the hypersensitivity induced by spinal cord ischemia in the rat. *Exp Neurol* 1991; 114:182–191.

Hao J-X, Xu X-J, Urban L, Wiesenfeld-Hallin Z. Repeated administration of systemic gabapentin alleviates allodynia-like behaviors in spinally injured rats. *Neurosci Lett;* in press.

Haley JE, Wilcox GL. Involvement for excitatory amino acids and peptides in the spinal mechanisms underlying hyperalgesia. In: Willis WD (Ed). *Hyperalgesia and Allodynia.* New York: Raven Press, 1992, pp 281–293.

Hayashi M, Ueyama T, Nemoto K, Tamaki T, Senba E. Sequential mRNA expression for immediate early genes, cytokines and neurotrophins in spinal cord injury. *J Neurotrauma* 2000; 17:203–218.

Hsu CY, Lin T-N, Xu J, Chao J, Hogan EL. Kinins and related inflammatory mediators in central nervous system injury. In: Salzman SK, Faden AL (Eds). *The Neurobiology of Central Nervous System Trauma.* New York: Oxford University Press, 1994, pp 145–154.

Hubscher CH, Johnson RD. Changes in neuronal receptive field characteristics in caudal brain stem following chronic spinal cord injury. *J Neurotrauma* 1999; 16:533–541.

Hulsebosch CE, Xu G-Y, Perez-Polo JR, et al. Rodent model of chronic central pain after spinal cord contusion and effects of gabapentin. *J Neurotrauma* 2000; 17:1205–1217.

Kakulas BA, Smith E, Gaekwad UF, Kaelan C, Jacobsen P. The neuropathology of pain and abnormal sensations in human spinal cord injury derived from the clinicopathological data base at the Royal Perth Hospital. In: Dimitrijevic MR, Wall PD, Lindblom U (Eds). *Recent Achievements in Restorative Neurology.* Basel: Karger, 1990, pp 37–41.

Lahuerta J, Bowsher D, Buxton PH, Lipton S. Percutaneous cervical cordotomy: a review of 181 operations in 146 patients, including a study on the location of pain fibers in the second cervical spinal cord segment of 29 cases. *J Neurosurg* 1994; 80:975–985.

Laughlin TM, Bethea JR, Yezierski RP, Wilcox GL. Involvement of the pro-inflammatory cytokine IL-1β in dynorphin-induced allodynia. *Pain* 2000; 84:159–167.

Lenz F. The thalamus and central pain syndromes: human and animal studies. In: Casey K (Ed). *Pain and Central Nervous System Disease: The Central Pain Syndromes.* New York: Raven Press, 1991, pp 171–182.

Levitt M. Postcordotomy spontaneous dysesthesias in macaques: recurrence after spinal cord transection. *Brain Res* 1989; 481:47–56.

Levitt M, Levitt JH. The deafferentation syndrome in monkeys: dysesthesias of spinal origin. *Pain* 1981; 10:129–147.

Mantyh PW, Rogers SD, Honore P, et al. Inhibition of hyperalgesia by ablation of lamina I spinal neurons expressing the substance P receptor. *Science* 1997; 275–278.

Milhorat T, Kotzen R, Harrison T, Capocelli A, Milhorat R. Dysesthetic pain in patients with syringomyelia. *Neurosurgery* 1996; 38:940–947.

Malmberg AB, Chen C, Tonegawa S, Basbaum AI. Preserved acute pain and reduced neuropathic pain in mice lacking PKC gamma. *Science* 1997; 278:275–279.

Morrow TJ, Paulson PE, Brewer KL, Yezierski RP, Casey KL. Chronic, selective forebrain responses to excitotoxic dorsal horn injury. *Exp Neurol* 2000; 161:220–226.

Melzack R, Loeser JD. Phantom body pain in paraplegics: evidence for a central "pattern generating mechanism" for pain. *Pain* 1978; 4:195–210.

Nag S, Riopelle RJ. Spinal neuronal pathology associated with continuous intrathecal infusion of *N*-methyl-D-aspartate in the rat. *Acta Neuropathol* 1990; 81:7–13.

Palecek J, Paleckova V, Willis WD. The effect of phorbol esters on spinal cord amino acid concentrations and responsiveness of rats to mechanical and thermal stimuli. *Pain* 1999; 80:597–605.

Pagni CA. *Central Pain: A Neurosurgical Challenge.* Torino: Edizioni Minerva Medica, 1998.

Pahl HL. Activators and target genes of Rel/NF-κB transcription factors. *Oncogene* 1998; 18:6853–6866.

Pollock LJ, Brown M, Boshes B, et al. Pain below the level of injury of the spinal cord. *AMA Arch Neurol Psychiatry* 1951; 65:319–322.

Piomelli D. Arachidonic acid in cell signaling. *Curr Opin Cell Biol* 1993; 5:274–280.

Plunkett JA, Yu C-G, Bethea JR, Yezierski RP. Effects of interleukin-10 (IL-10) on pain behavior and gene expression following excitotoxic spinal cord injury in the rat. *Exp Neurol* 2001; 169:144–154.

Qui J, Nesic O, Ye Z, et al. Bcl-x_L expression after contusion to the rat spinal cord. *J Neurotrauma* 2001; 18:1267–1278.

Regan R, Choi DW. Excitotoxicity and central nervous system trauma. In: Salzman SK, Faden AL (Eds). *The Neurobiology of Central Nervous System Trauma.* New York: Oxford University Press, 1994, pp 173–181.

Saade N, Ibrahim M, Atweh S, Jabbur S. Explosive autotomy induced by simultaneous dorsal column lesion and limb denervation: a possible model for acute deafferentation pain. *Exp Neurol* 1993; 119:272–279

Siddall P, Xu CL, Cousins M. Allodynia following traumatic spinal cord injury in the rat. *Neuroreport* 1995; 6:1241–1244.

Smith WL, Dewitt DL. Biochemistry of prostaglandin endoperoxide H synthase-1 and synthase-2 and their differential susceptibility to nonsteroidal anti-inflammatory drugs. *Semin Nephrol* 1995; 15:179–194.

Tator CH, Fehlings MG. Review of the secondary injury theory of acute spinal cord trauma with emphasis on vascular mechanisms. *J Neurosurg* 1991; 75:15–26.

Vierck CJ. Can mechanisms of central pain syndromes be investigated in animal models? In: *Pain and Central Nervous System Disease: The Central Pain Syndromes.* Casey K (Ed). New York: Raven Press, 1991, pp 129–141.

Vierck CJ, Light AR. Allodynia and hyperalgesia within dermatomes caudal to a spinal cord injury in primates and rodents. In: Sandkühler J, Bromm B, Gebhart GF (Eds). *Prog Brain Res* 2000; 129:411–428.

Vierck CJ Jr, Greenspan JD, Ritz LA, Yeomans DC. The spinal pathways contributing to the ascending conduction and the descending modulation of pain sensation and reactions. In: Yaksh T (Ed). *Spinal Systems of Afferent Processing.* New York: Plenum, 1986, pp 275–329.

Vierck CJ, Siddall P, Yezierski RP. Pain following spinal cord injury; animal models and mechanistic studies. *Pain* 2000; 89:1–5.

Watkins LR, Milligan ED, Maier SF. Glial activation: a driving force for pathological pain. *Trends Neurosci* 2001; 124:450–455.

Wiesenfeld-Hallin Z, Hao J-X, Aldskogius H, Seiger Å, Xu X-J. Allodynia-like symptoms in rats after spinal cord ischemia: an animal model of central pain. In: Boivie J, Hansson P, Lindblom U (Eds). *Touch, Temperature, and Pain in Health and Disease: Mechanisms and Assessments,* Progress in Pain Research and Management, Vol. 3. Seattle: IASP Press, 1994, pp 355–372.

Willis WD. Central sensitization and plasticity following noxious stimulation. In: Mayer EA, Raybould HE (Eds). *Basic and Clinical Aspects of Chronic Abdominal Pain.* Amsterdam: Elsevier, 1993, pp 201–217.

Woolf CJ. Excitability changes in central neurons following peripheral damage. In: Willis WD (Ed). *Hyperalgesia and Allodynia.* New York: Raven Press, 1992, pp 221–243.

Wrathall JR, Choiniere D, Teng YD. Dose dependent reduction of tissue loss and functional impairment after spinal cord trauma with the AMPA/kainate antagonist NBQX. *J Neurosci* 1994; 14:6598–6607.

Yakovlev AG, Faden AI. Sequential expression of c-fos protooncogene, TNF-alpha, and dynorphin genes in spinal cord following experimental traumatic injury. *Mol Chem Neuropathol* 1994; 23:179–190.

Yezierski RP. Pain following spinal cord injury: the clinical problem and experimental studies. *Pain* 1996; 68:185–194.

Yezierski RP. Pain following spinal cord injury: pathophysiology and central mechanisms. In: Sandkühler J, Bromm B, Gebhart GF (Eds). *Prog Brain Res* 2000; 129:429–448.

Yezierski RP, Park SH. The mechanosensitivity of spinal sensory neurons following intraspinal injections of quisqualic acid in the rat. *Neurosci Lett* 1993; 157:115–119.

Yezierski RP, Santana M, Park DH, Madsen PW. Neuronal degeneration and spinal cavitation following intraspinal injections of quisqualic acid in the rat. *J Neurotrauma* 1993; 10:445–456.

Yezierski RP, Liu S, Ruenes GL, Kajander KJ, Brewer KL. Excitotoxic spinal cord injury: behavioral and morphological characteristics of a central pain model. *Pain* 1998; 75:141–155.

Yezierski RP, Yu C-G, Wiley RG. Prevention and treatment of a spontaneous pain-like behavior following excitotoxic spinal cord injury by ablation of neurons expressing the substance P receptor. *Soc Neurosci Abstracts* 2000; 26(2):1959.

Young W. The post-injury responses in trauma and ischemia: secondary injury or protective mechanism? *CNS Trauma* 1987; 4:27–52.

Yu C-G, Bethea JR, Fairbanks CA, Wilcox GL, Yezierski RP. Effects of cyclosporin, interleukin-10 and agmatine on a spontaneous pain behavior following excitotoxic spinal cord injury in rats. *Soc Neurosci Abstracts* 2000; 26(2):1959.

Yu W, Hao X-J, Xu X-J, et al. Long-term alleviation of allodynia-like behaviors by intrathecal implantation of bovine chromaffin cells in rats with spinal cord injury. *Pain* 1998; 74:115–122.

Correspondence to: Robert P. Yezierski, PhD, Department of Orthodontics, University of Florida, 1600 S.W. Archer Road, Gainesville, FL 32610, USA. Tel: 352-392-4010; Fax: 352-392-3031; email: ryezierski@dental.ufl.edu.

Spinal Cord Injury Pain: Assessment, Mechanisms, Management. Progress in Pain Research and Management, Vol. 23, edited by Robert P. Yezierski and Kim J. Burchiel, IASP Press, Seattle, © 2002.

8

Assessment of Pain Sensitivity in Dermatomes Caudal to Spinal Cord Injury in Rats

Charles J. Vierck, Jr.,[a,b] and Alan R. Light[b]

[a]*Department of Neuroscience and McKnight Brain Institute, University of Florida College of Medicine, Gainesville, Florida, USA;* [b]*Department of Cell and Molecular Physiology, University of North Carolina School of Medicine, Chapel Hill, North Carolina, USA*

According to the taxonomy of spinal cord injury (SCI) pain presented in Chapter 2, chronic SCI pain that is felt in dermatomes caudal to the lesion is referred to as *below-level pain.* Chronic, below-level SCI pain occurs in some cases but not in others with apparently similar lesions (White and Sweet 1969). Usually its appearance is delayed by weeks, months, or even years (Laheuerta et al. 1994), and it waxes and wanes over time, varying both from day to day and from hour to hour (Ness 1998; Vierck and Light 2000). These features impose particularly difficult demands on models that seek to determine mechanisms and evaluate therapeutic approaches. For example, variability in incidence demands frequent testing over a long period to document the features of below-level pain and correlate them with lesion configuration. However, psychophysical testing of patients with chronic pain as a result of injury to the central nervous system (central pain) has shown a relationship between the distribution of spontaneous pain and a diminution or loss of naturally evoked pain and temperature sensations. These findings implicate interruption of the spinothalamic tract as a minimal or necessary condition for central, below-level pain (Boivie et al. 1989). Without consideration of additional factors that might determine whether interruption of the spinothalamic tract will or will not result in below-level pain (Chapter 9), this lesion can provide an appropriate animal model of below-level SCI pain.

An anterolateral spinal lesion that severs lateral spinothalamic tract axons originating in the contralateral gray matter spares other ascending pathways that might convey nociception rostrally (e.g., spinoreticular pathways or ventral and ipsilateral spinothalamic axons). Also, descending pathways to caudal spinal segments of pain referral are interrupted. An important first question, then, is whether below-level pain results from descending effects of a lesion on caudal neurons. That is, does central pain result from interruption of descending inhibitory pathways and/or from deafferentation effects on caudal neurons that convey nociceptive signals rostrally via spared pathways? If interruption of descending pathways is *entirely responsible* for the generation of chronic central pain, then *it might* be appropriate to utilize nociceptive reflexes as behavioral assays for changes in excitability that result in below-level pain. However, the use of nociceptive reflexes to assess pain sensitivity depends on the assumption that motoneurons and projection neurons for nociception will be affected alike by spinal lesions. This possibility can be addressed by comparing reflex responses that are organized segmentally with operant responses that rely upon conscious cerebral processing of nociceptive intensity.

Identification of behavioral responses that depend upon conscious evaluation of aversive properties of a stimulus is straightforward. Aversive qualities of a sensation provide the motivation to terminate stimulation, and consciously motivated responses to pain are inferred from occurrences of learned responses that escape the eliciting stimulus. Without such learning, a simple withdrawal response of a stimulated limb can terminate stimulation, but this often is reflexive and is not motivated escape. For example, in the Hargreaves test that has been used extensively to evaluate nociception (Hargreaves et al. 1988), the dependent measures are latency of withdrawal (for thermal stimulation) or frequency of withdrawal from mechanical stimuli. Withdrawal responses can occur at latencies shorter than those required for a conscious response, providing escape before a consciously motivated response can be formulated and actualized. The animal may subsequently attempt to move away and avoid further stimulation (LaBuda and Fuchs 2000), but such behaviors are not typically scored. Similar considerations apply to other presumed nociceptive assays, such as the hot-plate (Woolfe and MacDonald 1944), tail or paw immersion (Luttinger 1985), and tail-flick tests (D'Amour and Smith 1941). A response that is consciously motivated and directed to terminate a painful sensation must, at the minimum, employ movements involving spinal segments remote from the site of stimulation, and it must operate on the environment to escape the stimulus. For example, pressing a bar with a forelimb to terminate stimulation of a hindlimb represents an operant escape response (Vierck and Luck 1979; Vierck et al. 1990, 1995).

Operant learning to perform such a response is distinct from classical conditioning that can influence innate reflex responses with repetition of a stimulus.

There are various behaviors that can be elicited by nociceptive stimulation and appear to be purposive but are in fact unlearned, innate responses that do not depend upon conscious appreciation of pain. These innate responses are "hard wired" and occur automatically in certain circumstances. Such behaviors are frequently employed for nociceptive assays, both because they are organized supraspinally and because on intuitive grounds, they are appropriate for or specific to nociceptive stimulation. Licking, guarding, vocalizing, jumping, biting, and orienting require supraspinal processing, but experiments with long-term maintenance of decerebrate rats have shown that these behaviors are retained (Carroll and Lim 1960; Woolf 1984; Berridge 1989; Matthies and Franklin 1992; Table I) and do not depend upon conscious appraisal of nociception. These experiments raise an important question: Are all supraspinal responses to nociception comparable or adequate for evaluating the effects of spinal lesions (or other manipulations) on pain sensitivity? Similarly, are spinal projection neurons to brainstem and cerebral targets equally affected by a spinal lesion associated with development of chronic central pain?

To evaluate these questions, we compared the effects of lateral spinal lesions on behaviors representative of spinal, brainstem, and cerebral processing. These behaviors are flexion/withdrawal, vocalization, and operant escape, respectively. Six female Long Evans rats were adapted to handling and then to restraint in the apparatus schematically depicted in Fig. 1. They were suspended from rods inserted through loops in a custom-fitted cloth jacket, and their front paws rested on a fixed platform (on the left) and on a counter-weighted response lever (on the right). Their hindlimbs were tethered to force transducers for measurement of reflex force in response to electrocutaneous stimulation of either foot. A microphone supplied the signal for recording vocalizations emitted within 200 ms of the beginning of

Table I
Levels of processing required for behaviors that can be elicited in rats by nociceptive stimulation

Lesion Effect	Behaviors	Level of Processing
Lost after decerebration	Operant escape	Cerebrum
Preserved after decerebration; lost after spinalization	Licking, guarding, early vocalizations, flinching, jumping, biting, orienting	Brainstem
Preserved after spinalization	Stretch reflex, flexion reflex, withdrawal	Spinal cord

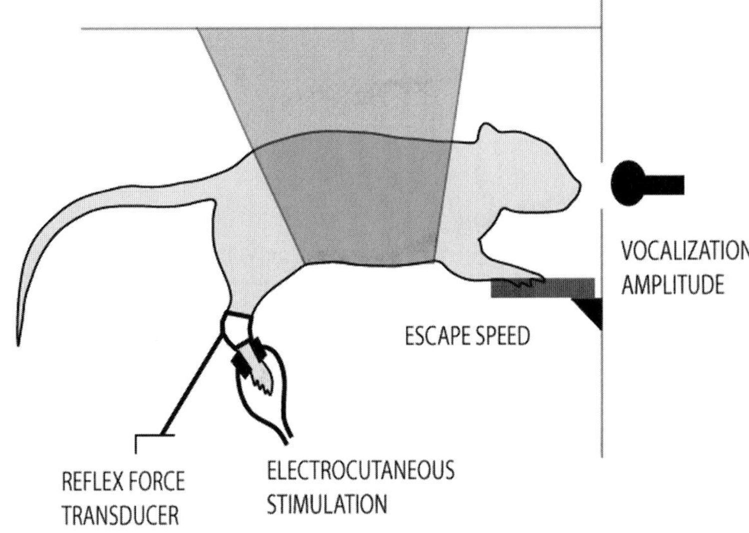

Fig. 1. Schematic representation of the testing setup for assessment of operant escape speed, flexion reflex amplitude, and vocalization amplitude in response to electrocutaneous stimulation of either foot. The rats were suspended from horizontal rods passed through vertical extensions of custom-fitted jackets. Constant current stimulation was passed between the dorsal and ventral surfaces of either foot. Flexion reflex amplitude was measured from leaf transducers tethered to anklets taped to each leg.

each trial. Preoperatively, the animals were trained to press the lever to escape electrocutaneous stimulation at progressively higher levels (across sessions), up to 0.80 mA/mm^2. Once an animal learned to escape reliably, intensities of 0.05, 0.1, 0.2, 0.4, and 0.8 mA/mm^2 were presented in eight series of ascending, then descending intensities that were alternated between sides, for a total of eight trials at each intensity per foot. Each trial consisted of up to 5 seconds of interrupted 60-Hz stimulation (50 ms on, 200 ms off). Stimulation was terminated (escaped) by the first bar-press that occurred after the first 50 ms of each trial period. Three response variables were digitized and stored for each trial: latency of operant escape, force of hindlimb flexion, and vocalization amplitude.

Averaged preoperative stimulus-response functions for escape speed and amplitudes of vocalization and hindlimb flexion are shown in Fig. 2. Escape speed is calculated as the inverse of latency, so that increased responsivity is depicted as higher values for each measure. It is apparent that the function relating operant sensitivity to the range of stimulus intensities delivered is linear or negatively accelerating and differs from the other response functions, which are positively accelerating. These features were similar for stimulation

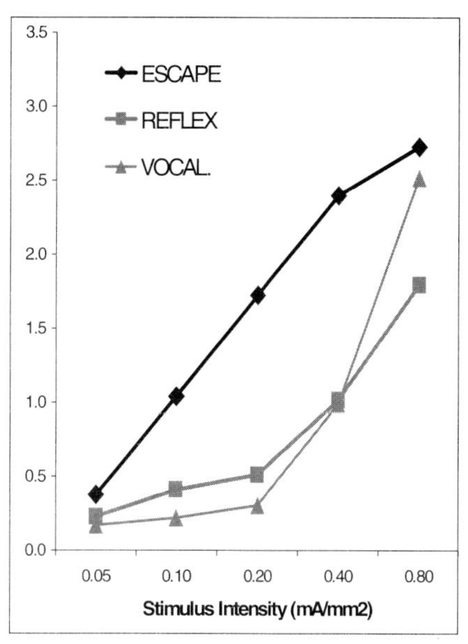

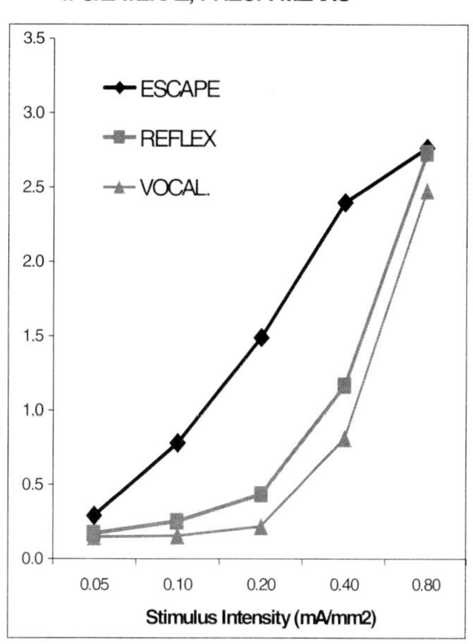

Fig. 2. Preoperative stimulus-response functions for stimulation of the left foot (left panel) and the right root (right panel). The ordinate represents seconds for operant speed (calculated as the maximal trial duration, 5 s, minus the response latency on each trial) and voltages obtained from the leaf transducers (flexion amplitude) and the amplified signal from the microphone (vocalization amplitude).

of either foot, as expected. The preoperative results show that sensation intensity becomes steadily more aversive over a range of intensities (0.1 to 0.4 mA/mm^2) that elicit minimal to no flexion reflex or vocalization. That is, the transfer functions for responses dependent upon spinal and brainstem circuits are distinct from the operant escape function that requires input to the cerebrum.

After stable preoperative performance was obtained, the six rats received a lesion of the right lateral column at the T2 vertebral level, under anesthesia (30 mg/kg ketamine and 10 mg/kg xylazine with supplementation). In order to standardize and maximize hemotoxic influences on the gray matter in the vicinity of the lesion (Vierck and Light 1999), each lesion cavity was packed with Gelfoam soaked in the animal's blood. Histological reconstructions of these lesions are shown in Fig. 3. Most of the lesions approximated a lateral hemisection, with variable involvement of the dorsal and ventral columns. These lesions interrupted the lateral spinothalamic tract substantially or completely on the right side. Behavioral testing continued for 6 months after surgery.

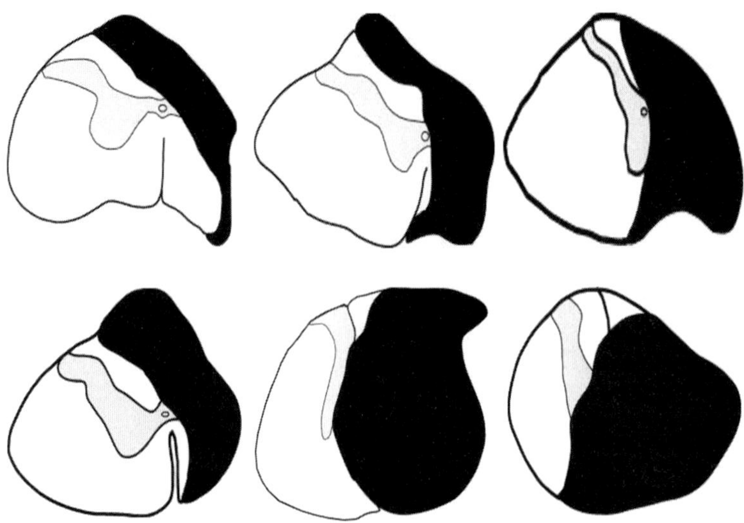

Fig. 3. Camera lucida reconstructions of the spinal lesions, drawn from histologically stained sections.

Averaged postoperative stimulus-response functions for stimulation contralateral to the lesions are shown in Fig. 4. It is apparent that contralateral responsivity was diminished for all three measures. Of particular interest, the stimulus-response function for operant speed was transformed to a positively accelerating form that resembles the preoperative functions for the innate responses (hindlimb flexion and vocalization). This result suggests that cerebral transmission of nociceptive information after a contralateral lesion depends on spared input to brainstem sites (e.g., via spinoreticular or spinoparabrachial pathways) that subserve innate responses and also project rostrally to the cerebrum (Willis and Westlund 1997).

Postoperative-preoperative difference scores for each measure are shown in Fig. 5, collapsed across all stimulus intensities delivered to the left and right hindlimbs. This figure reveals considerable differences between the ipsilateral and contralateral impact of the spinal lesions; also, differences between ipsilateral effects on the different measures are revealed. As shown previously (Vierck and Light 1999), introduction of blood into the unilateral lesion cavities uniformly produced an ipsilateral increase in operant escape responsivity, but flexion reflex force was not similarly increased ipsilaterally.

In apparent contrast to the dissociation between ipsilateral effects of unilateral spinal lesions on operant escape and reflex force, Fig. 5 shows that, overall, both operant escape speed and vocalizations decreased

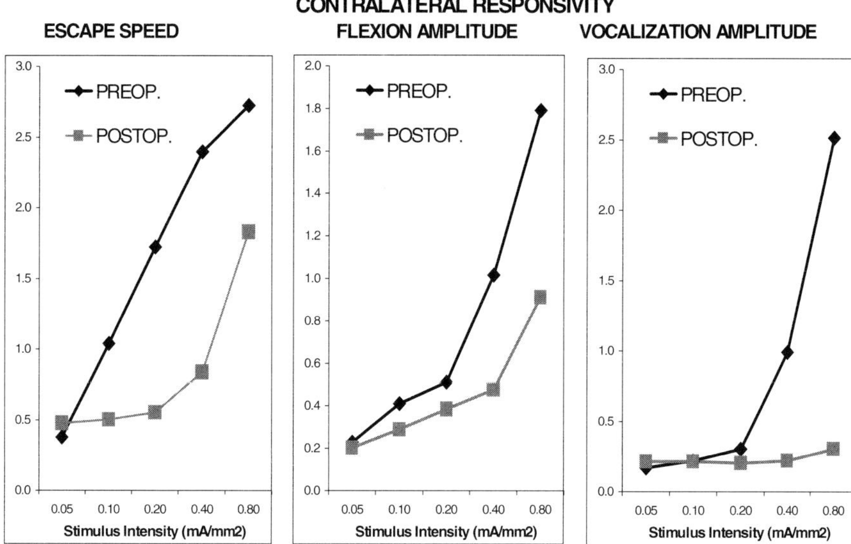

Fig. 4. Stimulus-response functions for stimulation of the left (contralateral) leg before and after the lesions shown in Fig. 3. The data are collapsed across all preoperative and postoperative testing sessions. Values on the ordinates are as in Fig. 2.

contralaterally and increased ipsilaterally. However, the postoperative time course of ipsilateral effects on escape speed and vocalization amplitudes differed considerably, as shown in Fig. 6. Operant speed was reliably enhanced soon after surgery and declined slightly over the postoperative period of testing. In contrast, vocalizations in response to ipsilateral stimulation were initially suppressed and then increased in amplitude to reliably exceed preoperative values. That is, the neural circuits subserving vocalization reflexes and conscious appreciation of nociceptive intensity reacted to SCI quite differently over time.

Another method of directly comparing nociceptive responses presumed to depend on spinal, brainstem, and cerebral processing is to correlate measurements of each response across the numerous trials presented postoperatively to each animal. If the presence or amplitude of vocalizations or flexion reflexes revealed sensation intensity, then trial-to-trial variations in response to each stimulus for individual animals should be highly correlated with the presence and speed of operant escape responses. However, Fig. 7 shows that the correlation coefficients for these comparisons were generally quite low, particularly for ipsilateral stimulation. They were also statistically insignificant in 21 of the 24 comparisons involving operant speed. These results are consistent with a demonstration that flexion reflexes and pain

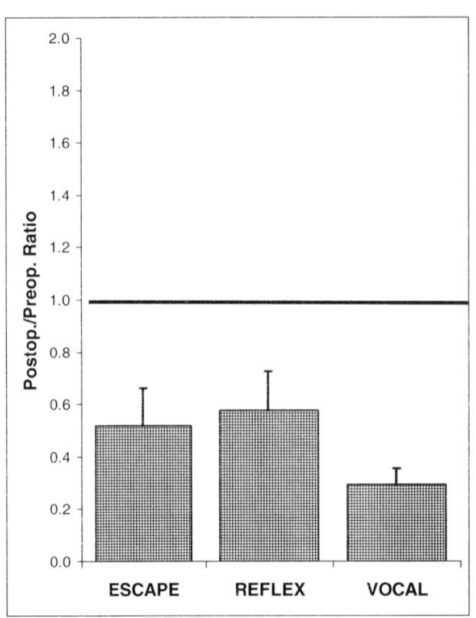

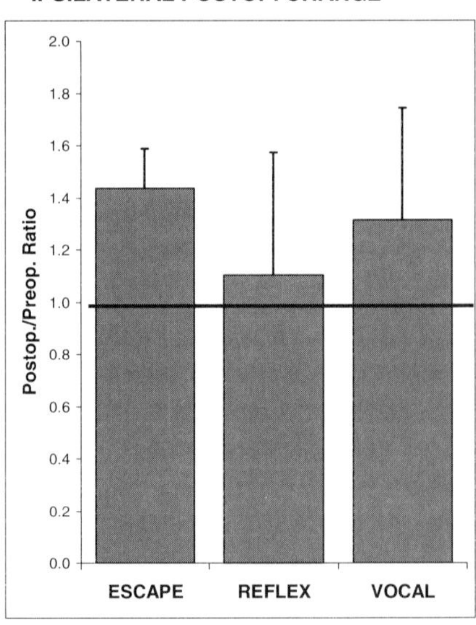

Fig. 5. Comparisons of ratios of average postoperative/preoperative values for the three measures of responsivity to stimulation of the left leg (left panel) or the right leg (right panel). Error bars show standard deviations.

sensations are dissociated after anterolateral cordotomy in humans (García-Larrea et al. 1993).

To this point, comparisons of different response measures failed to show that segmental flexion reflexes or supraspinally mediated vocalizations can be relied on to represent changes in nociceptive sensitivity after SCI. Examination of relationships between reflex and operant measures was aided by elicitation of each response on individual trials (i.e., to the same stimulus). However, the short latency flexion reflex elicited by electrocutaneous stimulation differs in form and neural substrate from the withdrawal responses to thermal or mechanical stimulation that are frequently used as a nociceptive assay (Hargreaves et al. 1988). Therefore, innate responses to thermal stimulation of the six animals with lateral column lesions were observed in parallel with the electrocutaneous stimulation paradigm. Each animal was tested in the morning on the electrocutaneous paradigm and was observed in the afternoon while on a thermally regulated hot plate.

Withdrawal responses to thermal stimulation are difficult to interpret because they can be elicited as a segmental spinal reflex or can represent a conscious escape response, and objective means of discriminating between these alternatives are not available. Also, withdrawal responses must be discriminated from locomotor movements and from elaborations of with-

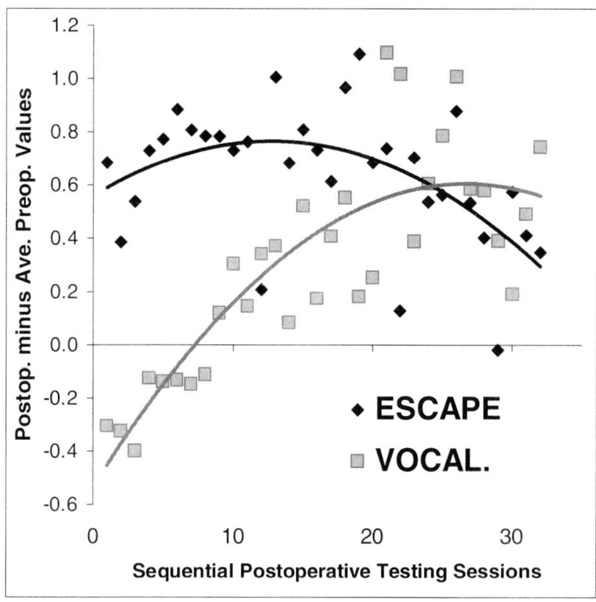

Fig. 6. Time course of postoperative changes in escape speed (filled symbols) and vocalization amplitude (shaded symbols). All values are derived from the group average of difference scores for individual animals, collapsed across stimulus intensities for single postoperative sessions minus a similarly collapsed average across all preoperative sessions for that animal.

drawal. Holding a hindpaw off the plate in an exaggerated flexion posture is categorized as a guarding response. However, withdrawal responses to heat often progress into licking episodes, and it is not clear whether these should be categorized separately from other withdrawals, such as guards. Thus, in practical terms, an observer can simply note the occurrence of withdrawal responses or can distinguish between withdrawal responses that progress to licking or do not.

In traditional hot-plate testing, the animal is placed on a surface preheated to 50°C or higher, and the measure of nociceptive sensitivity is latency to the first withdrawal response. These temperatures generate behavioral responses of very short latency, and thus it is difficult to observe hyperalgesia. Also, sensations evoked by high temperatures are dominated by input from myelinated (Aδ) nociceptors, and it could be important for understanding mechanisms of chronic pain to evaluate sensitivity to input from unmyelinated (C) nociceptors (Cooper et al. 1986). According to the results of a series of experiments in lightly anesthetized rats (Yeomans et al.

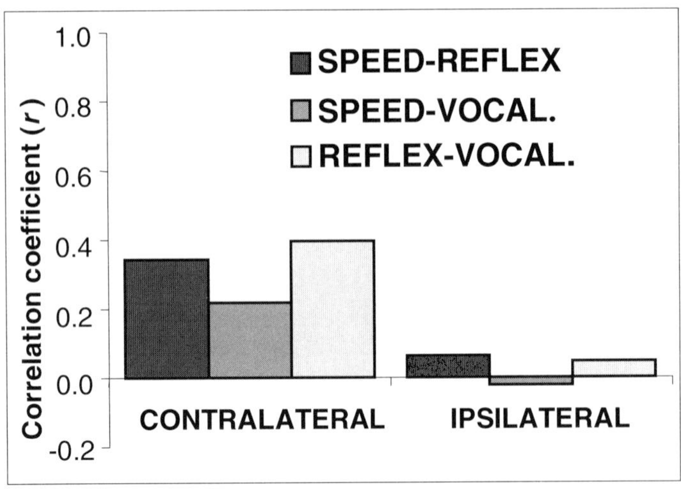

Fig. 7. Averaged correlation coefficients for postoperative responses of individual animals, comparing the response measures obtained on single trials of electrocutaneous stimulation. Speed-reflex = escape speed versus flexion reflex amplitude. Speed-vocal = escape speed versus vocalization amplitude. Reflex-vocal = flexion reflex amplitude versus vocalization amplitude.

1996), temperatures in the low nociceptive range that slowly increase skin temperature selectively activate C nociceptors and elicit withdrawal reflexes. Therefore, we tested each animal in separate sessions at temperatures of 43.7°C (6-minute trials) and 46°C (2-minute trials). The top panels in Fig. 8 show that latencies to the first response (either a guard or withdrawal and licking) for either temperature were not increased or decreased postoperatively. Based on latency measurements, innate licking and guarding responses to thermal stimulation were not depressed, but flexion reflexes elicited by electrocutaneous stimulation were attenuated after contralateral SCI. Also, the contralateral hypoalgesia and ipsilateral hyperalgesia revealed by operant escape responses in the same animals were not revealed by testing of licking and guarding responses.

Testing at low nociceptive temperatures permits trials that are long enough to obtain measures of innate response frequency and duration, in addition to the first response latency. The rationale for this approach is that the first latency is likely to be a reflex, but subsequent responses would be influenced (if not elicited) by conscious perception of nociceptive sensations experienced during the trial. However, the lower panels in Fig. 8 show that the duration of postoperative licking and guarding was not significantly influenced, either ipsilateral or contralateral to the lateral column lesions.

FIRST LATENCY TO LICK/GUARD

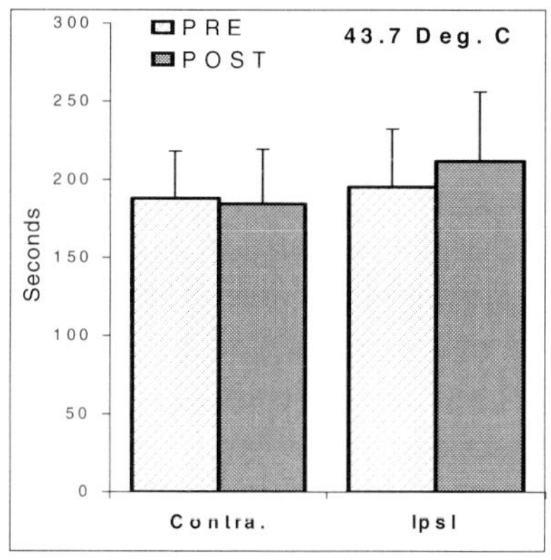

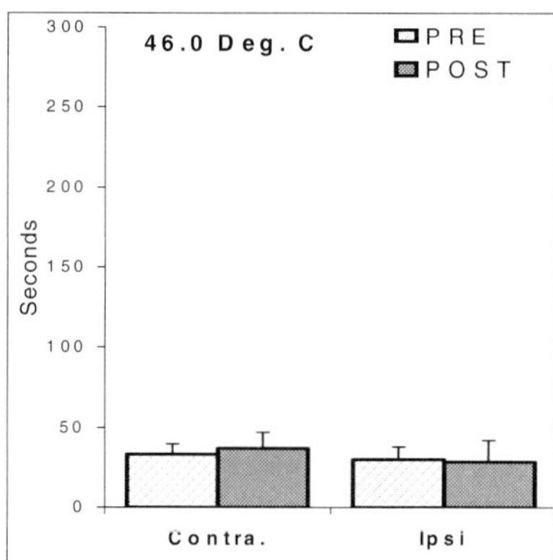

DURATION OF LICKS/GUARDS

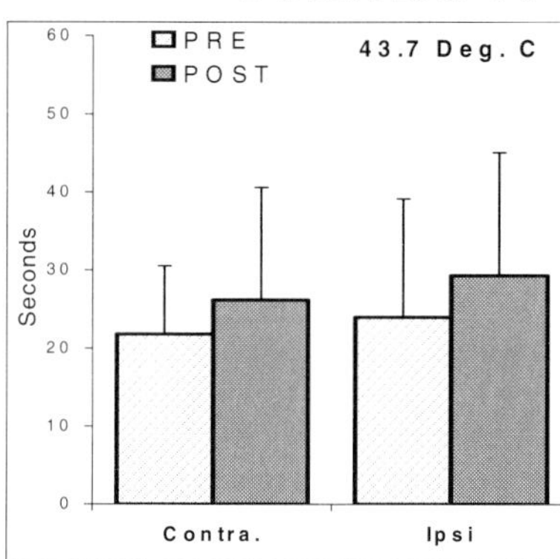

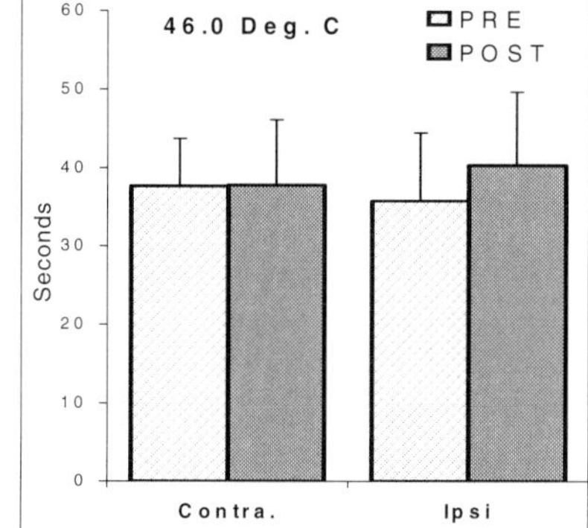

Fig. 8. Averaged preoperative and postoperative latencies of the first innate response observed after animals were placed on a surface preheated to 43.7° or 46.0°C. The first latencies were separately noted for the left and right hindlimbs, but licking and guarding responses were not differentiated for this measure. Error bars show standard deviations.

Unfortunately, the software used to collect these data accumulated all response durations, regardless of category. However, frequencies of licking and guarding responses were separately tabulated, as shown in Fig. 9. Consistent with the measures of latency and duration, the number of innate responses (combined licks and guards) was not altered postoperatively. However, an interesting change in response preference did occur for the hindlimb ipsilateral to the lesion. Preoperatively, most of the responses were licks, and this did not change for the contralateral hindlimb. In contrast, most of the postoperative responses of the ipsilateral hindlimb were classified as guards. Thus, postoperative counts of licks or guards did not reveal the pronounced contralateral hypoalgesia shown by operant escape testing, but

LATERAL COLUMN LESION + HEMOGLOBIN

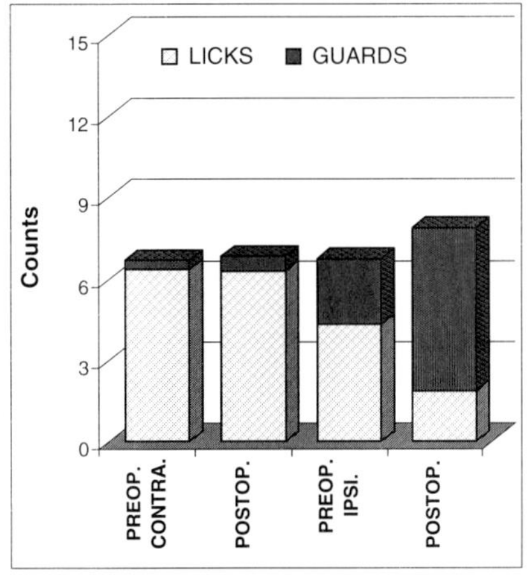

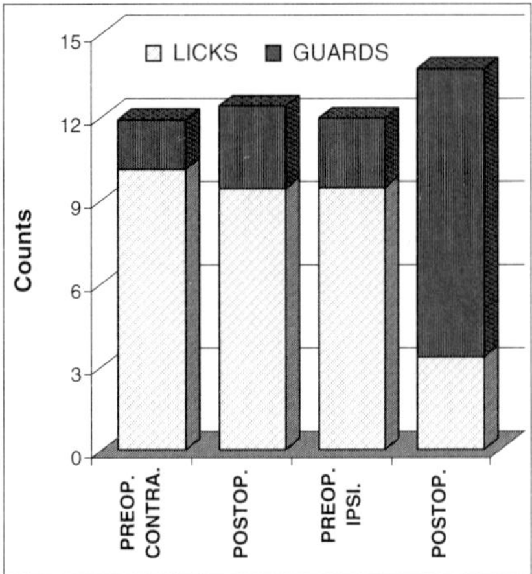

Fig. 9. Average counts of preoperative and postoperative innate responses categorized as licks (open bars) or guards (shaded bars) in response to 43.7° or 46.0°C thermal stimulation. These responses were separately noted for the left and right legs.

the ipsilateral hyperalgesia was accompanied by increased numbers of guard responses on the hot plate.

A general conclusion with important implications for modeling changes in below-level pain sensitivity after SCI is that observation of behaviors other than operant escape is misleading. This result is not surprising for behaviors such as the limb withdrawal that can be observed in spinally transected animals (Franklin and Abbott 1989; Borszcz et al. 1992; Kauppila 1998), because below-level chronic pain clearly depends upon effects of a spinal lesion on rostral projections of the pain pathways (Vierck and Light 2000). Thus, investigation of below-level pain sensitivity places demands on a behavioral model that may or may not apply to at-level pain from SCI or from trauma to peripheral nerves. In the latter cases, if abnormalities in neural processing are confined to the dorsal horn in a limited segmental distribution, observation of innate responses might reveal changes related to pain processing.

A more surprising result of comparisons between innate behaviors and operant escape is that all responses dependent on supraspinal processing were not similarly dependent on nociceptive stimulation and were not affected alike by spinal lesions. Unfortunately, evidence that a response is elicited by nociceptive input to supraspinal structures is not sufficient to conclude that modulation of this response will reflect a change in nociceptive sensations. For example, early vocalizations to electrocutaneous stimulation appeared, superficially, to suffice as a measure of nociception. Similar to operant escape responses, vocalization amplitude decreased with contralateral and increased with ipsilateral stimulation when averaged across the postoperative testing period of 6 months. However, there were several differences between these responses to identical stimuli—the stimulus-response functions differed markedly, vocalizations to stimulation contralateral to the spinal lesion were essentially eliminated when escape responses were present, and the postoperative time course of ipsilateral changes was *opposite* for the two measures. The neural circuits responsible for vocalization and operant escape were affected differently over time after SCI. Early vocalization to nociceptive stimulation is most likely triggered by spinal input to the periaqueductal gray matter—a brainstem structure involved in organization of output to the vocal apparatus (Kelly et al. 1946; Jurgens and Pratt 1979). Apparently this brainstem circuit is affected uniquely by interruption of input from the spinal cord, just as segmental nociceptive input to flexor motoneurons is influenced by SCI uniquely, compared to effects on systems of nociceptive projection to the cerebral cortex.

Although used almost universally as measures of nociception in laboratory animal models, variations of withdrawal responses are particularly difficult to interpret in terms of nociception. Simple withdrawal, as exemplified by electrocutaneous flexor reflexes, is a segmental spinal response that cannot be used to investigate manipulations that affect all levels of nociceptive projection. Additional, apparently purposeful elaborations of withdrawal responses, namely licking and guarding, must depend on brainstem circuits because they are preserved after decerebration (Carroll and Lim 1960; Woolf 1984; Berridge 1989; Matthies and Franklin 1992). These innate responses are not elicited as a result of consciously perceived aversion that is integrated with learned environmental adaptations. Accordingly, neither licking nor guarding responses revealed the contralateral hypoalgesia that occurs after interruption of the spinothalamic tract (King 1957; Vierck et al. 1986; Laheuerta et al. 1994). This failure to reveal hypoalgesia cannot be attributed to a lack of sensitivity to the stimulus, because a 2.3°C difference in temperature of the hot plate had a substantial effect on the innate response measures (Figs. 8 and 9).

The stereotyped licking response is particularly problematic as a measure of nociception because it is likely to occur in response to sensations of warmth (Mauderli et al. 2000). Thus, the commonly used latency measure for licking often does not clearly represent a nociceptive response. Guarding behavior is more likely a response to nociception, and it revealed the ipsilateral hypersensitivity detected by operant escape. But can these apparently comparable effects on innate and operant measures be attributed to the same mechanism(s)? The ipsilateral increase in guard responses might represent a below-level effect of the spinal lesion on withdrawal reflexes. Prolongation of withdrawal responses (guarding) that has been interpreted as evidence of conscious aversion (Hargreaves et al. 1988) can occur as a manifestation of spastic changes after SCI (Dimitrijevic and Nathan 1967). Alternatively, the enhanced guarding may have represented escape responses that occurred because of supraspinal influences of the lesion. Therefore, inclusion of guarding as a measure adds little to interpretation of the operant escape responses, because the nature of guard responses (reflex or operant) is ambiguous.

Fig. 10 provides a schematic summary of rostral and caudal influences expected to result from interruption of one lateral column of the spinal cord. A well-documented effect is partial deafferentation of somatosensory nuclei

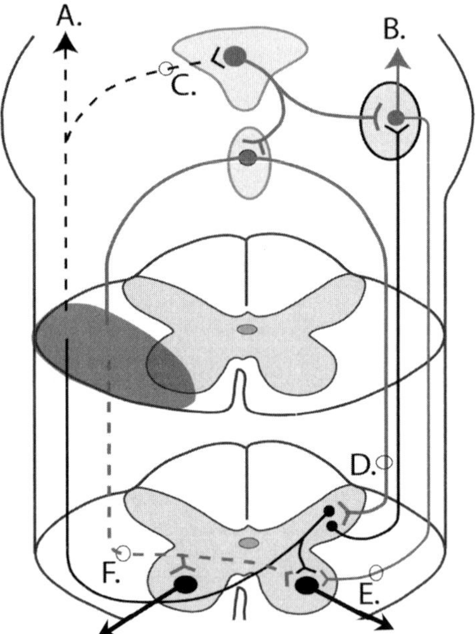

Fig. 10. Schematic diagram of expected effects of a lesion involving one lateral column of the thoracic spinal cord. (A) Spinothalamic input to the thalamus would be interrupted on the side of the lesion, contralateral to the source of input. (B) Spinoreticular input to the brainstem would be partially spared, at least for the side opposite the lesion. (C) Some of the spinoreticular input to the brainstem would be interrupted, as shown for afferents to the periaqueductal gray. (D,E) Descending reticulospinal pathways to the spinal gray matter would be spared on the side opposite the lesion but could be altered functionally, because of partial deafferentation of brainstem structures such as the periaqueductal gray. (F) Descending reticulospinal pathways would be partially interrupted by the lesion, affecting spinal gray matter on both sides, including motoneurons.

in the thalamus after interruption of the spinothalamic tract (A in Fig. 10). Spared inputs to the thalamus and cortex include the spinal lemniscal pathways and relays from the brainstem that could be indirectly affected by the lesion (B in Fig. 10). Because of adaptations to the partial loss of input (Ralston et al. 2000), thalamocortical projection cells become abnormally active "spontaneously," and sensitivity to remaining inputs is altered (Weng et al. 2000). These effects can only be assessed by operant measures of pain sensitivity that depend upon cerebral processing.

Additional ascending effects of a spinal lesion that are important to recognize are schematized by C in Fig. 10. A lateral column lesion interrupts substantial projection systems to the brainstem reticular formation, shown only in part as reduced input to the periaqueductal gray. Important effects of a partial loss of spinoreticular projections will be (1) to alter innate behaviors that depend upon circuits through the brainstem and (2) to modify descending influences on the dorsal and the ventral horns of the spinal cord. It might be expected that these influences would be diffuse and would similarly affect different innate responses that depend on brainstem circuits, but this appears not to be the case. For example, vocalizations and licking and guarding responses were differentially affected by the lateral column lesions, both for ipsilateral and contralateral stimulation. Thus, not only does SCI differentially affect reflex and operant responses, but different innate responses to nociceptive stimulation are altered in different ways.

In addition to influences on functional pathways connecting the spinal cord and brainstem, lateral column lesions interrupt descending pathways that terminate in the dorsal and ventral horns on both sides of the spinal cord (D and E in Fig. 10). The combined below-level effect will be to influence motoneurons and cells of origin of ascending spinal pathways and interneurons acting separately on these output systems. It is highly unlikely that motoneurons and projection neurons will be affected identically. Therefore, use of a segmental spinal reflex to evaluate effects of a spinal lesion on sensory projection systems is risky and, similar to use of other innate responses, can lead to false negative and false positive findings. For example, the contralateral diminution of flexion reflex amplitude probably resulted from interruption of descending spinal pathways, in contrast to the contralateral reduction of escape speed, which is expected from interruption of nociceptive input to the cerebrum. The lack of ipsilateral changes for flexion and withdraw responses (combining licks and guards) is regarded as a false negative, in comparison to the ipsilateral enhancement of operant escape speed.

In summary, our study addressed the use of innate behavioral responses to nociceptive stimulation in experiments directed at understanding mechanisms of pain coding and modulation. The validity of any such method for pain assessment should be established by directly comparing experimental manipulations of these measures with effects on aversively motivated and consciously directed operant escape responses. This is the case for any experimental manipulation that can affect central neural processing (i.e., that cannot be ascribed completely to peripheral effects on nociceptors). For these comparisons, a distinction must be made between responses that depend on segmental spinal circuitry, on supraspinal projections to the brainstem, and on cerebral processing of sensory information. When unilateral interruption of the lateral spinal column was used as the experimental manipulation, operant escape responses were affected in accordance with human clinical reports of chronic pain and pain sensitivity after anterolateral cordotomy (King 1957; White and Sweet 1969; García-Larrea et al. 1993; Laheuerta et al. 1994). These results encourage the use of operant escape testing to reflect abnormal central processing of pain after SCI. However, innate responses characterized as segmental spinal or brainstem dependent were not affected over time in a manner comparable to escape responses. Effects on these innate response measures (limb flexion, withdrawal, guarding or licking, and vocalization) have frequently been regarded as evidence for manipulation of pain and have been referred to in terms such as analgesia, allodynia, or hyperalgesia, depending on the direction of change. At least for the case of below-level effects of unilateral lesions of the spinal white matter, we believe that these terms should not be used for alterations of innate responses. Neural circuits responsible for innate responses are affected differently from the pathways that subserve escape responses to nociceptive stimulation.

ACKNOWLEDGMENTS

Supported by NIH grants NS 14899, NS 16433, NS 07261 and the State of Florida Brain and Spinal Cord Injury and Rehabilitation Trust Fund. The technical support of Ivy McManus and Kirk McNaughton is gratefully acknowledged.

REFERENCES

Berridge KC. Progressive degradation of serial grooming chains by descending decerebration. *Behav Brain Res* 1989; 33:241–253.

Boivie J, Leijon G, Johansson I. Central post-stroke pain—a study of the mechanisms through analyses of the sensory abnormalities. *Pain* 1989; 37:173–185.

Borszcz GS, Johnson CP, Anderson ME, Young BJ. Characterization of tailshock elicited withdrawal reflexes in intact and spinal rats. *Physiol Behav* 1992; 52:1055–1062.

Carroll MN, Lim RKS. Observations on the neuropharmacology of morphine and morphine-like analgesia. *Arch Int Pharmacodyn* 1960; 125:383–403.

Cooper BY, Vierck Jr CJ, Yeomans DC. Selective reduction of second pain sensations by systemic morphine in humans. *Pain* 1986; 24:93–116.

D'Amour FE, Smith DL. A method for determining loss of pain sensation. *J Pharmacol Exp Ther* 1941; 72:74–79.

Dimitrijevic MR, Nathan PW. Studies of spasticity in Man. *Brain* 1967; 90:1–29.

Franklin KBJ, Abbott FV. Techniques for assessing the effects of drugs on nociceptive responses. In: Boulton AA, Baker GB, Greenshaw AJ (Eds). *Neuromethods*, Psychopharmacology, Vol. 13. Clifton: Humana Press, 1989, pp 145–216.

García-Larrea L, Charles N, Sindou M, Mauguière F. Flexion reflexes following anterolateral cordotomy in man: dissociation between pain sensation and nociceptive reflex RIII. *Pain* 1993; 55:139–149.

Hargreaves K, Dubner R, Brown F, Flores C, Joris J. A new and sensitive method for measuring thermal nociception in cutaneous hyperalgesia. *Pain* 1988; 32:77–88.

Jurgens U, Pratt R. Role of the periaqueductal grey in vocal expression of emotion. *Brain Res* 1979; 167:367–378.

Kauppila T. Influence of spinalization on spinal withdrawal reflex responses varies depending on the submodality of the test stimulus and the experimental pathophysiological condition in the rat. *Brain Res* 1998; 797:234–242.

Kelly AH, Beaton LE, Magoun HW. A midbrain mechanism for facio-vocal activity. *J Neurophysiol* 1946; 9:181–189.

King RB. Postchordotomy studies of pain threshold. *Neurology* 1957; 7:610–614.

LaBuda CJ, Fuchs PN. A behavioral test paradigm to measure the aversive quality of inflammatory and neuropathic pain in rats. *Exper Neurol* 2000; 163:490–494.

Laheuerta J, Bowsher D, Lipton S, Buxton PH. Percutaneous cervical cordotomy: a review of 181 operations on 146 patients with a study on the location of "pain fibers" in the C-2 spinal cord segment of 29 cases. *J Neurosurg* 1994; 80:975–985.

Luttinger D. Determination of antinociceptive efficacy of drugs in mice using different water temperatures in a tail immersion test. *J Pharmacol Methods* 1985; 13:351–357.

Mauderli AP, Acosta-Rua A, Vierck CJ. An operant assay of thermal pain in conscious, unrestrained rats. *J Neurosci Meth* 2000; 97:19–29.

Matthies BK, Franklin KBJ. Formalin pain is expressed in decerebrate rats but not attenuated by morphine. *Pain* 1992; 51:199–206.

Ness TJ. A case of spinal cord injury-related pain with baseline rCBF brain SPECT imaging and beneficial response to gabapentin. *Pain* 1998; 78:139–143.

Ralston DD, Dougherty PM, Lenz FA, et al. Plasticity of the inhibitory circuitry of the primate ventrobasal thalamus following lesions of the somatosensory pathways. In: Devor M, Rowbotham MC, Wiesenfeld-Hallin Z (Eds). *Proceedings of the 9th World Congress on Pain*, Progress in Pain Research and Management, Vol. 16. Seattle: IASP Press, 2000, pp 427–434.

Vierck CJ, Light AR. Effects of combined hemotoxic and anterolateral spinal lesions on nociceptive sensitivity. *Pain* 1999; 83:447–457.

Vierck CJ Jr, Light AR. Allodynia and hyperalgesia within dermatomes caudal to a spinal cord injury in primates and rodents. *Prog Brain Res* 2000; 129:411–428.

Vierck CJ Jr, Luck MM. Loss and recovery of reactivity to noxious stimuli in monkeys with primary spinothalamic chordotomies, followed by secondary and tertiary lesions of other cord sectors. *Brain* 1979; 102:233–248.

Vierck CJ Jr, Greenspan JD, Ritz LA, Yeomans DC. The spinal pathways contributing to the ascending conduction and the descending modulation of pain sensations and reactions. In: Yaksh TL (Ed). *Spinal Systems of Afferent Processing*. New York: Plenum Press, 1986, pp 275–329.

Vierck CJ Jr, Greenspan JD, Ritz LA. Long term changes in purposive and reflexive responses to nociceptive stimulation in monkeys following anterolateral chordotomy. *J Neurosci* 1990; 10:2077–2095.

Vierck CJ Jr, Lee CL, Willcockson HH, et al. Effects of anterolateral spinal lesions on escape responses of rats to hindpaw stimulation. *Somatosens Motor Res* 1995; 12:163–174.

Weng H-R, Lee JI, Lenz FA, et al. Functional plasticity in primate somatosensory thalamus following chronic lesion of the ventral lateral spinal cord. *Neuroscience* 2000; 101:393–401.

White JC, Sweet WH. *Pain and the Neurosurgeon: A Forty-Year Experience*. Springfield: Charles C. Thomas, 1969.

Willis WD, Westlund KN. Neuroanatomy of the pain system and of the pathways that modulate pain. *J Clin Neurophysiol* 1997; 14:2–31.

Woolf CJ. Long term alterations in the excitability of the flexion reflex produced by peripheral tissue injury in the chronic decerebrate rat. *Pain* 1984; 18:325–343.

Woolfe G, MacDonald AD. The evaluation of the analgesic action of pethidine hydrochloride (Demerol). *J Pharmacol Exp Ther* 1944; 80:300–307.

Yeomans DC, Pirec V, Proudfit HK. Nociceptive responses to high and low rates of noxious cutaneous heating are mediated by different nociceptors in the rat: behavioral evidence. *Pain* 1996; 86:141–150.

Correspondence to: Charles J. Vierck, PhD, Department of Neuroscience, University of Florida College of Medicine, Gainesville, FL 32510-0244, USA. Tel: 352-392-6555; Fax: 352-392-8513; email: vierck@mbi.ufl.edu.

Spinal Cord Injury Pain: Assessment, Mechanisms, Management. Progress in Pain Research and Management, Vol. 23, edited by Robert P. Yezierski and Kim J. Burchiel, IASP Press, Seattle, © 2002.

9

Mechanisms of Increased Pain Sensitivity within Dermatomes Remote from an Injured Segment of the Spinal Cord

Charles J. Vierck, Jr., Richard L. Cannon, Kristin A. Stevens, Antonio J. Acosta-Rua, and Edward D. Wirth, III

Department of Neuroscience and McKnight Brain Institute, University of Florida College of Medicine, Gainesville, Florida, USA

This chapter describes changes in sensitivity to sensory input that can occur within spinal segments rostral and caudal to a spinal cord injury (SCI). We will describe relationships between lesion configuration and changes in sensitivity of neurons within spinal segments remote from the injury. In addition, we will distinguish between alterations in responsivity that are revealed by tests of spinal reflexes and by assessments of sensory quality and intensity. This chapter focuses on incomplete injuries of the spinal cord, when some pathways are spared that are capable of transmitting activity around a spinal lesion. Chronic pain and reflex abnormalities following complete transection of the spinal cord probably result from mechanisms similar to those revealed by partial lesions, but we focus on incomplete SCI because evaluation of chronic pain is facilitated by sensory testing, which is not instructive for stimulation caudal to a spinal transection.

Common assumptions concerning the functional consequences of SCI are (1) that spinal reflexes and conscious sensations are globally and similarly affected, (2) that these effects only involve spinal segments at and caudal to the lesion, and (3) that both the reflex and sensory consequences of SCI result from interruption of long spinal pathways in the white matter. Vierck and Light challenged the first assumption in Chapter 8, and we will elaborate further with a distinction between spasticity and the spastic syndrome.

We will question the second and third assumptions using data from animal models and psychophysical observations of humans with SCI.

MECHANISMS OF BELOW-LEVEL HYPERREFLEXIA AFTER SCI

Spasticity has been rigorously defined as a velocity-dependent enhancement of stretch reflexes (Lance 1980). It can occur as a result of lesions throughout the length of the neuraxis, from motor cortex to spinal cord (Brown 1994). For some time, lateral hemisection was the lesion of choice for modeling spasticity from SCI (Carter et al. 1991), but lesions restricted to the ipsilateral dorsolateral column also produce spasticity (Taylor et al. 1997, 1999). Descending reticulospinal pathways are implicated (Engberg et al. 1968). These findings confirm a long-standing assumption that spinal hyperexcitability results from interruption of long descending pathways (Bucy et al. 1966), but this principle should not be generalized to mechanisms of SCI effects on all spinal neurons and circuits.

After a dorsolateral spinal lesion, spasticity can be observed within several days and persists indefinitely. In contrast, a more comprehensive increase in excitability, the spastic syndrome, can develop slowly over time within segments caudal to SCI. The spastic syndrome is characterized by exaggerated flexion and withdrawal reflexes that can radiate spatially to be characterized as mass reflexes involving muscles not normally associated with responses to a local nociceptive stimulus (Dimitrijevic and Nathan 1967). With time after SCI, a non-nociceptive cutaneous or proprioceptive stimulus can elicit flexion and clonus, and the clasp-knife reflex can be observed. The spastic syndrome occurs only after spinal lesions and can occur without exaggeration of stretch reflexes (Schmit et al. 2000). Although spasticity can be regarded as beneficial to recovery of locomotor skills, particularly in comparison to flaccidity (Zehr and Stein 1999), the spastic syndrome is a disruptive and disturbing consequence of SCI.

The spastic syndrome shares certain features with chronic pain, but these forms of hyperexcitability can occur independently or together. Chronic pain or the spastic syndrome or both can develop slowly over time after SCI, and once present, pain and flexion reflexes can be elicited by non-nociceptive stimulation. Also, abnormal characteristics of spatial radiation and persistence are shared. Therefore, although thresholds and amplitudes of flexion or withdrawal reflex circuits cannot be used to reveal the presence of chronic central pain following SCI (Vierck et al. 1990; see also Chapter 8), some aspects of reflex transformation apparently result from mechanisms common to the development of chronic SCI pain.

We propose that extensive lesions involving spinal gray and white matter produce a combination of effects that are conducive to development of the spastic syndrome and/or chronic central pain, depending upon which neural circuits are affected. First, we present evidence to establish the lesion configuration that is required to produce the spastic syndrome. The flexion reflex will be used as an assay for the spastic syndrome. Then, we will make comparisons with effects of spinal lesions on pain sensitivity.

We conducted experiments with monkeys involving measurement of flexion reflex amplitude and duration to address the possibility that the spastic syndrome results from interruption of spinal white matter. We applied electrocutaneous stimulation to the mid-lateral calf of either leg of monkeys comfortably seated in restraining chairs while receiving food reinforcement. The stimulation on each trial consisted of a short (10-ms) burst of alternating, constant current, applied through wells of electrode paste separated by 1 cm. Amplified reflex responses were derived from force transducers tethered to ankle cuffs.

The first consideration in these experiments was to determine whether interruption of the ipsilateral dorsolateral column produces a generalized hyperreflexia that includes stretch and flexion reflexes. Fig. 1A shows the form of flexion reflex responses to 1.5 mA/mm^2, averaged over testing sessions early in the preoperative period of testing. The principal peak of force occurred 130 ms after the onset of stimulation, and a trailing activation of flexor motoneurons was evident until approximately 500 ms. The persistence of the flexion response contrasts with reactive resistance to muscle stretch that does not appreciably outlast the stimulus for normal animals (Taylor et al. 1997). The flexion response was similar for stimulation of either leg and was consistent over time, with slight attenuation as the animals became acclimated to the daily testing regimen (Fig. 1C).

In dramatic contrast to the exaggeration of stretch reflexes produced by small lesions of the ipsilateral dorsolateral column (Taylor et al. 1999), panels B and D of Fig. 1 reveal a virtual elimination of flexion reflexes produced by ipsilateral electrocutaneous stimulation. Also, the depression of flexion reflexes persisted over time (e.g., Fig. 1D). Contradictory to the expectation that nociceptive flexion reflexes would be particularly enhanced by interruption of descending reticulospinal pathways in the dorsolateral column (Basbaum and Fields 1979), the opposite effect was obtained reliably. This result shows that modulatory effects on stretch and flexion reflexes differ considerably. Such a dissociation could have been anticipated, because spasticity can occur as a result of lesions at all levels of the neuraxis, but the spastic syndrome is uniquely associated with SCI and results from lesions involving regions of the spinal cord other than the dorsolateral columns.

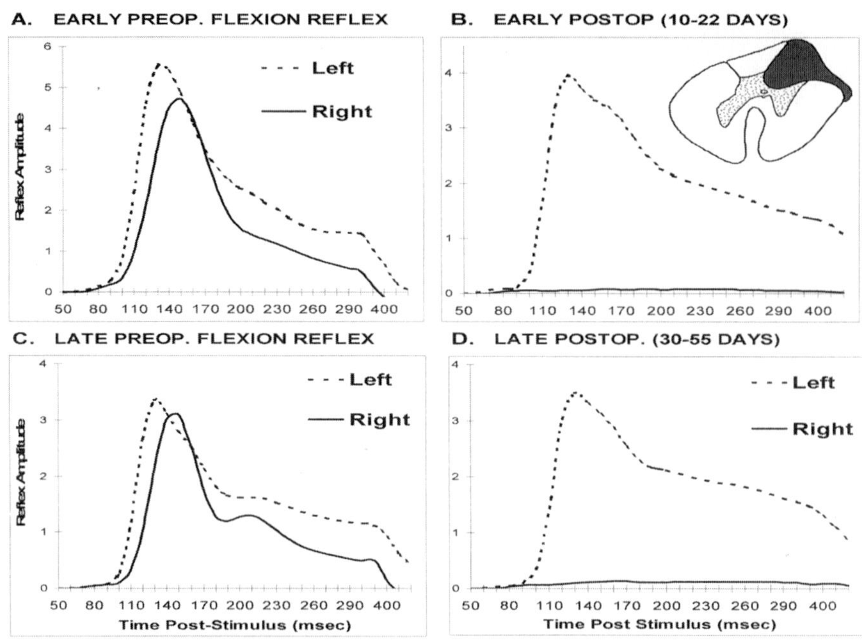

Fig. 1. Digitized tracings of the output of force transducers tethered to the legs of a monkey stimulated on the lateral calf. A and C: Preoperative tracings of flexion reflex force during 10-day periods of testing reveal consistent response forms for the left and right legs, with some attenuation of peak force over time. The preoperative responses consisted of a prominent peak at 120–140 ms after stimulus onset, followed by a low level of flexion force that persisted through 400 ms. The output of the transducers was linear within the range of forces generated and is expressed in millivolts on the ordinate. B and D: Postoperative recordings averaged over 10 days of testing early and late after administration of a thoracic lesion of the right dorsolateral column (inset). For this animal, the flexion reflex was eliminated ipsilateral to the lesion.

Numerous studies have shown an association between interruption of the spinothalamic tract and development of contralateral chronic pain in segments caudal to the lesion (Boivie et al. 1989). Therefore, if the spastic syndrome and chronic central pain are linked and are associated with interruption of spinal white matter, interruption of the anterolateral column should produce hyperactive flexion reflexes over time. However, chronic pain results from involvement of the spinothalamic tract at any point in its course to the thalamus and beyond (Cassinari and Pagni 1969), in contrast to the spastic syndrome, which is unlikely to result from interruption of an ascending spinal pathway. Interruption of descending pathways in the anterolateral spinal column could deprive motoneurons of inhibitory influences and exaggerate reflexes (Jankowska et al. 1993), but the opposite result is demonstrated in Fig. 2. Bilateral attenuation of flexion reflexes was observed after interruption of one anterolateral column of the spinal cord in a monkey tested for 5 months postoperatively. This result confirms previous investigations of flexion reflex excitability of monkeys and humans after anterolateral cordotomy (Vierck et al. 1990; García-Larrea et al. 1993).

If both dorsolateral and anterolateral spinal lesions result in depression of flexion reflexes, how is it that SCI can cause substantial increases in flexion reflex amplitude and duration, as a prominent component of the spastic syndrome? One possibility is that a massive caudal deafferentation from extensive interruption of spinal white matter is required, and that the spastic syndrome results from extensive reorganization of segmental input to ventral horn interneurons and motoneurons (Goldberger and Murray 1978). The spastic syndrome commonly develops after complete or nearly complete spinal transection, suggesting that the amount of white matter damage might be a critical factor. For example, transection of the sacrocaudal spinal cord results in gradual development of exaggerated withdrawal reflexes of the tails of cats in response to electrocutaneous stimulation (Friedman et al.

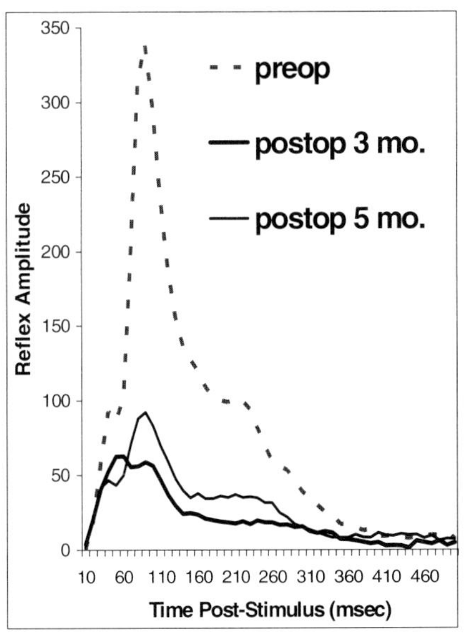

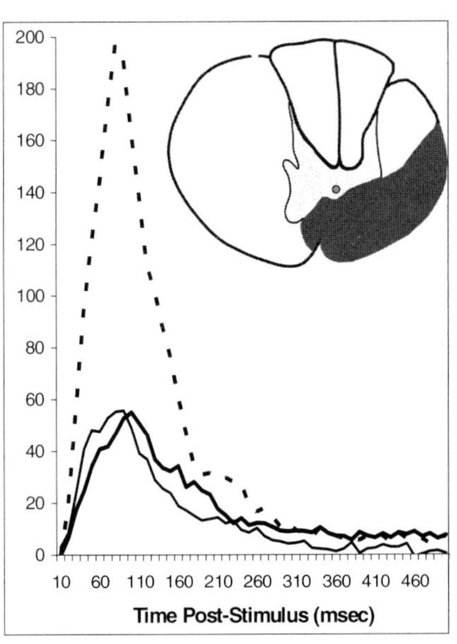

Fig. 2. Digitized tracings of flexion reflexes, averaged over 10 testing sessions before and after a thoracic right anterolateral spinal lesion in a monkey. The preoperative response form was sharply peaked for this animal and was consistently greater in amplitude on the left. Transducer output is converted to grams of force on the ordinate. Postoperative testing revealed a substantial bilateral reduction in the amplitude of flexion reflexes over testing periods that began at 90 and 150 days after surgery.

2001). This model of SCI permits evaluation of segmental reflexes without disruption of autonomic control or locomotor capabilities of the animals (Ritz et al. 1992). These features facilitated the design of an experiment with monkeys that investigated the effects of spinal lesions that interrupted long pathways but preserved some propriospinal control over segmental reflexes.

Bilateral propriospinal networks of connections between spinal segments are difficult to study, but they apparently make up the bulk of intraspinal axons (Chung et al. 1984) and exert modulatory effects on segmental reflexes (Sandkühler et al. 1991; Jones 1998). These extensive systems of interconnected interneurons are presumed to be critical for intersegmental coordination of reflex and locomotor patterns (Kato et al. 1985) and for spatial summation of pain (Wall et al. 1999). However, the contributions of propriospinal systems to functional plasticity after SCI have rarely been considered. One strategy for investigating propriospinal influences on recovery from SCI is to make right and left lateral hemisections at different segmental levels of the spinal cord (Fig. 3). Although long spinal pathways will be severed by these lesions, including long propriospinal pathways (Miller et al. 1999), there should be partial sparing of short propriospinal connections between segments rostral and caudal to the lesions (Petro and Antal 2000). When the hemisections are made at upper sacrocaudal levels, effects of conditioning hindlimb stimulation on subsequent responses to tail stimulation would show that functional propriospinal connections have been spared. That is, stimulation of a leg (A in Fig. 3) can theoretically activate the bilateral system of propriospinal interneurons and influence withdrawal reflexes elicited by test stimulation of tail segments caudal to the staggered hemisections (B to C in Fig. 3).

Three *Macaca fascicularis* monkeys were trained to accept restraint in a monkey chair and receive electrocutaneous stimulation of either lateral calf or the tail. Early in the preoperative period of testing, thresholds for elicitation of reflex flexion and withdrawal were obtained by varying the intensity of 5-ms square wave pulses at each site of stimulation. All subsequent testing was conducted with stimulation at three times the established preoperative threshold intensities. Within a testing session, stimuli were delivered to either leg and then to the tail at different condition-test intervals, or single stimuli were delivered to the tail. Fifteen seconds elapsed between trials of single or paired stimulation. After stable preoperative data were obtained over several months of testing, each animal received staggered right and left lesions of spinal white matter at sacrocaudal segments Ca1 and Ca3. These lesions are shown in Fig. 4. In each case, the combined effect of the two lesions was to interrupt all dorsal spinal pathways but spare some portion of ventral spinal cord, either unilaterally (#1 and #3) or bilaterally (#2). The

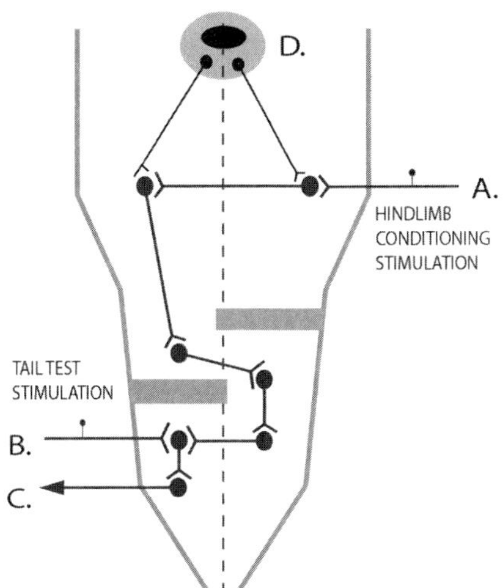

Fig. 3. Schematic diagram of the rationale for testing intersegmental reflex modulation before and after staggered sacrocaudal spinal lesions. Electrocutaneous stimulation at distal sites on the tail (B) polysynaptically activates flexor motoneurons of the tail (C). Conditioning stimulation of either hindlimb (A) modulates tail reflexes via bilateral, multisynaptic propriospinal connections that bypass the staggered lesions of long spinal pathways. Introduction of quisqualic acid into the spinal gray matter at a thoracic level (D) affects condition-test modulation of tail reflexes by leg stimulation.

animals were then tested for more than 1 year before receiving a second surgical procedure, as described below.

Fig. 5 shows amplitudes of conditioned tail reflexes (preceded by leg stimulation) in relation to the magnitude of unconditioned responses to tail stimulation in the same testing sessions. Preoperatively, conditioning leg stimulation reduced the amplitude of tail-withdrawal reflexes over condition-test intervals of 25–800 ms. Thus, tail reflexes of intact animals were consistently inhibited by preceding stimulation of a leg. The duration of this inhibition was quite long, and the maximum effect approached a 30% reduction in amplitude of the tail reflex. In distinct contrast, after long spinal pathways were interrupted by lesions placed between segments receiving input from the legs and the tail, conditioning leg stimulation reliably increased the amplitude of tail reflexes relative to unconditioned responses. This result shows that some propriospinal modulation has been spared by the staggered spinal lesions. Also, the reversal of caudally directed intersegmental modulation after the lateral spinal lesions indicates that a facilitatory role of short propriospinal systems is unmasked or released by interruption of long spinal pathways. This result is supported by reports of unique intersegmental evocation of reflexes in human SCI patients (Calancie et al. 1996). In intact animals, intersegmental modulation most likely includes influences from spinobulbospinal pathways (Shimamura et al. 1980) that were interrupted by the lateral spinal lesions.

An important question raised by the demonstration of altered intersegmental influences concerns tonic versus phasic influences on reflexes. The reversal from stimulus-locked (phasic) inhibition to facilitation of caudal

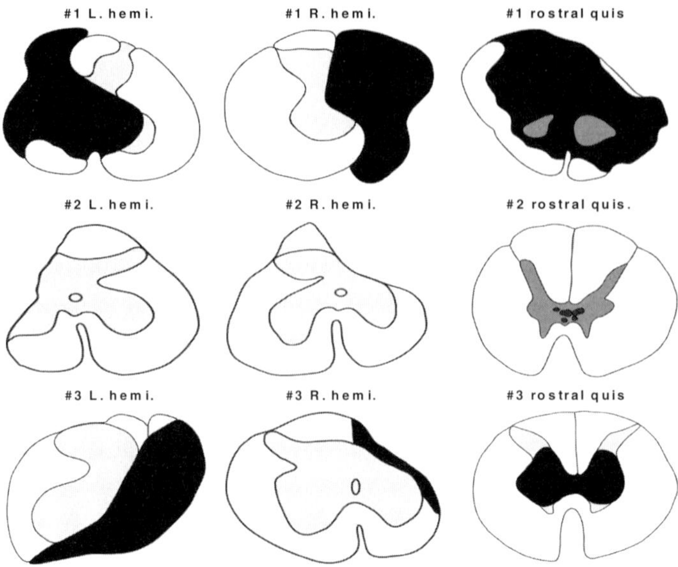

Fig. 4. Camera lucida drawings of the lateral spinal and quisqualic acid lesions for three *Macaca fascicularis* monkeys. Lesions are denoted by absence of tissue (#2) or by blackened areas corresponding to scar tissue or cystic cavities.

reflexes after interposed lesions of spinal white matter indicates that postoperative tail responses to single stimuli might be enhanced relative to preoperative amplitudes, if the propriospinal system is tonically active. However, this was not unambiguously the case, as shown in Fig. 6. The maximal amplitude of tail reflexes to single pulse stimulation was reduced postoperatively, but the duration of the reflex was increased. Thus, extensive interruption of long spinal pathways did not produce clear evidence of the spastic syndrome. The prolonged duration of caudal reflexes could result from long-lasting facilitation by spinal pattern generators for locomotion (Viala et al. 1974), but the large-amplitude withdrawal responses characteristic of the spastic syndrome were not produced. This result confirms the effects of restricted dorsal and ventral lesions on flexion reflexes of monkeys and reinforces doubts that the spastic syndrome can be attributed solely to interruption of long spinal pathways.

Other experiments indicate that ischemic damage in the vicinity of a spinal lesion can determine whether increased pain sensitivity will develop over time (Vierck 1991; Vierck and Light 1999, 2000). We thus extended our experiment with staggered hemisections to include a second surgical procedure. Rostral to the lateral spinal lesions, within segments T12 to L1, each animal received six injections of 120 mM quisqualic acid into the

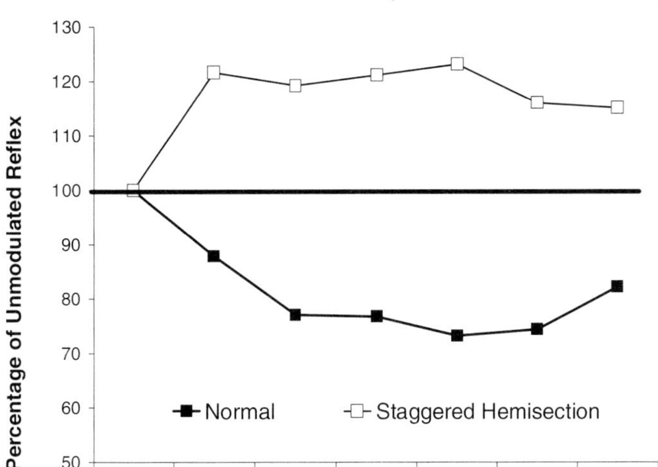

Fig. 5. Percentage change in the maximal amplitude of tail reflexes conditioned by prior stimulation of either leg, averaged across 10 sessions for three monkeys, before and after staggered sacrocaudal lesions of spinal white matter. Preoperatively, conditioning stimulation reduced the amplitude of withdrawal reflexes of the tail. Postoperatively, conditioning stimulation increased the amplitude of tail reflexes.

spinal gray matter. At three injection sites on each side, spaced 1 mm apart rostrocaudally, we injected 1.0 μL of quisqualic acid at each of three depths in the gray matter, using a Hamilton syringe fitted with a micropipette. The intent of this procedure was to introduce excitotoxicity within the gray matter. The reflex tests were then repeated to determine whether abnormal activity among spinal interneurons near the injections (Yezierski and Park 1993; see also Chapter 7) would influence caudal spinal segments via propriospinal conduction past the lateral spinal lesions (see Fig. 3). The extent of observable damage on histological reconstruction at T12–L1 varied considerably among the three animals, ranging from small clusters of cavities in the gray matter (#2) to extensive loss of neurons (#3) to a large lesion that extended throughout the gray and white matter (#1). The large lesion must have resulted from disruption of the blood supply to the region injected.

The effect of quisqualic acid injection on tail reflexes is shown in Fig. 6. Overall, and for each animal, the amplitude of tail reflexes was increased beyond preoperative levels, and reflex durations remained excessive. The reduction in withdrawal reflex amplitude produced by staggered spinal lesions was transformed by the rostral quisqualic acid lesions into an enhancement. It

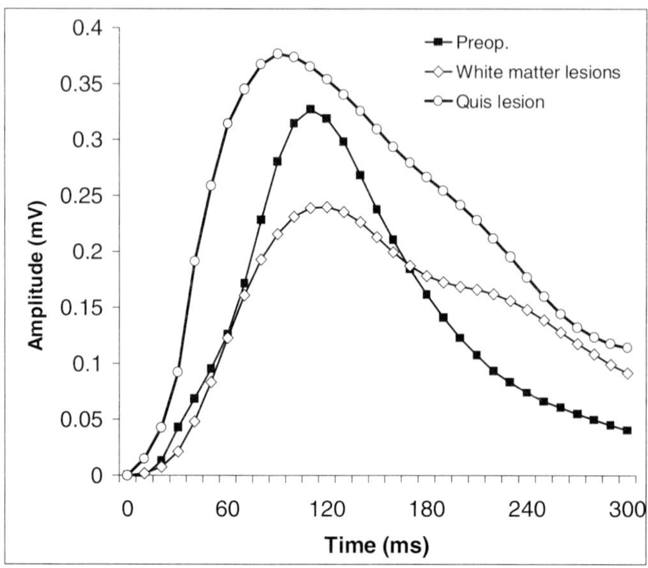

Fig. 6. Digitized averages of unconditioned tail-withdrawal reflexes before surgery (normal), after staggered sacrocaudal lesions of spinal white matter, and after subsequent thoracic injection of quisqualic acid into spinal gray matter (quis lesion). The white matter lesions decreased the amplitude of tail reflexes, but addition of rostral quisqualic acid lesions of gray matter exaggerated tail reflexes above normal values.

is unlikely that reflex facilitation for the monkeys after the second surgery resulted from interruption of descending input to caudal segments beyond that produced by the lateral spinal lesions. An explanation consistent with clinical findings and the present study is that descending propriospinal systems are tonically activated by excitotoxic influences near the site of spinal injuries that include ischemic and excitotoxic involvement of gray matter. Tonic hyperexcitability as a consequence of spinal ischemia or syringomyelia in humans has been documented (Nogués and Stålberg 1999; Nogués et al. 2000).

The overall conclusion from the results presented to this point is that the spastic syndrome results not from long tract interruption alone but from a combination of long tract damage and excitatory influences on gray matter. Involvement of gray matter has previously been regarded as unimportant for below-level functional disorders for two main reasons: (1) Damage to gray matter has been viewed in terms of negative signs (loss of function), rather than position signs (e.g., exaggerated reflexes). However, current models of at-level phenomena have shown that neuronal hyperactivity is an important consequence of insult to the gray matter (Yezierski and Park 1993). (2) Effects of a gray-matter lesion have been assumed to be restricted to dermatome(s) directly affected, due to a lack of evidence for remote transmission of neuronal activity from the site of a lesion via the propriospinal system. Also, we do not yet fully understand the interactions between deafferentation from section of long spinal pathways and changes in propriospinal function over time.

MECHANISMS OF BELOW-LEVEL ALLODYNIA/HYPERALGESIA AFTER SCI

Chronic pain, allodynia, and hyperalgesia do not result reliably from interruption of spinal white matter (Vierck et al. 1986; Vierck and Light 2000). Therefore, it is important to determine whether pain sensitivity is enhanced by combined influences of gray and white matter damage in a manner similar to SCI that eventuates in the spastic syndrome. An affirmative answer is provided by experiments involving measurement of escape behavior before and after administration of surgical lesions involving one anterolateral column. In these experiments, evidence for postoperative development of increased sensitivity to nociceptive stimulation was derived from (1) periods of recovery from a contralateral decrease in sensitivity presumed to result from interruption of the lateral spinothalamic tract, and (2) a persistent ipsilateral enhancement of escape behavior. In experiments with monkeys, these effects did not depend only on interruption of anterolateral white matter but were more likely to occur if the lesion was medially extensive, intruding on gray matter (Vierck et al. 1990). In subsequent experiments with rats, development of allodynia and hyperalgesia was apparent only when blood was introduced into the lesion cavity during the surgical procedure (Vierck and Light 1999). Blood in proximity to the gray matter would have elicited ischemia (Sadrzadeh et al. 1987) and is likely to have generated excitotoxic cascades and associated hyperactivity of spinal neurons (Yezierski 1996). In contrast, interruption of spinothalamic axons by superficial lesions of anterolateral white matter that do not invade the gray matter do not appear to be associated with development of chronic pain or hypersensitivity to nociceptive stimulation (Nathan and Smith 1979).

Because the propriospinal system conducts both rostrally and caudally (Kusmirek 1997; Jones 1998; Petko and Antal 2000), we might expect to find above-level chronic pain after SCI involving gray matter. However, such pain has not been reported in cases where peripheral pathology can be ruled out. A possible reason is that deafferentation from interruption of white matter would be much less extensive at rostral spinal levels than at caudal spinal segments. That is, chronic pain (and the spastic syndrome) appear to depend in part on deafferentation, which is less extensive for spinal segments rostral to a thoracic lesion and minimal to absent for brainstem and cerebral targets of projection from forelimb segments. However, there is some evidence for abnormal sensitivity to afferent drive of above-level spinal segments.

After lateral hemisection of the thoracic spinal cord of rats, withdrawal responses of both forelimbs to thermal and mechanical stimulation are enhanced (Christensen et al. 1996). These lesions are medially extensive and involve the gray matter. Also, studies in humans have shown altered sensitivity for stimulation rostral to functionally complete spinal lesions. A widespread increase in detection thresholds on the thorax of SCI patients extended well beyond a band near the lesion that was insentient to touch (Saddiki-Traki et al. 1999). However, the magnitude of elicited sensations was increased by 58% over responses of normal subjects within a region of up to 33 cm from the at-level dermatome. These patients did not experience chronic pain. Similarly, Cohen et al. (1996) observed that pain sensitivity and stimulus detection were enhanced within segments rostral to SCI, but only for patients with below-level pain. Defrin et al. (1999) obtained the opposite results—elevated pain thresholds for rostral stimulation only for patients with below-level pain. The latter effect was attributed to the phenomenon of diffuse noxious inhibitory control (DNIC; LeBars et al. 1979). Finally, a neurophysiological confirmation of altered sensitivity rostral to thoracic lesions of one lateral spinal column has revealed abnormal bursting and enhanced sensitivity for cells in the forelimb region of the thalamic nucleus ventralis posterolateralis (Weng et al. 2000).

These results indicate that the nature of above-level changes in sensitivity depends on the testing methods and on the presence of abnormal sources of activity that generate at-level and/or below-level pain. Further evidence for the importance of these factors comes from a long-term investigation of eight patients with progressive syringomyelia by Wirth and colleagues (Chapter 18). In addition to the observations reported in Chapter 18, each patient was trained to verbally rate the magnitude of evoked sensations, using a paradigm that produces temporal summation of cold or heat pain sensations (Vierck et al. 1997). These ratings were compared with those of similarly trained controls. The cystic cavitations revealed by magnetic resonance imaging (MRI) were extensive rostrocaudally for most of the patients, but the rostral extent of damage to the spinal cord did not reach the stimulated segment (C6, the thenar eminence). Temporal summation of pain was substantially increased over normal values for stimulation of one or both hands for eight subjects. The enhanced sensitivity to repetitive thermal stimulation was observed for patients that did and did not report chronic pain in an upper or lower extremity. Therefore, for segments above a spinal lesion, increased sensitivity to nociceptive input was observed but was not necessarily associated with chronic pain. However, because of altered sensitivity, it is expected that these patients would be especially prone to experience above-level pain from any source of nociceptive input (e.g., muscle strain).

Facilitation of input to segments both rostral and caudal to a spinal lesion was well demonstrated by testing for temporal summation of cold pain in a patient with a cystic cavity restricted to T5–T6 (Fig. 7). Psychophysical ratings for temporal summation of heat and cold pain during repetitive stimulation of the hands and feet of this patient were clearly elevated beyond normal levels, and cold pain was dramatically enhanced. For normal subjects repetitive stimulation of the skin with a cold probe (0.2°C) produces sensations of cold during contact that does not progress to painful levels, but a deep aching pain sensation gradually builds up and radiates well beyond the site of skin contact. Unlike the distinct second pain sensation that summates with repetitive heat stimulation, the ache from cold stimulation is continuous, once established. The deep sensation is clearly perceived by all subjects but does not attain high levels (approximately 40 on a scale in which 20 represents pain threshold and 100 represents unbearable pain). As shown in Fig. 7, the rate of temporal summation of the aching sensation is quite slow for normal subjects. In contrast, the syringomyelia patient rated the sensation during the first contact of the cold probe with the skin as painful, and the intensity of the cold pain sensation quickly escalated to high ratings. The patient terminated each series of cold stimulation before normal subjects rated the aching sensation as clearly painful. Other functional effects of this lesion extended to segments above and below the cystic cavitation revealed by nuclear magnetic resonance (NMR). Bilateral weakness in the wrists and aching sensations in the hands slowly developed over years. The legs were similarly affected, with weakness and a low level of chronic pain.

SUMMARY

The results presented here challenge the assumption that the spastic syndrome and chronic central pain with allodynia and hyperalgesia can be ascribed only to interruption of certain pathways in the spinal white matter. For example, in contrast to spasticity (a velocity-dependent exaggeration of monosynaptic stretch reflexes), which results from interruption of pathways

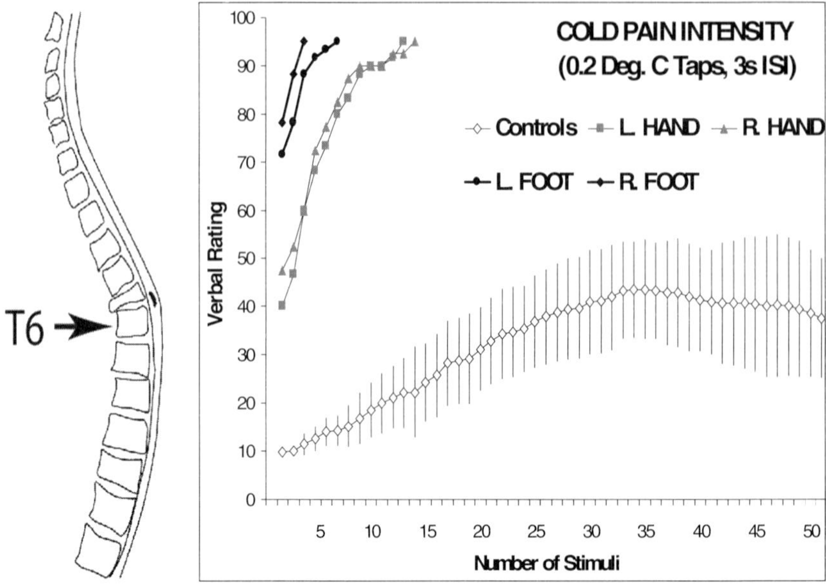

Fig. 7. Left panel: A drawing from longitudinal MRI images of the spinal cord of a patient with a syringomyelia cavity at the site of a prior injury at the T6–T7 vertebral level. Evidence of damage to the spinal cord was restricted to that level. However, this subject was hypersensitive to cold stimulation of the hands and feet (right panel), as shown by enhanced temporal summation with repetitive stimulation (ISI = interstimulus interval). For comparison, averaged temporal summation of an aching cold sensation for seven normal controls is shown, with standard deviation bars.

in the dorsolateral white matter, polysynaptic flexion reflexes are depressed by lesions primarily involving spinal white matter. Exaggeration of flexion reflexes, exemplary of the spastic syndrome, appears to require spinal lesions that invade the gray matter to the extent that ischemia sets up excitotoxic cascades which generate abnormal neural activity among neurons near the lesion (Fig. 8). Traumatic injury to the spinal cord from vertebral displacement (the most common cause of SCI) begins with traumatic and ischemic damage to the gray matter and progresses with time to involve white matter. Thus, progressive excitotoxic destruction of gray matter is a primary and a prominent feature of clinical SCI. Selective destruction of white matter is an experimental strategy for modeling SCI that appears to have missed the mark in terms of certain disruptive positive consequences of SCI (development of mass reflexes and chronic pain).

If our assumptions are correct, the emphasis on gray matter damage has important clinical implications for preventative management of the sequelae of SCI. Early treatments directed at limiting ischemia, inflammation, and

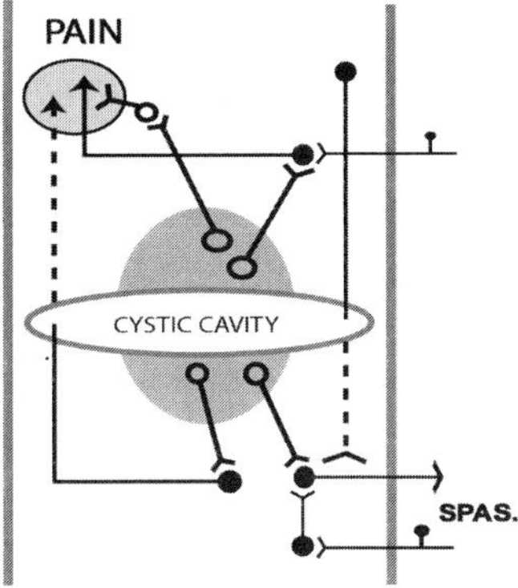

Fig. 8. Schematic representation of factors contributing to development of chronic central pain or the spastic syndrome ("spas.") after SCI. Lateral extension of a cystic cavity at the site of spinal injury interrupts axons (dashed lines) and partially deafferents neuronal systems rostral and caudal to the lesion. Ischemic/excitotoxic damage rostral and caudal to the lesion is presumed to modulate (facilitate) input to reflex and pain transmission cells rostral and caudal to the lesion, particularly in combination with partial deafferentation of the neuronal system. The most tentative aspect of this proposal is whether ascending propriospinal activity exerts effects on supraspinal systems.

excitotoxicity can curtail the typical progression of gray matter damage that occurs over time after the injury (Yezierski 2000). Depending on the pattern of initial injury (e.g., preservation of blood supply in the vicinity of spinal trauma), pathological destruction of white matter could also be reduced, because much of this occurs progressively with formation of cystic cavities. Preservation of white matter is obviously advantageous for sparing of adaptive sensory and motor capabilities. Also, curtailment of gray matter deterioration could remove a critical determinant of disruptive and disturbing symptoms such as chronic pain and the spastic syndrome.

The therapeutic potential of early treatment has been demonstrated by an experiment involving transplantation of fetal spinal tissue into sacrocaudal transection cavities of cats at the time of surgery (Friedman et al. 2001). Without transplantation, exaggerated withdrawal reflexes of the tail developed after spinal transection. In contrast, transplantation of fetal spinal tissue prevented the expected increases in magnitude and duration of withdrawal reflexes. In these animals, the fetal spinal tissue integrated with host gray matter but probably did not restore conduction past the lesion in white matter. A parsimonious interpretation of this result is that the fetal tissue prevented development of the spastic syndrome by attenuating neuronal hyperexcitability at the borders of what would have been a transection cavity in the absence of the graft.

Evidence reviewed here indicates that it is not destruction of spinal tissue per se that promotes development of positive symptoms after SCI. Rather, we offer the hypothesis that abnormal activity within the spinal gray matter propagates rostrally and caudally via the propriospinal system to exert excitatory or facilitatory influences on neural circuits remote to the injury. Demonstrations of extensive rostral and caudal increases in metabolic activity after SCI support this possibility (Schwartzman et al. 1983; Scremin et al. 1990).

These and related findings raise a number of questions concerning properties of propriospinal systems. For example, do ascending and descending propriospinal systems exert similar effects in terms of sensory and reflex modulation of remote spinal segments? Propriospinal connections differ for long and short axon components, for rostral, caudal, ipsilateral, and contralateral projections from a given site, for dorsal and ventral horns, and even for medial and lateral divisions of the spinal gray matter (Szentagothai 1951; Petko and Antal 2000). Does propriospinal conduction have influences on cerebral processing of pain, contributing to perceptions of chronic below-level pain after spinal lesions that include complete transection? What are the sensory and/or modulatory functions of Lissauer's tract, a propriospinal component that receives nociceptive input? These are fundamentally important questions concerning a primitive and extensive system of control over spinal processing.

A related set of questions concerns the relative or interactive participation of gray and white matter lesions in the development of central pain, allodynia, hyperalgesia, and the spastic syndrome. Do the facilitatory effects of propriospinal activity depend on removal of other systems of modulation, as suggested by the reversal from intersegmental inhibition to facilitation of withdrawal reflexes that was observed (Fig. 5) after opposed lateral spinal lesions? In the experiments reviewed here, white matter damage was found to be insufficient, whereas injury to both gray and white matter produced reflex exaggeration and heightened sensitivity to nociceptive stimulation. Gray matter insult alone was not evaluated. In experiments dealing with at-level phenomena resulting from excitotoxic injury to gray matter, the pattern and amount of cellular destruction are critical factors (Vierck et al. 2000; Gorman et al. 2001), and these may also be determinants of positive symptoms at rostral and caudal dermatomes following SCI. The often delayed appearance of chronic pain and the spastic syndrome may result from progression of a spinal lesion to a certain configuration or size, rather than (or in addition to) progressions of neural reorganization from loss of white matter connections. The association or dissociation of chronic pain and the spastic syndrome could then depend on relative effects of a lesion and/or on excitatory effects on dorsal and ventral propriospinal systems that preferentially modulate sensory and motor spinal processing.

ACKNOWLEDGMENTS

Supported by NIH grants NS 07261, NS 35702 and the State of Florida Brain and Spinal Cord Injury and Rehabilitation Trust Fund. The technical support of Jean Kaufman and Anwarul Azam is gratefully acknowledged.

REFERENCES

Basbaum AI, Fields H. The origin of descending pathways in the dorsolateral funiculus of the spinal cord of the cat and rat: further studies of the anatomy of pain modulation. *J Comp Neurol* 1979; 187:513–532.

Boivie J, Leijon G, Johansson I. Central post-stroke pain—a study of the mechanisms through analyses of the sensory abnormalities. *Pain* 1989; 37:173–185.

Brown P. Pathophysiology of spasticity. *J Neurol Neurosurg Psychiatry* 1994; 57:773–777.

Bucy PC, Ladpli R, Ehrlich A. Destruction of the pyramidal tract in the monkey. *J Neurosurg* 1966; 25:1–20.

Calancie B, Lutton S, Broton JG. Central nervous system plasticity after spinal cord injury in man: interlimb reflexes and the influence of cutaneous stimulation. *Electroencephalogr Clin Neurophysiol* 1996; 101:304–315.

Carter RL, Ritz LA, Shank CP, Scott EW, Sypert GW. Correlative electrophysiological and behavioral evaluation following L5 lesions in the cat: a model of spasticity. *Exp Neurol* 1991; 114:206–215.

Cassinari V, Pagni CA. *Central Pain: A Neurosurgical Survey*. Cambridge, MA: Harvard University Press, 1969.

Christensen MD, Everhart AW, Pickelman JT, Hulseboch CE. Mechanism and thermal allodynia in chronic central pain following spinal cord injury. *Pain* 1996; 86:97–108.

Chung K, Kevetter GA, Willis WD, Coggeshall RE. An estimate of the ratio of propriospinal to long tract neurons in the sacral spinal cord of the rat. *Neurosci Lett* 1984; 44:173–177.

Cohen MJ, Song Z-K, Schandler SL, Ho W-H, Vulpe M. Sensory detection and pain thresholds in spinal cord injury patients with and without dysesthetic pain, and in chronic low back pain patients. *Somatosens Motor Res* 1996; 13:29–38.

Defrin R, Ohry A, Blumen N, Urca G. Acute pain threshold in subjects with chronic pain following spinal cord injury. *Pain* 1999; 83:275–282.

Dimitrijevic MR, Nathan PW. Studies of spasticity in man. *Brain* 1967; 90:1–29.

Engberg I, Lundberg A, Ryall RW. Reticulospinal inhibition of transmission in reflex pathways. *J Physiol* 1968; 194:201–223.

Friedman RM, Ritz LA, Reier PJ, Vierck CJ Jr. Effects of sacrocaudal spinal cord transection and transplantation of fetal spinal tissue on withdrawal reflexes of the tail. *Neurorehabil Neural Repair* 2001; 14:333–345.

García-Larrea L, Charles N, Sindou M, Mauguière F. Flexion reflexes following anterolateral cordotomy in man: dissociation between pain sensation and nociceptive reflex RIII. *Pain* 1993; 55:139–149.

Goldberger ME, Murray M. Recovery of movement and axonal sprouting may obey some of the same laws. In: Cotman CW (Ed). *Neuronal Plasticity*. New York: Raven Press, 1978, pp 73–96.

Gorman AL, Yu C-G, Ruenes GR, Daniels L, Yezierski RP. Conditions affecting the onset, severity, and progression of a spontaneous pain-like behavior after excitotoxic spinal cord injury. *J Pain* 2001; 2:229–240.

Jankowska E, Riddell JS, Skoog B, Noga BR. Gating of transmission to motoneurones by stimuli applied in the locus coeruleus and raphe nuclei of the cat. *J Physiol* 1993; 461:705–722.

Jones SL. Noxious heat-evoked *fos*-like immunoreactivity in the rat lumbar dorsal horn is inhibited by glutamate microinjections in the upper cervical spinal cord. *Brain Res* 1998; 788:337–340.

Kato M, Murakami S, Hirayama H, Hikino K. Recovery of postural control following chronic bilateral hemisections at different spinal cord levels in adult cats. *Exp Neurol* 1985; 90:350–364.

Kusmirek J. Lumbar but not cervical intrathecal DAMGO suppresses extrasegmental nociception in awake rats. *Brain Res* 1997; 767:375–379.

Lance JW. Symposium synopsis. In: Feldman RG, Young RR, Koella WP (Eds). *Spasticity: Disordered Motor Control.* Chicago: Year Book, 1980, pp 485–494.

LeBars D, Dickenson AH, Besson JC. Diffuse noxious inhibitory control (DNIC). I. Effects on dorsal horn convergent neurons in the rat. *Pain* 1979; 6:283–304.

Miller KE, Douglas VD, Richards,AB, Chandler MJ, Foreman RD. Propriospinal neurons in the C1–C2 spinal segments project to the L5–S1 segments of the rat spinal cord. *Brain Res Bull* 1999; 47:43–47.

Nathan PW, Smith MC. Clinico-anatomical correlation in anterolateral cordotomy. In: Bonica JJ, Liebeskind JC, Albé-Fessard DG (Eds). *Proceedings of the Second World Congress on Pain,* Advances in Pain Research and Therapy, Vol. 3. New York: Raven Press, 1979, pp 921–926.

Nogués M, Stålberg E. Electrodiagnostic findings in syringomyelia. *Muscle Nerve* 1999; 22:1653–1659.

Nogués M, Cammarota A, Solá C, Brown P. Propriospinal myoclonus in ischemic myelopathy secondary to a spinal dorsal arteriovenous fistula. *Mov Disord* 2000; 15:355–358.

Petro M, Antal M. Propriospinal afferent and efferent connections of the lateral and medial areas of the dorsal horn (laminae I–IV) in the rat lumbar spinal cord. *J Comp Neurol* 2000; 422:312–325.

Ritz LA, Friedman RM, Rhoton EL, Sparkes ML, Vierck Jr CJ. Lesions of cat sacrocaudal spinal cord: a minimally-disruptive model of injury. *J Neurotrauma* 1992; 9:219–230.

Saddiki-Traki F, Tremblay N, Dykes RW, et al. Differences between the tactile sensitivity on the anterior torso of normal individuals and those having suffered complete transection of the spinal cord. *Somatosens Mot Res* 1999; 16(4):391–401.

Sadrzadeh SM, Anderson DK, Panter, SS, Hallaway PE, Eaton SA. Hemoglobin potentiates central nervous system damage. *J Clin Invest* 1987; 79:662–664.

Sandkühler J, Stelzer B, Fu Q-G. Propriospinal neurones are involved in the descending inhibition of lumbar spinal dorsal horn neurones from the mid-brain. In: Bond MR, Charlton JE, Woolf CJ (Eds). *Proceedings of the VIth World Congress on Pain.* Amsterdam: Elsevier Science, 1991, pp 313–318.

Schmit BD, McKenna-Cole A, Rymer WZ. Flexor reflexes in chronic spinal cord injury triggered by imposed ankle rotation. *Muscle Nerve* 2000, 23:793–803.

Schwartzman RJ, Eidelberg E, Alexander GM, Yu J. Regional metabolic changes in the spinal cord related to spinal shock and later hyperreflexia in monkeys. *Ann Neurol* 1983; 14:33–37.

Scremin OU, O'Neal M, Scremin AME. Glucose utilization and reflex activity of the transected rat spinal cord. *Brain Res* 1990; 531:203–210.

Shimamura M, Kogure I, Wada S. Three types of reticular neurons involved in the spino-bulbo-spinal reflex of cats. *Brain Res* 1980; 186:99–113.

Szengothai J. Short propriospinal neurons and intrinsic connections of the spinal gray matter. *Acta Morphol Acad Sci Hung* 1951; 1:81–94.

Taylor JS, Friedman RF, Munson JB, Vierck Jr CJ. Stretch hyperreflexia of triceps surae muscles in the conscious cat after dorsolateral spinal lesions. *J Neurosci* 1997; 17:5004–5015.

Taylor J, Munson J, Vierck CJ. Effects of dorsolateral spinal lesions on stretch reflex threshold and stiffness in awake cats. *Eur J Neurosci* 1999; 11:363–368.

Viala D, Valin A, Buser P. Relationship between the "late reflex discharge" and locomotor movements in acute spinal cats and rabbits treated with DOPA. *Arch Ital Biol* 1974; 112:299–306.

Vierck CJ Jr. Can mechanisms of central pain syndromes be investigated in animal models? In: Casey KL (Ed). *Pain and Central Nervous System Disease: The Central Pain Syndromes.* New York: Raven Press, 1991, pp 129–141.

Vierck CJ, Light AR. Effects of combined hemotoxic and anterolateral spinal lesions on nociceptive sensitivity. *Pain* 1999; 83:447–457.

Vierck CJ Jr, Light AR. Allodynia and hyperalgesia within dermatomes caudal to a spinal cord injury in primates and rodents. *Prog Brain Res* 2000; 129:411–428.

Vierck CJ Jr, Greenspan JD, Ritz LA, Yeomans DC. The spinal pathways contributing to the ascending conduction and the descending modulation of pain sensations and reactions. In: Yaksh TL (Ed). *Spinal Systems of Afferent Processing*. New York: Plenum Press, 1986, pp 275–329.

Vierck CJ Jr, Greenspan JD, Ritz LA. Long term changes in purposive and reflexive responses to nociceptive stimulation in monkeys following anterolateral chordotomy. *J Neurosci* 1990; 10:2077–2095.

Vierck CJ Jr, Cannon RL, Fry G, Maixner WL. Characteristics of temporal summation of second pain sensations elicited by brief contact of glabrous skin by a preheated thermode. *J Neurophysiol* 1997; 78:991–1002.

Vierck CJ Jr, Siddall PJ, Yezierski RP. Pain following spinal cord injury: animal models and mechanistic studies. *Pain* 2000; 89:1–5.

Wall PD, Lidierth M, Hillman P. Brief and prolonged effects of Lissauer tract stimulation on dorsal horn cells. *Pain* 1999; 83:579–589.

Weng H-R, Lenz FA, Schwartz A, et al. Functional plasticity in primate somatosensory thalamus following chronic lesion of the ventral lateral spinal cord. *Neuroscience* 2000; 101:393–401.

Yezierski RP. Pain following spinal cord injury: the clinical problem and experimental studies. *Pain* 1996; 68(2):185–194.

Yezierski RP. Pain following spinal cord injury: pathophysiology and central mechanisms. *Prog Brain Res* 2000; 129:429–449.

Yezierski RP, Park S-H. The mechanosensitivity of spinal sensory neurons following intraspinal injections of quisqualic acid in the rat. *Neurosci Lett* 1993; 157:115–119.

Zehr EP, Stein RB. What functions do reflexes serve during human locomotion? *Prog Neurobiol* 1999; 58:185–203.

Correspondence to: Charles J. Vierck, Jr., PhD, Department of Neuroscience, University of Florida College of Medicine, Gainesville, FL 32510-0244, USA. Tel: 352-392-6555; Fax: 352-392-8513; email: vierck@mbi.ufl.edu.

Spinal Cord Injury Pain: Assessment, Mechanisms, Management. Progress in Pain Research and Management, Vol. 23, edited by Robert P. Yezierski and Kim J. Burchiel, IASP Press, Seattle, © 2002.

10

Physiological and Pharmacological Characterization of a Rat Model of Spinal Cord Injury Pain after Spinal Ischemia

Xiao-Jun Xu, Jing-Xia Hao,
and Zsuzsanna Wiesenfeld-Hallin

Department of Medical Laboratory Sciences and Technology, Division of Clinical Neurophysiology, Karolinska Institute, Huddinge University Hospital, Huddinge, Sweden

Photochemically induced spinal cord ischemia in rats is a useful model of spinal cord injury (SCI) pain. Following the ischemic insult, rats develop hypersensitivity to mechanical stimulation in the dermatome of the affected spinal segments. Rats that sustain prolonged ischemia and severe spinal tissue damage involving dorsal gray matter develop a chronic phase of pain-like behaviors characterized by a marked allodynia-like phenomenon to mechanical or cold stimulation in skin areas related to the injured spinal segment. Some rats also exhibit signs of spontaneous pain and dysesthesia. In some respects this chronic phase resembles SCI pain as seen in the clinic. This chapter reviews acute and chronic pain-like responses to spinal cord ischemia in rats, considers possible mechanisms of the allodynia-like phenomenon, and describes pharmacological studies conducted with this model with the aim of identifying effective new treatment strategies for chronic pain following SCI.

PHOTOCHEMICALLY INDUCED SPINAL CORD ISCHEMIA

The photochemical technique was used initially to generate vascular thrombosis and focal brain ischemia (Watson et al. 1988; Dietrich et al. 1996). The method involves a photochemical reaction between a photosensitizing dye circulating in the bloodstream and a focused light source, which produces large quantities of free oxygen that damages the endothelial layer of the vessel. The subsequent initiation of thrombosis leads to localized ischemia and tissue injury (Watson et al. 1988). In the early 1990s, in collaboration with Prof. Å. Seiger, we adapted this method at the Karolinska Institute to produce ischemic spinal cord injury (SCI). We showed that spinal cord ischemic injury can be produced with laser irradiation of the spinal cord after intravenous administration of erythrosin B in rats (Hao et al. 1991, 1992a). The extent of the injury can be controlled by varying the duration of laser irradiation, which produces variable and controllable reduction in spinal cord blood flow (Hao et al. 1991, 1994). Such graded degree of injury can be verified both morphologically and behaviorally (by examining motor performance).

While conducting these experiments, we soon realized that the vast majority of rats exhibited agitation to handling after irradiation, a phenomenon similar to that seen after intrathecal (i.t.) delivery of strychnine or bicuculline, drugs that block the action of the inhibitory transmitters glycine and GABA (Beyer et al. 1985; Yaksh 1989). Subsequent careful examination further revealed that some spinally injured rats also exhibited chronic pain-related behaviors. We have since conducted extensive morphological, behavioral, physiological, and pharmacological studies to characterize this rat model of SCI pain, with the aim of exploring the underlying neuronal mechanisms and seeking effective treatments for this difficult clinical condition (Tables I–III).

ACUTE PAIN-LIKE BEHAVIORS

Within 24 hours of spinal ischemia, about 90% of rats developed hypersensitivity to mechanical stimuli (Hao et al. 1991, 1992a) (Fig. 1). Acute allodynia affected animals both with mild and severe ischemic injury (Fig. 1). In rats with mild and transient ischemia, motor deficits were minor and we detected little or no morphological damage to the spinal cord using light microscopy (Hao et al. 1991, 1992a). Severe ischemia producing marked motor deficits and spinal injury caused similar acute hypersensitivity, often followed by a chronic phase of allodynia (Fig. 1).

The behavioral abnormalities during the acute phase primarily involved mechanical hypersensitivity to brushing and pressure (Table I). We detected some cold hypersensitivity, but found no increased responsiveness to heat stimuli. The allodynic area was usually fairly large, including both flanks and the whole back region (Fig. 2A). At the time of our initial experiments, using Sprague-Dawley rats, this acute phase of allodynia lasted less than a week.

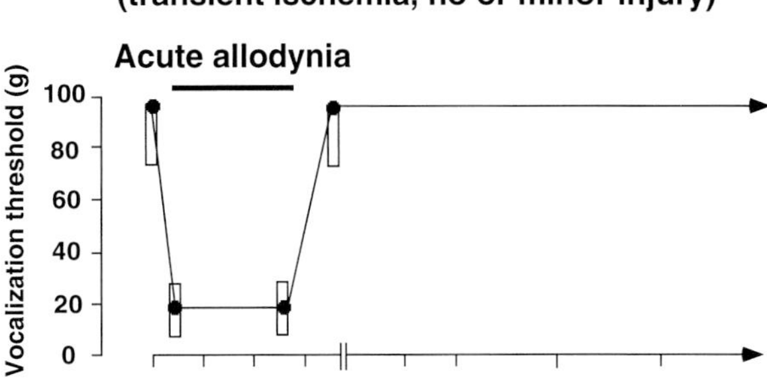

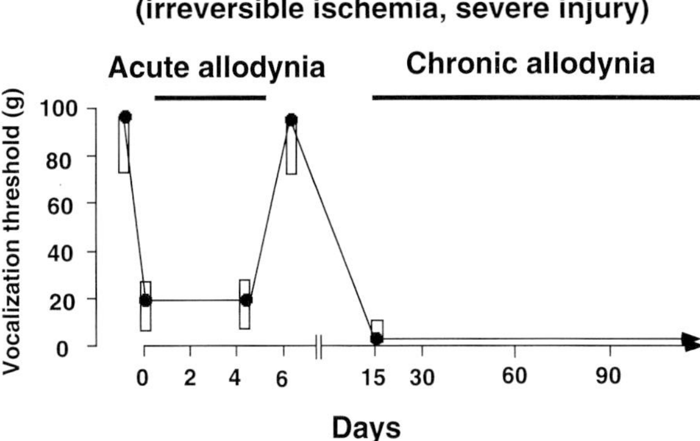

Fig. 1. Illustration of the time course of acute vs. chronic allodynia in spinally injured rats. The filled dots indicate the median vocalization threshold to mechanical stimulation with von Frey hairs, and the edge of the box indicates variability. The maximal stimulus intensity used is 95 g. Rats with transient ischemia that have no or minor injury to the spinal cord have only acute allodynia, whereas rats with severe injury have acute followed by chronic allodynia.

PHYSIOLOGICAL MECHANISMS OF ACUTE ALLODYNIA

We studied the neuronal mechanisms underlying acute allodynia by recording the activity of single wide-dynamic-range (WDR) neurons in the dorsal horn and comparing their response characteristics in normal and allodynic animals (Hao et al. 1992b,c). The receptive field sizes and background activity were similar in the two groups. In normal rats, electrical stimulation of the cutaneous receptive field that activated both A and C afferents evoked a biphasic response, with a short-latency A-fiber-mediated response and a long-latency C-fiber-mediated response. In contrast, in allodynic animals the stimulus evoked a prolonged burst, with no separation between A- and C-fiber-mediated activity. The overall response magnitude

Table I
Comparison of differences between acute and chronic allodynia-like behaviors in spinally injured rats

	Acute	Chronic
Laser irradiation	1–20 minutes	10–20 minutes
Morphological lesion	none or minor	severe
Occurrence	>90% of rats	about 50%
Latency to symptom	hours	14–60 days
Duration of pain	days	months to years
Area of allodynia	large	initially small
Vocalization threshold	usually >10 g	usually <1 g
Cold allodynia	present	prominent
Relief by baclofen	yes	no
AMPA antagonist	yes	no
NMDA antagonist	no	yes

Abbreviations: AMPA = α-amino-3-hydroxy-5-methyl-4-isoxazolepropionic acid; NMDA = *N*-methyl-D-aspartate.

was increased in the allodynic rats, and in particular the A-fiber-mediated response was much greater than normal.

The response of the WDR neurons to mechanical stimulation with calibrated von Frey hairs in normal animals increased linearly with increased pressure. In contrast, the response in the allodynic animals had a significantly lower threshold than normal, and the response magnitude increased

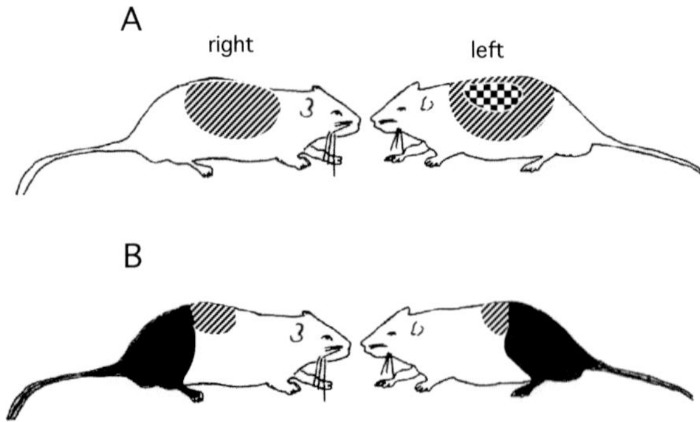

Fig. 2. Illustration of the typical allodynic area in a rat with (A) acute and (B) chronic allodynia. In panel A, the injury is at spinal segment T11–T12, whereas in panel B the injury is at L4–L5. Note the widespread allodynia in the acute stage; this rat had a vocalization threshold of 27.5 g at the shaded area and 13.0 g at the checkerboard-patterned area. In the rat with chronic allodynia, the initial allodynic area is more discrete. This rat had a vocalization threshold of 0.6 g at the shaded area. The area with sensory loss, autotomy, and excessive scratching is shown in black.

exponentially, reaching maximal discharge frequencies at lower stimulus intensities than in normal animals. Interestingly, the responses of the WDR cells to noxious thermal stimuli applied with a CO_2 laser were indistinguishable in the normal and allodynic animals. Thus, the responses of single neurons clearly reflected the rats' behavioral abnormalities, where we observed allodynia to mechanical stimulation, but not to heat.

Systemic or i.t. administration of low doses of baclofen, a GABA-B-receptor agonist, was effective in alleviating acute allodynia in behavioral experiments, whereas muscimol, a GABA-A-receptor agonist, had no effect (Hao et al. 1991). Similarly, baclofen also normalized the response pattern of dorsal horn WDR neurons recorded from allodynic rats to electrical stimulation and increased the response threshold of these neurons to mechanical stimulation (Hao et al. 1992c), indicating an important role for activation of the GABA-B receptors in controlling the expression of mechanical allodynia. We have subsequently demonstrated that the number of dorsal horn neurons exhibiting GABA-like immunoreactivity was temporarily decreased after spinal cord ischemia when acute allodynia was observed (Zhang et al. 1994).

Taken together, these results indicate that in this model acute allodynia is predominantly mediated by abnormal input from myelinated afferents. The sensory abnormality is primarily due to disinhibition, involving a loss of GABAergic presynaptic control of input via myelinated afferents (Game and Lodge 1975; Price et al. 1987), which may result from a high susceptibility of GABAergic neurons to excitotoxicity (Sloper et al. 1986). The results suggest that inhibition not only of input mediated by nociceptors (Melzack and Wall 1965), but also of large-diameter afferents, is important for maintaining normal sensory function.

CHARACTERIZATION OF CHRONIC ALLODYNIA-LIKE BEHAVIOR IN SPINALLY INJURED RATS

A chronic syndrome, with more severe sensory abnormalities than in the acute condition, develops in about 50% of animals following severe, irreversible spinal cord ischemia (Xu et al. 1992a; Fig. 1). The main symptoms of this chronic syndrome are strong mechanical and cold allodynia referred to relatively small skin areas located in the transitional zone (Fig. 2B). The allodynic area tends to increase in size with time, but remains at the level of injury. A minority of these animals display autotomy and excessive scratching in areas with sensory loss, which may indicate phantom pain or dysesthesia (Fig. 2B).

Chronic allodynia developed only in animals with severe SCI, although the extent of injury was quite variable. Injury to dorsal gray matter appeared to be essential for the development of allodynia. There was usually a variable delay of 2–8 weeks from the time of injury to the appearance of chronic allodynia. Once present, allodynia usually persisted without signs of remission for the entire lifetime of the animal. Interestingly, not all rats with a similar degree of SCI developed chronic allodynia, possibly due to different levels of endogenous inhibitory control exerted by opioids. Thus, systemic or i.t. naloxone or selective μ-opioid-receptor antagonists could trigger the appearance of typical allodynia-like responses in nonallodynic, spinally injured rats (Hao et al. 1998). Finally, the level of endogenous inhibitory control may be set by anti-opioid systems, such as the neuropeptide cholecystokinin (CCK) (Xu et al. 1994, 2001).

PHYSIOLOGICAL MECHANISMS OF CHRONIC ALLODYNIA-LIKE BEHAVIORS

To determine the neuronal basis of the observed allodynia-like behaviors, we conducted electrophysiological studies examining the responses of single units recorded from the thoracic and lumbar dorsal horn in spinal-cord-injured allodynic rats. We found several abnormalities in the distribution and response characteristics of dorsal horn neurons in these rats. In allodynic rats, 17% of the units had no receptive field, compared to 0% in control rats (Fig. 3). Most of these units were located at or close to the lesioned spinal segment, and they discharged spontaneously at high frequencies. Furthermore, allodynic rats showed a significant change in the relative proportion of low-threshold (LT), WDR, and high-threshold (HT) neurons recorded, the proportion being 16%, 63%, and 21%, respectively, in allodynic rats vs. 43%, 36%, and 21% in controls (Fig. 3). The rate of ongoing activity of HT neurons was significantly higher in allodynic rats (Fig. 4), and these rats showed increased neuronal responses to mechanical stimulation (Fig. 5). WDR neurons in allodynic rats responded with higher discharge rates to innocuous mechanical stimuli compared to control rats, and the percentage of WDR and HT neurons showing afterdischarges to noxious pinch increased significantly in allodynic rats. Finally, the proportion of WDR and HT neurons responding to innocuous cold stimulation increased from 53% and 25%, respectively, in control rats to 91% and 83% in allodynic animals (Fig. 6).

These results show that spinally injured rats exhibiting chronic pain-related behaviors have numerous abnormalities in the response pattern of dorsal horn interneurons rostral to the lesion; some of these abnormalities correlate with the behavioral manifestations of allodynia. It is likely that the area adjacent to the lesion contains a zone clustered with spontaneously active neurons, some of which lack an identifiable receptive field, indicating deafferentation. These discharges may give rise to painful sensations and/or dysesthesias that are referred to the body area caudal to the lesion and that manifest as autotomy and excessive scratching. Furthermore, neurons located up to three segments rostral to the lesion developed mechanical and cold hypersensitivity, which may account for the allodynia to mechanical and cold stimuli.

PHARMACOLOGY OF THE ACUTE AND CHRONIC ALLODYNIA-LIKE BEHAVIORS

Systemic or i.t. morphine appeared to have a limited effect on acute allodynia (Table II), probably due to a reduction in the density of μ-opioid receptors in the spinal cord after ischemia (Hao et al. 1991; Yu et al. 1999). In contrast, during chronic allodynia i.t. morphine was effective, but systemic morphine was not (Yu et al. 1998a; Table III). The potency of the antiallodynic effect of i.t. morphine was, however, reduced compared to its

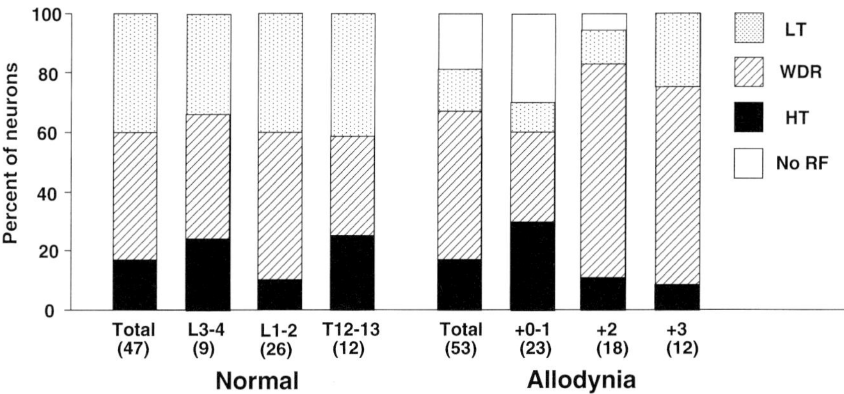

Fig. 3. Distribution of different types of neurons recorded in normal or allodynic rats. The percentage of low-threshold (LT, gray), wide-dynamic-range (WDR, hatched), high-threshold (HT, black) neurons, or neurons with no receptive field (no RF, open) is shown for both the total sample and different recording levels. The number of neurons in each group is shown below each column. The χ^2 test indicated a significant overall difference between normal and allodynic rats regarding the distribution of LT, WDR, and HT neurons ($\chi^2 = 6.5$, df = 2, $P < 0.05$). There was also a significant difference in the distribution in recording level for allodynic rats ($\chi^2 = 13.9$, df = 6, $P < 0.05$), but not for normal rats ($\chi^2 = 4.1$, df = 4, $P > 0.05$).

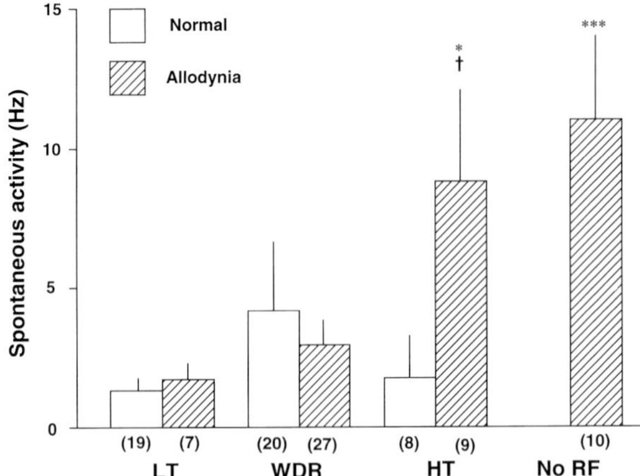

Fig. 4. The average rate of ongoing activity recorded from normal (open columns) or allodynic (shaded columns) rats classified by cell types (see Fig. 3 legend for abbreviations). The data are expressed as mean ± SEM, and the number of neurons is indicated below each column. ANOVA indicated a significant difference for the rate of activity among different types of neurons in allodynic rats ($F_{3,47} = 8.3$, $P < 0.001$), but not in normal rats ($F_{2,43} = 1.8$, $P > 0.05$). The post hoc test was with the Fisher protected least significant difference (PLSD) test, * = $P < 0.05$ and *** = $P < 0.001$ compared to either LT or WDR neurons in the allodynic rats; † = $P < 0.05$ compared to HT neurons in normal rats with unpaired t test.

antinociceptive effect, and spinally injured rats rapidly developed tolerance to its effects (Yu et al. 1998b). Thus, morphine is clearly less potent in alleviating central pain-like behaviors in spinally injured rats. Although spinal

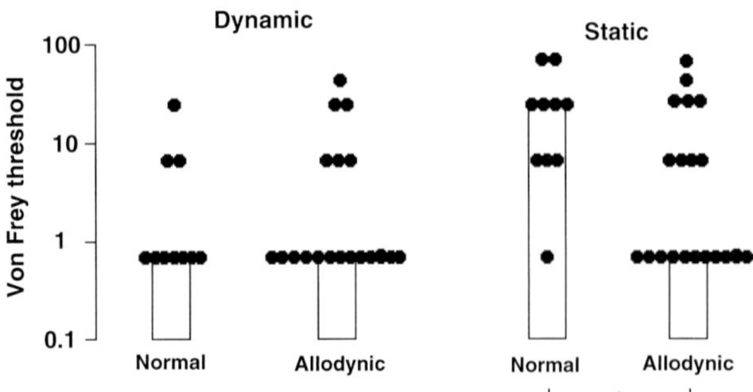

Fig. 5. Response threshold of individual dorsal horn WDR neurons to dynamic or static mechanical stimulation. Each neuron is represented by a circle, and the median value for each group is indicated by the height of the columns. * = $P < 0.05$ between normal and allodynic rats with the Mann-Whitney U-test. The intensity of stimulation (measured in micronewtons) is illustrated on a log scale on the y axis.

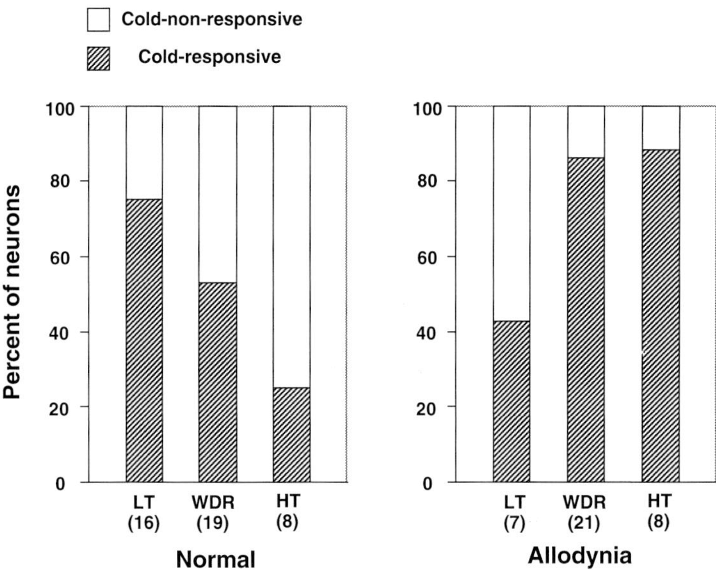

Fig. 6. Percentage of neurons responding (hatched) or not responding (open) to cold in normal or allodynic rats. The number of neurons included in each group is indicated under each column. The χ^2 test indicated that the frequency of cold-responsive cells was significantly increased for both WDR and HT neurons in allodynic rats compared to normal rats ($\chi^2 = 5.2$ and 6.4, df = 1, $P < 0.05$).

Table II
Summary of the effect of drugs on acute allodynia in spinally injured rats

Drug	Systemic	Intrathecal
Morphine	–	±
Clonidine	n.t.	±
R-PIA	n.t.	±
Baclofen	+	+
Muscimol	–	–
Tocainide	+	n.t.
NBQX (AMPA antagonist)	+	n.t.
MK-801 (NMDA antagonist)	+	n.t.

Symbols: + = good effect; ± = limited effect; – = no effect; n.t. = not tested. R-PIA = R-phenyl-isopropyladenosine; other abbreviations are as in Table I.

Table III
Summary of the effect of systemically or intrathecally applied drugs on chronic allodynia in spinally injured rats

Drug	Systemic	Intrathecal
Morphine	– (sedation)	+
CI977, U50488 (κ-opioid agonists)	– (sedation)	– (increased pain)
DAMGO (μ-opioid agonist)	n.t.	+
DPDPE (δ-opioid agonist)	n.t.	+
Clonidine	– (sedation)	+
R-PIA	n.t.	+
Baclofen	–	n.t.
Muscimol, THIP (GABA-A agonist)	–	n.t.
Tocainide, mexiletine	+	n.t.
Carbamazepine	– (sedation)	n.t.
Gabapentin	+	n.t.
Diazepam	– (sedation)	n.t.
NBQX (AMPA antagonist)	– (sedation)	n.t.
MK-801, CGS 19755 (NMDA antagonist)	± (stereotypic behavior)	–
Dextromethorphan (NMDA antagonist)	+ (hyperactivity)	n.t.
L-NAME (NOS inhibitor)	+ (hypertension)	–
7-Nitroindazole (nNOS inhibitor)	+	n.t.
CP-96,345 (NK-1-receptor antagonist)	–	n.t.
CI-988 (CCK-2-receptor antagonist)	+	–
Galanin, neuropeptide Y (inhibitory peptides)	n.t.	–

Note: Side effects are listed in parentheses. Symbols are as in Table II.
Abbreviations: AMPA = α-amino-3-hydroxy-5-methyl-4-isoxazolepropionic acid; CCK-2 = cholecystokinin-2; GABA = γ-aminobutyric acid; NK1 = neurokinin-1; NMDA = *N*-methyl-D-aspartate; nNOS = neuronal nitric oxide synthase; NOS = nitric oxide synthase; R-PIA = R-phenyl-isopropyladenosine.

administration of morphine is effective initially, it is unclear whether monotherapy with i.t. morphine could provide long-term relief in patients with SCI pain because the development of tolerance may present a problem.

Adenosine is an endogenous purine nucleotide with extensive distribution intra- and extracellularly in the nervous system (Fredholm 1995). Activation of spinal adenosine A1 receptors produces antinociception (Sawynok et al. 1998). In a recent series of studies we have shown that i.t. R-phenylisopropyladenosine (R-PIA), an adenosine A1-receptor agonist, effectively alleviated chronic allodynia in spinally injured rats (Sjölund et al. 1998; von Heijne et al. 1998). The antiallodynic effect of R-PIA persisted considerably longer than that of morphine upon repetitive administration (von Heijne et al. 1998), and there was a synergistic interaction between R-PIA and morphine (von Heijne et al. 2000). Interestingly, i.t. R-PIA appears to have only limited effect against acute allodynia (von Heijne et al. 2001), possibly indicating that the strong antiallodynic effect of R-PIA against chronic allodynia depends on structural and/or functional plasticity after injury.

Several other differences are interesting in the pharmacology of acute vs. chronic allodynia. While baclofen is effective in treating acute allodynia (Hao et al. 1991), chronic allodynia does not respond to this drug (Xu et al. 1992a). This finding suggests that GABAergic mechanisms may not play such an important role in the pathophysiology of chronic allodynia as they do immediately after injury. Moreover, acute allodynia is sensitive to blockade of the α-amino-3-hydroxy-5-methyl-4-isoxazolepropionic acid (AMPA) receptor for glutamate (Xu et al. 1993), but not to blockade of the *N*-methyl-D-aspartate (NMDA) receptor, whereas the opposite is true for chronic allodynia (Hao and Xu 1996). Again, this finding suggests the involvement of central nervous system plasticity in the mechanisms of chronic pain, in which the activation of NMDA receptors may play an important role. Systemically applied local anesthetics, such as tocainide and mexiletine, are effective in both the acute and chronic conditions (Hao et al. 1992d; Xu et al. 1992a,b).

CONCLUSIONS

Significant advances have been made in the development of clinically relevant animal models for pain following SCI (Yezierski 1996; Yezierski et al. 1998). Although critics may argue that no ground-breaking developments in treatment have resulted from studies based on animal models, it is undeniable that we have gained considerable knowledge regarding the physiology and pharmacology of this pain condition. The accumulation of such knowledge will undoubtedly contribute to the quest to effectively treat SCI pain, a task that has largely eluded pain management so far.

ACKNOWLEDGMENTS

The studies conducted by the authors were supported by the Swedish Medical Research Council (07913 and 12168) and by Astra Pain Control. We would like to thank our collaborators throughout the years for their contributions.

REFERENCES

Beyer C, Roberts LA, Komisaruk BR. Hyperalgesia induced by altered glycinergic activity at the spinal cord. *Life Sci* 1985; 37:875–882.

Dietrich WD, Ginsberg MD, Busto R, Watson BD. Photochemically induced cortical infarction in the rat. 1. Time course of hemodynamic consequences. *J Cereb Blood Flow Metab* 1996; 6:184–194.

Fredholm BB. Adenosine receptors in the central nervous system. *Physiol Sci* 1995; 10:122–128.

Game CJA, Lodge D. The pharmacology of the inhibition of dorsal horn neurones by impulses in myelinated cutaneous afferents in the cat. *Exp Brain Res* 1975; 23:75–84.

Hao J-X, Xu X-J. Treatment of chronic allodynia-like symptoms in rats after spinal cord injury: effects of systemic glutamate receptor antagonists. *Pain* 1996; 66:279–286.

Hao J-X, Xu X-J, Aldskogius H, Seiger Å, Wiesenfeld-Hallin Z. Allodynia-like effect in rat after ischemic spinal cord injury photochemically induced by laser irradiation. *Pain* 1991; 45:175–185.

Hao J-X, Xu X-J, Aldskogius H, Seiger Å, Wiesenfeld-Hallin Z. Photochemically induced transient spinal ischemia induces behavioral hypersensitivity to mechanical and cold, but not to noxious heat, stimuli in the rat. *Exp Neurol* 1992a; 118:187–194.

Hao J-X, Xu X-J, Yu Y-X, Seiger Å, Wiesenfeld-Hallin Z. Transient spinal cord ischemia induces temporary hypersensitivity of dorsal horn wide dynamic range neurons to myelinated, but not unmyelinated, fiber input. *J Neurophysiol* 1992b; 68:384–391.

Hao J-X, Xu X-J, Yu Y-X, Seiger Å, Wiesenfeld-Hallin Z. Baclofen reverses the hypersensitivity of dorsal horn wide dynamic range neurons to mechanical stimulation after transient spinal cord ischemia: implications for a tonic GABAergic inhibitory control of myelinated fiber input. *J Neurophysiol* 1992c; 68:392–396.

Hao J-X, Yu Y-X, Seiger Å, Wiesenfeld-Hallin Z. Systemic tocainide relieves mechanical hypersensitivity and normalizes the responses of hypersensitive dorsal horn wide dynamic range neurons after transient spinal cord ischemia in rats. *Exp Brain Res* 1992d; 91:229–235.

Hao J-X, Herregodts P, Lind G, et al. Photochemically induced spinal cord ischaemia in rats: assessment of blood flow by laser Doppler flowmetry. *Acta Physiol Scand* 1994; 151:209–215.

Hao J-X, Yu W, Xu X-J. Evidence that spinal endogenous opioidergic systems control the expression of chronic pain-related behaviors in spinally injured rats. *Exp Brain Res* 1998; 118:259–268.

Melzack R, Wall PD. Pain mechanisms: a new theory. *Science* 1965; 150:971–979.

Price GW, Kelly JS, Bowery NG. The location of GABA-B receptor binding sites in mammalian spinal cord. *Synapse* 1987; 1:530–538.

Sawynok J. Adenosine receptor activation and nociception. *Eur J Pharmacol* 1998; 347:1–11.

Sjölund K-F, von Heijne M, Hao J-X, et al. Intrathecal administration of R-phenylisopropyladenosine reduces presumed pain behavior in a rat model of central pain. *Neurosci Lett* 1998; 243:89–92.

Sloper JJ, Johnson P, Powell TPS. Selective degeneration of interneurons in the motor cortex of infant monkeys following controlled hypoxia: a possible cause of epilepsy. *Brain Res* 1986; 198:204–209.

von Heijne M, Hao J-X, Yu W, et al. Tolerance to the anti-allodynic effect of intrathecal R-phenylisopropyladenosine in a rat model of ischemic spinal cord lesion: lack of cross-tolerance with morphine. *Anesth Analg* 1998; 87:1367–1371.

von Heijne M, Hao J-X, Sollevi A, Xu X-J, Wiesenfeld-Hallin Z. Marked enhancement of anti-allodynic effect by combined intrathecal administration of the adenosine A-1 receptor agonist R-phenylisopropyladenosine and morphine in a rat model of central pain. *Acta Anaesthesiol Scand* 2000; 44:665–671.

von Heijne M, Hao J-X, Sollevi A, Xu X-J. Effects of intrathecal morphine, baclofen, clonidine and R-PIA on the acute allodynia-like behaviors after spinal cord ischemia in rats. *Eur J Pain* 2001; 5:1–10.

Watson BD, Dietrich WD, Prado R, Green BA. Photochemically induced vascular thrombosis (photothrombosis): central nervous system consequences and clinical possibilities. In: Gorio T (Ed). *Neural Development and Regeneration.* Berlin: Springer-Verlag, 1988, pp 507–524.

Xu X-J, Hao J-X, Aldskogius H, Seiger Å, Wiesenfeld-Hallin Z. Chronic pain-related syndrome in rats after ischemic spinal cord lesion: a possible animal model for pain in patients with spinal cord injury. *Pain* 1992a; 48:279–290.

Xu X-J, Hao J-X, Seiger Å, et al. Systemic mexiletine relieves chronic allodynia-like symptoms in rats with ischemic spinal cord injury. *Anesth Analg* 1992b; 74:649–652.

Xu X-J, Hao J-X, Seiger Å, Wiesenfeld-Hallin Z. Systemic excitatory amino acid receptor antagonist of the α-amino-3-hydroxy-5-methyl-4-isoxazolepropionic acid (AMPA) receptor, but not of *N*-methyl-D-aspartate (NMDA) receptor, relieves the mechanical hypersensitivity in rats after transient spinal cord ischemia. *J Pharmacol Exp Ther* 1993; 267:140–144.

Xu X-J, Hao J-X, Seiger Å, et al. Chronic pain-related behaviors in spinally injured rats: evidence for functional alterations of the endogenous cholecystokinin and opioid systems. *Pain* 1994; 56:271–277.

Xu X-J, Alster P, Wu W-P, Hao J-X, Wiesenfeld-Hallin Z. Increased level of cholecystokinin in the cerebrospinofluid is associated with the chronic pain-like behavior in spinally injured rats. *Peptides* 2001; in press.

Yaksh TL. Behavioral and autonomic correlates of the tactile evoked allodynia produced by spinal glycine inhibition: effect of modulatory receptor systems and excitatory amino acid antagonists. *Pain* 1989; 37:111–123.

Yezierski RP. Pain following spinal cord injury: the clinical problem and experimental studies. *Pain* 1996; 68:185–194.

Yezierski RP, Liu S, Ruenes GL, Kajander KL, Brewer K. Behavioral and morphological characteristics of a central pain model. *Pain* 1998; 75:141–155.

Yu W, Hao J-X, Xu X-J, Wiesenfeld-Hallin Z. Comparison of the anti-allodynic and antinociceptive effects of systemic, intrathecal and intracerebroventricular morphine in a rat model of central neuropathic pain. *Eur J Pain* 1997a; 1:17–29.

Yu W, Hao J-X, Xu X-J, Wiesenfeld-Hallin Z. The development of morphine tolerance and dependence in rats with chronic pain. *Brain Res* 1997b; 756:141–146.

Yu W, Hao J-X, Xu X-J, et al. Spinal cord ischemia reduces mu-opioid receptors in rats: correlation with morphine insensitivity. *Neuroreport* 1999; 10:87–91.

Zhang A-L, Hao J-X, Seiger Å, Xu X-J, et al. Decreased GABA immunoreactivity in spinal cord dorsal horn neurons after transient spinal cord ischemia in the rat. *Brain Res* 1994; 656:187–190.

Correspondence to: Zsuzsanna Wiesenfeld-Hallin, PhD, Division of Clinical Neurophysiology, Huddinge University Hospital, S-141 86 Huddinge, Sweden. Tel: 46-8-58587085; Fax: 46-8-58587050; email: zsuzsanna.wiesenfeld-hallin@neurophys.hs.sll.se.

Spinal Cord Injury Pain: Assessment, Mechanisms, Management. Progress in Pain Research and Management, Vol. 23, edited by Robert P. Yezierski and Kim J. Burchiel, IASP Press, Seattle, © 2002.

11

Pharmacology of Chronic Pain after Spinal Cord Injury: Novel Acute and Chronic Intervention Strategies

Claire E. Hulsebosch

Department of Anatomy and Neurosciences, The University of Texas Medical Branch at Galveston, Galveston, Texas, USA

Spinal cord injury (SCI) results in a devastating loss of function below the level of the lesion in which motor recovery varies. Chronic central pain syndromes develop in most cases (Christensen et al. 1996; Christensen and Hulsebosch 1997), usually within several months to years after injury (Richards et al. 1980; Christensen and Hulsebosch 1997; Rintala et al. 1998).

The development of various pain states after SCI continues to present a significant challenge to physicians. Embarrassingly little is known concerning the pathophysiology of pain following trauma to the central nervous system. Clearly, the attention devoted to the treatment of chronic central pain (CCP) is under-represented in terms of research, and thus treatment options are limited. The definition of central pain, according to the International Association for the Society of Pain, is "pain initiated or caused by a primary lesion or dysfunction in the central nervous system" (Merskey and Bogduk 1994). Chronic pain is pain that persists beyond the period of wound healing (Bonica 1953). Thus, CCP after SCI is pain that persists long after the initial injury site has healed.

Central pain syndromes and dysesthesias (an unpleasant abnormal sensation that may or may not be painful) can be divided into two broad categories based on the dependency of the pain to peripheral stimuli: (1) persistent pain, which occurs independently of peripheral stimuli, has spontaneous onset, increases intermittently, and is described as numbness, burning, cutting, piercing, or electrical sensations (Davidoff and Roth 1991); and (2) peripherally evoked pain, which occurs in response to either normally non-noxious or noxious stimuli. Where the peripherally evoked pain occurs in response to normally non-noxious stimuli, the pain state developed is considered to be allodynia, and where it occurs as an exaggerated response to normally noxious stimuli, the pain state developed is termed hyperalgesia. A subtle but important definition is the state of increased sensitivity to stimulation that may or may not be painful, which is considered to be hyperesthesia (Merskey and Bogduk 1994). CCP syndromes are characterized by persistent pain (Vierck 1991; Lenz et al. 1994), with concomitant changes in peripheral somatosensory responses (Vierck 1991).

The failure of therapeutic strategies to treat dysesthesias of SCI is due in large part to the difficulty in modeling such injuries in mammalian models with similar pathophysiological mechanisms to the clinical symptomology. In this regard, several challenges face the pain investigator. For example, it is not possible to directly and objectively test the presence of pain in animal subjects, and therefore it is impossible to test an animal model for a subjective, emotional experience. A fundamental question is, "Can central pain syndromes be investigated in animal models?" Animal models have the advantage that objective and unemotional responses can be measured reliably. In CCP syndromes, the assumption is that the level of activity of some portion of the nociceptive pathway changes, and that such changes persist chronically and alter thresholds to stimuli from the periphery (Vierck 1991). The peripheral changes are clinically characterized by "over-reactivity" to somatosensory stimulation, a classical clinical feature that has been associated with central pain syndromes (Head and Holmes 1911; Riddoch 1938). Therefore, when reflex threshold changes are accompanied by changes in whole-body posturing to avoid or stop further stimuli (avoidance posturing) and by vocalizations, writhing, and other behaviors consistent with the experience of a nociceptive stimulus, then the model becomes better validated for pain studies. As an illustration, we empirically determined that after hemisection, all animals became exquisitely sensitive to handling, would turn and bite the handler, vocalize, and writhe, and would continue to evoke behaviors consistent with the experience of nociceptive stimuli for weeks to months after surgery (until sacrifice). Based on these observations, we carefully characterized the development of both mechanical and thermal hyperalgesia and allodynia that persisted for months and suggested the value of this model for chronic pain studies (Christensen et al. 1996).

To our knowledge, there are only a few models of chronic pain after SCI: (1) The ischemic model, in which an intravascular photochemical reaction occludes blood vessels, thereby producing spinal cord ischemia that results in a band of mechanical allodynia on the trunk at the lesion site (the "girdle" region) (Hao et al. 1991; Xu et al. 1992; see Chapter 10). (2) Unilateral quisqualate injection, which results in overgrooming and mechanical allodynia (Yezierski et al. 1998). (3) The spinal contusion model, which results in changes in spontaneous activity (Mills and Hulsebosch 2001) as well as thermal and mechanical allodynia (Siddall et al. 1995; Hulsebosch et al. 2000c; see Chapter 12), and demonstrates "girdle" allodynia (Hulsebosch et al. 2000c). (4) Anterolateral lesions in monkeys and rats, which produce overgrooming and mechanical allodynia (Ovelmen-Levitt et al. 1995; Vierck and Light 2000). (5) Hemisection in rats, which results in bilateral "girdle" allodynia, thermal and mechanical allodynia (Christensen and Hulsebosch 1997), and alterations in spontaneous activity (Hulsebosch et al. 2000b). This chapter focuses on the use of the hemisection model and the contusion model for the study of chronic pain.

The spinal contusion rat model has the obvious advantage of presenting the pathophysiological profile that most closely approximates the clinical pathophysiology after SCI and is thus thought to be the most clinically relevant model (Bunge et al. 1993; Bunge 1994; Hulsebosch et al. 2000c). However, this model cannot be used to study below-level pain because the animal's hindlimbs are profoundly affected by the lesion. However, it is excellent for the analysis of at-level or above-level pain using evoked stimuli. In addition, the contusion lesion, in which the damage to the spinal cord is progressive, has some variability in the extent to which specific neural circuits and spinal tracts are involved over time. Spontaneous measures of animal activity may offer an opportunity to indirectly measure spontaneous components of CCP in this model. By contrast, the hemisection model offers other advantages: (1) all animals develop allodynia, as compared to only 44% of spinal ischemic rats (Hao et al. 1991; Xu et al. 1992), 50% of quisqualate rats (Abraham et al. 2001), and 80% of spinal contused rats (Mills et al. 2001a); (2) both spontaneous and evoked components of central neuropathic pain occur; (3) the model offers surgical ease and reproducibility, and no weight drop apparatus is needed; (4) "twice-daily" bladder expressions are not required for up to 2 weeks; (5) no accompanying bladder infections occur; and (6) hindlimb recovery is better, allowing for spontaneous and evoked testing. The most important of these advantages is that all of the animals develop allodynia (Mills et al. 2001a). In both of these models, (1) we avoid the variability of vascular-dependent lesions; (2) we can examine responses to a variety of somatic stimuli because pharmacological interventions may selectively alter one quality of sensation (e.g., thermal and not tactile); (3) we can assess changes in locomotion using the open field test scale (Basso et al. 1995) to reveal alterations in motor control that might affect the nociceptive tests; and (4) we can investigate spontaneous changes in behavior.

The data presented in this chapter are taken from the forelimbs in both hemisection and contusion SCI models and thus represent above-level SCI pain (Siddall et al. 2000; see Chapter 2). The hindlimbs were too compromised in the SCI contusion model to produce meaningful data and so comparisons in hindlimb data could not be made for the contusion model versus the hemisection models. For all the spinal hemisection data, the hindlimbs behaved similarly to the forelimbs, but the responses were different in absolute values (see Fig. 3, bottom graphs). We previously reported a persistent state of hyperexcitability in dorsal horn neurons recorded below the level of injury in the hemisection models both ipsilateral and contralateral to the injured side (Christensen and Hulsebosch 1997). Thus, membrane properties of wide-dynamic-range neurons are changed permanently and dramatically by SCI. Intrathecally applied compounds can be used to modulate specific membrane or ion receptor populations and thus alter membrane excitability. By examining the effects of pharmacological interventions on the mechanical and thermal allodynia that develops after hemisection (Christensen et al. 1996) and contusion injuries to the cord (Siddall et al. 1995; Hulsebosch et al. 2000c; Mills et al. 2000), we can begin to characterize the behavioral and electrophysiological properties of receptor/ion channel agonists and antagonists, thus paving the way for more efficacious clinical treatments for CCP.

Fig. 1 presents a schematic diagram of a projection neuron, such as a spinothalamic tract neuron, showing the input from primary afferents, interneurons, and descending systems (Dougherty and Staats 1999). In all three of these systems, putative transmitter substances can either facilitate or inhibit the excitability of the projection neurons by causing receptor-mediated alterations in membrane potential. Equally important in projection neuron excitability is the presence of ion channels and a variety of second-messenger and transsynaptic signaling cascades. Thus, by pharmacological interventions using antagonists of excitatory receptors or agonists of inhibitory receptors, or by appropriate manipulation of ion channel permeability, it is possible to alter the hyperexcitability that is present after SCI. The accompanying figures show examples of pharmacological interventions with the rat spinal hemisection model after development of mechanical and thermal allodynia. Fig. 2 displays inhibition of peptide primary afferent transmission by a calcitonin gene-related peptide (CGRP) antagonist (after Bennett et al. 2000a), and shows inhibition of excitatory amino acid (EAA) receptors by an *N*-methyl-D-aspartate (NMDA) antagonist and a non-NMDA antagonist (after Bennett et al. 2000b). Fig. 3 demonstrates application of exogenous catecholamines (Hains et al. 2000a) or serotonin (Hains et al. 2000b), which are both found in descending inputs that provide tonic inhibition on projection neurons, and Fig. 4 shows examples of evoked and spontaneous allodynia

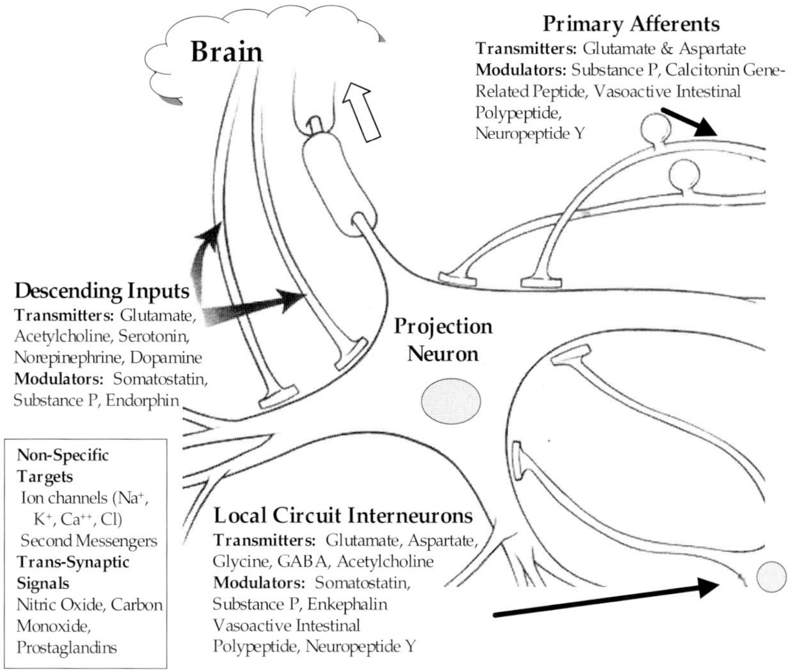

Fig. 1. Diagram (after Dougherty and Staats 1999) representing the inputs onto projection neurons in nociceptive circuits. This diagram illustrates the variety of receptors and ion channels that contribute to the membrane potential and to substances that can alter membrane potentials at points along the cell surface. Projection neurons are known to become hyperexcitable after SCI, and consequently the resting membrane potential is closer to threshold. An understanding of the receptors and ion channels involved in the hyperexcitability allows appropriate therapeutic interventions such as intrathecal delivery of antagonists or agonists to the "foci" that are hyperexcitable, which can return the membrane potential (and consequently the nociceptive circuit) to preinjury potentials and lessen hyperexcitability. Site-specific deliveries of such compounds could be targeted to centers of hyperexcitability in the cord or to the ventral posterior lateral thalamus or higher centers, to attenuate the sensation of pain after SCI.

behaviors with gabapentin, an L-type calcium channel blocker (Hulsebosch et al. 2000b). Behavioral measures of both mechanical and thermal allodynia are described in detail elsewhere (Christensen et al. 1996); they include frequency or latency measures of brisk paw withdrawals, accompanied by active attention of the rat to the stimulus by head turning and biting attacks on the stimulus, and by whole-body escape posturing to avoid a repeated stimulus. The inclusion of these complex behaviors excludes simple hyperreflexia, which is a segmental response (Woolf 1984; Vincler et al. 2001). Briefly, all the above interventions attenuated both mechanical and thermal allodynia, with the exception of the NMDA antagonist D-AP5 and the

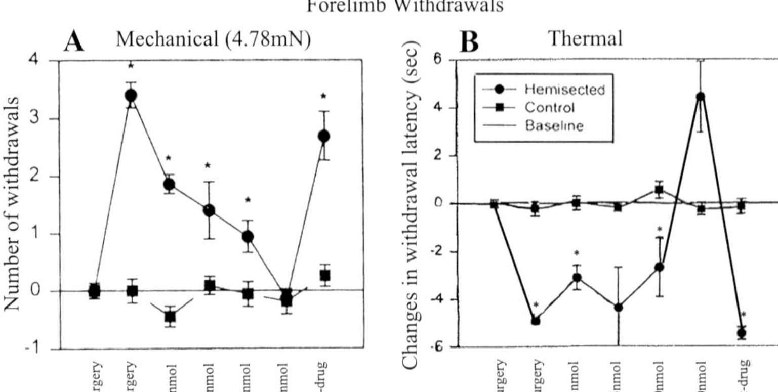

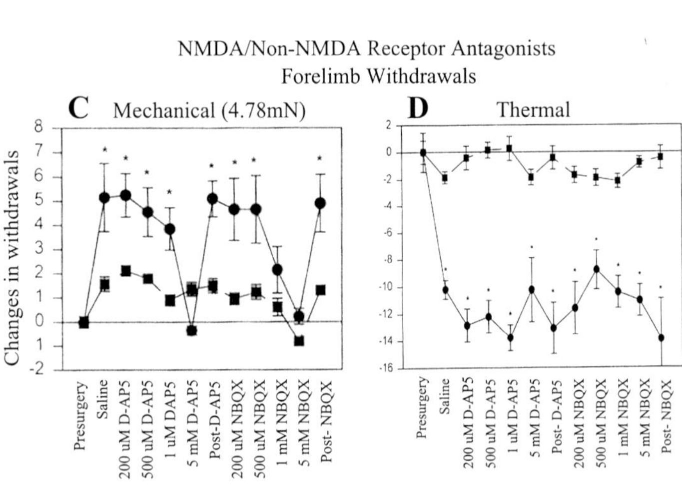

Fig. 2. Data from behavioral experiments are presented in two general groupings showing forelimb withdrawals of T13 spinal hemisected rats and sham surgery control rats 30 or more days after surgery, in response to intrathecal application of compounds that are antagonists to excitatory transmitters or peptides onto projection neurons. These substances should aid in attenuating the supersensitivity to evoked stimuli, i.e., the mechanical and thermal allodynia that develops after SCI. These compounds, which act differentially to attenuate allodynia, were the CGRP antagonist $CGRP_{8\text{-}37}$, which binds to the CGRP receptor but does not activate its cytoplasmic domain; D-AP5, a competitive antagonist for the NMDA receptor; and NBQX sodium salt, a water-soluble, competitive AMPA/kainate receptor antagonist. $CGRP_{8\text{-}37}$ attenuates both mechanical and thermal allodynia, while D-AP5 and NBQX attenuate only mechanical allodynia in dose-response-related manners. T13 spinal hemisection data are plotted as solid circles, sham surgery data are plotted as solid squares. Data are shown as means ± standard deviations. Asterisks indicate statistically significant differences compared to presurgical behavior ($P < 0.05$).

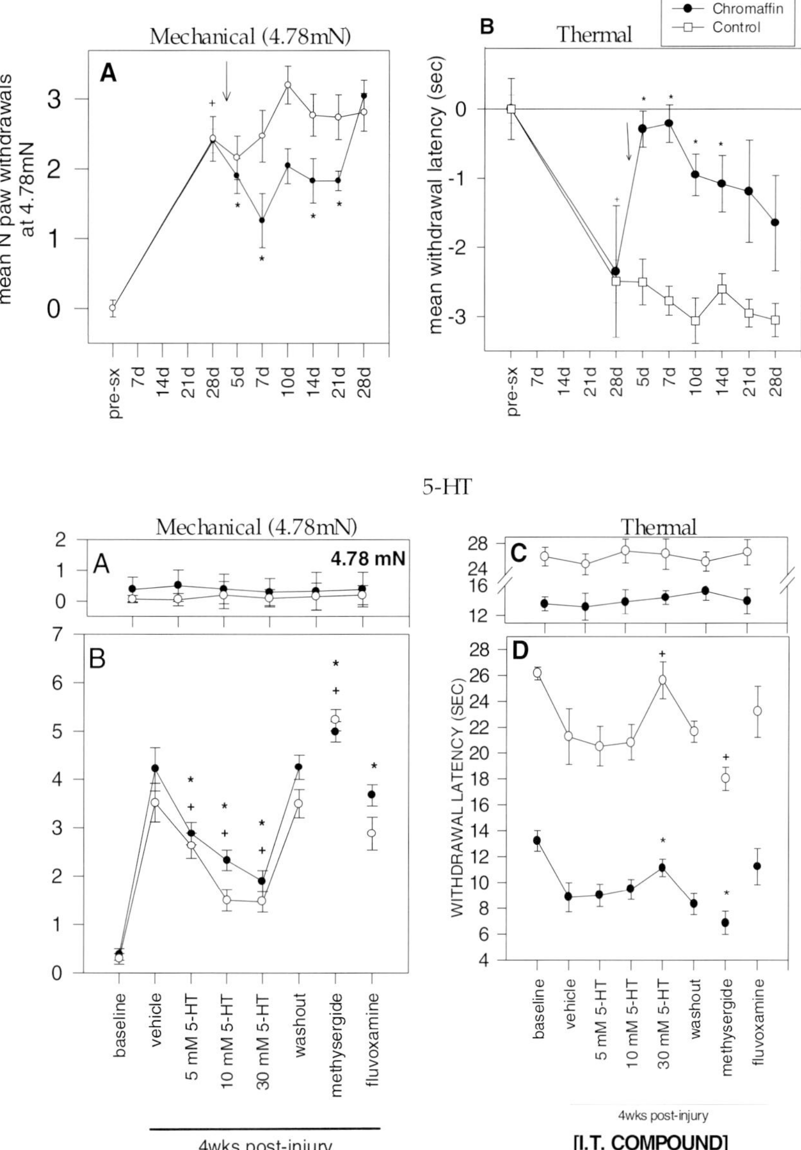

Fig. 3. Data from behavioral experiments are presented in two general groupings for T13 spinal hemisected rats and sham surgery control rats 30 or more days after surgery, in response to intrathecal application of compounds that are known inhibitory transmitters of descending systems onto projection neurons. *(Legend continues on next page.)*

non-NMDA antagonist NBQX, which attenuated mechanical but not thermal allodynia.

The acute pathophysiology of SCI includes a sudden increase in EAA concentrations (Faden and Simon 1988; Liu et al. 1991; Tator and Fehlings 1991), and any intervention that is given acutely may alter the conditions that set up central sensitization. Thus, another promising approach to CCP treatment is to use agents in the acute stages of SCI that prevent hyperexcitability from developing in the chronic stages. Researchers are beginning to understand specific EAA subtype activation in the pathophysiology of excitotoxicity in SCI (Faden and Simon 1988; Liu et al. 1991; Tator and Fehlings 1991). The three major classes of EAA receptors are (1) ionotropic non-NMDA receptors (selectively sensitive to adenosine monophosphate [AMPA] or kainate); (2) ionotropic NMDA receptors (selectively activated by NMDA, and by a voltage-gated ionic channel for cations); and (3) metabotropic receptors that are coupled to G-protein second messenger systems that play direct roles in maintained hyperexcitability or central sensitization, a proposed mechanism for CCP (Coderre 1992; Willis 1993; Woolf 1983; Chen and Huang 1992; Ma and Woolf 1995). NMDA, non-NMDA, and metabotropic EAA receptors are clearly major components of the SCI sequelae. Following injections of NMDA (Liu et. al. 1997), AMPA, and quisqualate, which is an agonist of both the metabotropic (Schoepp et al. 1990; McDonald and Schoepp 1992) and AMPA glutamate receptors (Monaghan et al. 1989; Koh et al. 1990; Mayer and Miller 1990), histopathological analysis in rodent SCI models demonstrated the formation of spinal cavities similar to those

---

(Continued from previous page.) These substances not only should aid in attenuating the supersensitivity to evoked stimuli, but also may inhibit the dysesthetic, persistent component of the chronic pain syndrome. Shown are responses to evoked stimuli, i.e., the mechanical and thermal allodynia that develops after SCI. The compounds used were catecholamines, produced by adrenal chromaffin cell transplants; and 5-HT, delivered by indwelling intrathecal catheters that terminate at the lesioned segment. These compounds attenuate both mechanical and thermal allodynia. The top row shows T13 spinal hemisection data with adrenal chromaffin cell transplants plotted as solid circles and T13 spinal hemisection data with skeletal muscle cell transplants (controls) plotted as open squares or circles. The bottom row shows sham surgery control data plotted in graphs A and C where the closed circles represent the forelimb responses and the open circles represent the hindlimb responses. T13 spinal hemisection data are plotted in graphs B and C, where the closed circles represent the forelimb responses and the open circles represent the hindlimb responses. Graphs A–D of 5-HT data support the development of denervation supersensitivity to 5-HT after chronic SCI. Data are shown as means ± standard deviations. In the top row, plus signs indicate statistically significant differences compared to presurgical behavior, and asterisks indicate statistically significant differences compared to presurgical behavior. In the bottom row, asterisks (forelimbs) or plus signs (hindlimbs) indicate statistically significant differences compared to postsurgical behavior ($P < 0.05$).

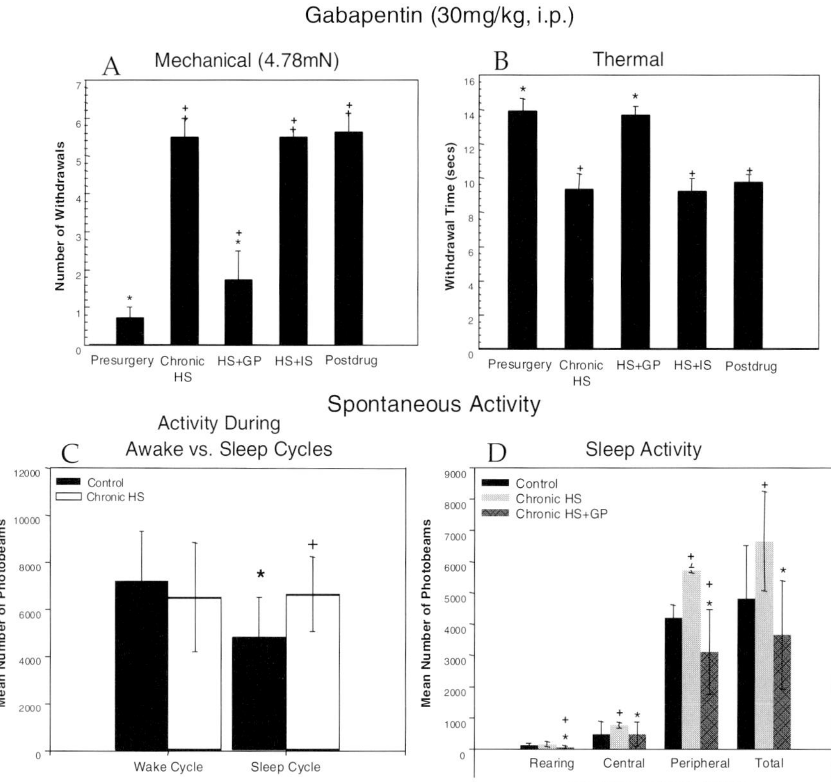

Fig. 4. Injections of 30 mg/kg gabapentin (GP) were given by intraperitoneal injection after which von Frey stimulation (4.78 mN strength) and thermal heat stimulation were given to the glabrous surface of both forelimbs and hindlimbs before surgery, and again at least 30 days after spinal hemisection surgery (Chronic HS). Shown in the top row are the number of paw withdrawal responses for the forelimbs that are accompanied by complex behaviors consistent with the receipt of a noxious stimulus (A) or the withdrawal time after radiant heat exposure (B). The responses are statistically significant (plus signs) after Chronic HS compared to presurgery ($P < 0.05$) and that gabapentin treatment returned the behaviors to presurgical conditions (HS + GP), whereas the inactive isomer (HS + IS) had no effect. The gabapentin effect lasted for up to 6 hours, after which the behavior returned to values similar to Chronic HS (Postdrug). As an alternate test, because spinally injured patients do not sleep well (Rintala et al. 1998), we measured spontaneous activity by testing the rats' movements within a flexfield system using the San Diego Activity boxes (see Mills and Hulsebosch 2001). The Chronic HS group demonstrated no significant difference in activity in recordings made during the first 2 hours of the wake and the first 2 hours of the sleep cycle, indicating abnormally increased activity in the sleep cycle when compared to the sham surgery control group. Treatment with GP attenuated the increased activity in the sleep cycle and returned the values to sham surgery control values (plus signs indicate statistically significant data compared to control, and asterisks indicate statistically significant data compared to Chronic HS, where $P < 0.05$).

observed in SCI patients (Liu et al. 1997; Yezierski et al. 1998; Mills et al. 2002). In another study, blockade of the NMDA receptor with dextrorphan reduced the release of amino acids following spinal cord ischemia (Rokkas et al. 1994); however, no behavioral or histologic assessment was done. In addition, intraspinal or intrathecal injections of NBQX, an AMPA/kainate antagonist, after SCI resulted in a significant decrease in neural damage that was correlated to the dose: the greater the dose, the less tissue was damaged. The increased rescue of neural tissue corresponded to both increases in locomotor function and decreases in abnormal somatosensory scores (Wrathall et al. 1994, 1996). Thus, reduction in tissue loss after SCI improves outcome. In fact, studies that included dermatome CCP measures (Hao et al. 1991; Xu et al. 1992; Christensen and Hulsebosch 1997; Liu et al. 1997; Yezierski et al. 1998; Hulsebosch et al. 2000c) indicate that the larger the lesion, the greater the area of "at-level" allodynia. Thus, interventions that reduce lesion size should improve functional outcome.

In the case of SCI-induced central sensitization, an increase in the activation state of EAA receptors may occur by a variety of mechanisms. The EAA receptor state may change, receptor upregulation may occur, and spinal circuit reorganization may contribute to increased excitability, any of which can contribute to hyperexcitability of STT cells. For example, activation of the NMDA and AMPA/kainate receptors by EAA produces membrane depolarization, resulting in an increased open channel state that is followed by Ca^{2+} influx intracellularly. EAA-mediated activation of the metabotropic glutamate receptor and the increased intracellular Ca^{2+} levels activate phospholipase C, which catalyzes the production of protein kinase C through the metabotropic glutamate receptor and the inositol triphosphate

---

Fig. 5. Shown in the top panel is the proportion of spared tissue 1 hour after a spinal contusion injury compared to 60 days after a contusion produced by the NYU device, with a 10-g, 12.5-mm drop that produces a moderate level of injury. Considerable white and grey matter is spared after 1 hour, and a characteristic central necrotic core is present. By 60 days after the injury, the lesion has progressively spread so that only a thin rim of white matter is spared. The progressive spread of the contusion lesion in the rat model parallels human SCI pathology and has been well described for many decades. Recently the progression has been attributed to the glutamate/aspartate spread of excitotoxicity, which results in a progressive secondary cell loss and sets up the conditions for persistent hyperexcitability (Hulsebosch et al. 2000a). Thus, early interventions that inhibit glutamate receptor action may be useful in rescuing cells at risk of secondary injury and may attenuate chronic pain syndromes. The bottom panel demonstrates three such interventions injected in the epicenter of the contusion injury beginning 15 minutes after injury over a 25-minute interval. The substances tested were AIDA (a selective metabotropic glutamate receptor [mGluR] group 1 antagonist), LY 367385 (a selective mGluR1 antagonist), and MPEP (a selective mGluR5 antagonist). Representative photomicrographs of spinal cord cross-sections from each treatment group were stained with Luxol blue and cresyl violet at sections 2.4 mm rostral (left),

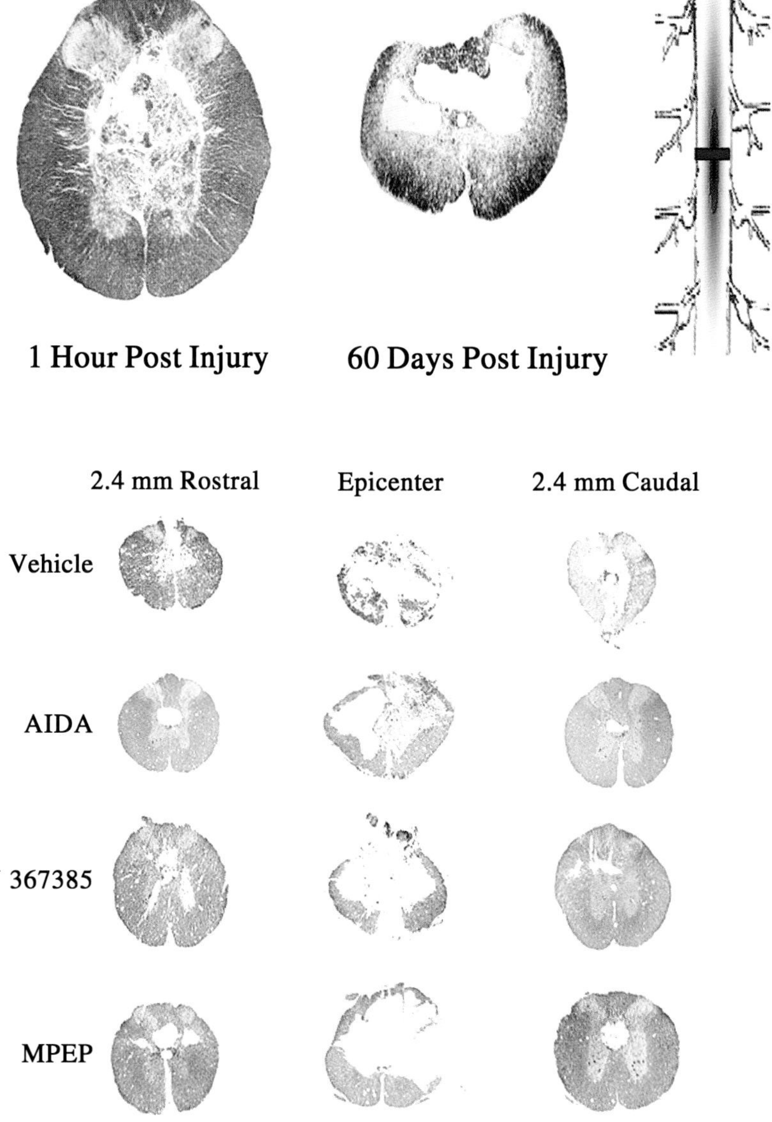

2.4 mm caudal (right), and through the epicenter of injury (middle) for groups treated with artificial cerebrospinal fluid (ACSF) (row 1), 200 nmol AIDA (row 2), LY 367385 (row 3), and 250 nmol MPEP (row 4). All sections at the epicenter are reduced in diameter and are characterized by a small rim of white matter sparing. A rostrocaudal gradient of reduced tissue loss is evident in all treatment groups. However, AIDA, LY 367385, and MPEP treatments increased the amount of spared white matter at the epicenter compared to the vehicle-treated group.

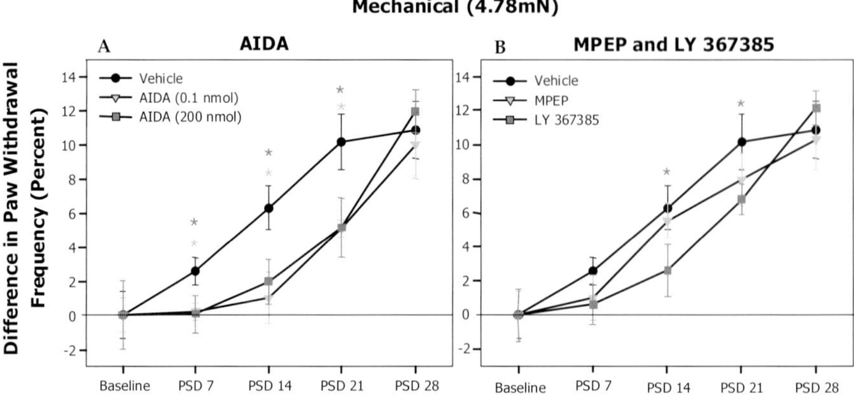

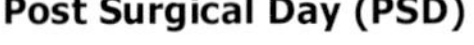

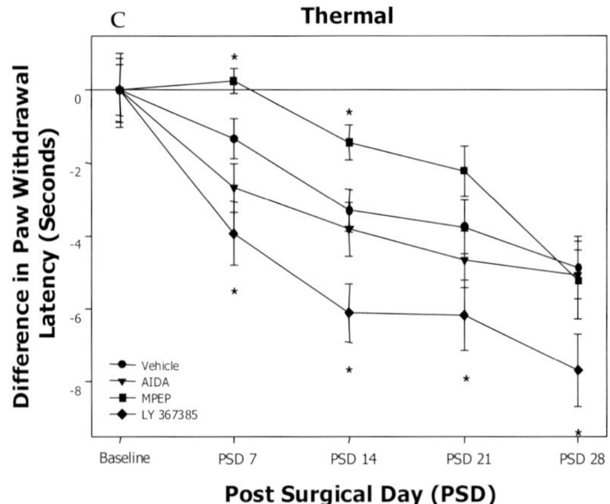

Fig. 6. Forelimb paw withdrawal responses to mechanical (A and B) and thermal (C) stimuli in the groups treated with AIDA, LY 367385, and MPEP compared to the vehicle-treated group described in Fig. 5. A single treatment with AIDA or LY 367385 attenuated the development of mechanical allodynia through day 21 but MPEP had no effect. In the thermal behavioral tests, LY 367385 exacerbated the thermal allodynia while MPEP attenuated the development of thermal allodynia and AIDA had no effect. An asterisk indicates a statistically significant difference ($P < 0.05$) compared to the vehicle-treated group.

pathway. Many subsequent pathways are proposed to sustain the NMDA-receptor ion channel open state and allow increased calcium influx, which may result in maintained hyperexcitability or, if intracellular levels of Ca^{2+} are high, in cell death (Chen and Huang 1992; Coderre 1992). In the case of sustained central sensitization, such as occurs in CCP after SCI (Christensen and Hulsebosch 1997), the changes in secondary intracellular pathways are presumably sustained and maintain the hyperexcitability of the cell, including both metabotropic and ionotropic glutamate receptors (Coderre 1992; Ma and Woolf 1995; Mills et al. 2002). Thus, the basis for neural excitability in CCP is shifted from ionotropic receptors to an activation or sensitization mediated by a combination of ionotropic and metabotropic glutamate receptors. Interventions targeted at ionotropic and metabotropic glutamate receptors should be developed to prevent CCP. However, many blockers of the NMDA receptor are psychotomimetic, and therefore unsuitable for use in a conscious patient, as might be the situation following SCI. Substantial problems are encountered with high-affinity, noncompetitive inhibitors such as MK-801, while the least detrimental effects are found with blockers of the glycine binding site, the polyamine binding site, and glutamate release blockers (Muir and Lees 1995). Therefore, for maximum clinical relevance, we recommend studies of competitive blockers that offer a broad therapeutic window of efficacy. Acute interventions in a rat spinal contusion model of agents that block the metabotropic glutamate receptor, which is the only G-protein-coupled EAA receptor (the rest being ionotropic receptors), are demonstrated in Figs. 5 and 6 (after Mills and Hulsebosch 2001; Mills et al. 2001, 2002).

In summary, CCP appears to be a product of a variety of mechanisms that contribute to a sustained and altered hyperexcitability of neurons in nociceptive circuits (Loeser et al. 1968; Melzack and Loeser 1978). Only two decades ago, most treating physicians viewed CCP after SCI as a clinical entity suitable for psychiatric referrals, the general dogma being that there was no pathophysiological substrate that could adequately account for the persistent pain syndromes. We now have animal models, promising therapeutic interventions that may be successfully applied clinically, and well-designed clinical trials for management of CCP after SCI based on data gleaned from animal studies (Hulsebosch et al. 2000c; see Chapter 22). As neurosurgeons become more aggressive with intervention techniques, we can design preclinical animal trials for acute intervention in the SCI patient population to rescue tissue in the lesion area and to prevent the development of CCP. Finally, with the advent of molecular interventions, it is now possible to think of genetically engineered cellular delivery systems for eventual clinical use (Hains et al. 2001). Thus, in terms of incremental functional recovery in patients by advances in therapeutic interventions (Hulsebosch et al. 2000a), chronic central pain may well be among the first of the SCI-related dysfunctions to be "cured."

ACKNOWLEDGMENTS

The author wishes to acknowledge the valuable contributions of collaborators of the UTMB SCI consortium and the excellent administrative assistance of our Program Coordinator, Ms. Debbie Pavlu. This work was supported by the Kent Waldrep National Paralysis Foundation, the RGK Foundation, the Spinal Cord Research Foundation, Mission Connect of The Institute for Rehabilitation and Research (TIRR), and NIH grants NS 11255 and NS 39161.

REFERENCES

Abraham KE, McGinty JF, Brewer KL. The role of kainic acid/AMPA and metabotropic glutamate receptors in the regulation of opioid mRNA expression and the onset of pain-related behavior following excitotoxic spinal cord injury. *Neuroscience* 2001; 104:863–874.

Basso M, Beattie MS, Bresnahan JC. A sensitive and reliable locomotor rating scale for open field testing in rats. *J Neurotrauma* 1995; 12:1–21.

Bennett AD, Chastain KM, Hulsebosch CE. Alleviation of mechanical and thermal allodynia by $CGRP_{8\text{-}37}$ in a rodent model of chronic central pain. *Pain* 2000a; 86:163–175.

Bennett AD, Everhart AW, Hulsebosch CE. Intrathecal administration of an NMDA or a non-NMDA receptor antagonist reduces mechanical but not thermal allodynia in a rodent model of chronic central pain after spinal cord injury. *Brain Res* 2000b; 859:72–82.

Bonica JJ. Central pain. In: Bonica JJ (Ed). *The Management of Pain*. Philadelphia: Lea and Febiger, 1953, pp 1014–1022.

Bunge RP. Clinical implications of recent advances in neurotrauma research. In: Salzman SK, Faden AI (Eds). *The Neurobiology of Central Nervous System Trauma*. New York: Oxford University Press, 1994, pp 328–339.

Bunge RP, Puckett WR, Becerra JL, Marcillo A, Quencer RM. Observations on the pathology of human spinal cord injury. A review and classification of 22 new cases with details from a case of chronic cord compression with extensive focal demyelination. In: Seil FJ (Ed). *Advances in Neurology*, Vol. 59. New York: Raven Press, 1993, pp 75–89.

Chen L, Huang LY. Protein kinase C reduces Mg^{2+} block of NMDA-receptor channels as a mechanism of modulation. *Nature* 1992; 356:521–523.

Christensen MD, Hulsebosch CE. Chronic central pain after spinal cord injury. *J Neurotrauma* 1997; 14:517–537.

Christensen MD, Everhart AW, Pickelmann JT, Hulsebosch CE. Mechanical and thermal allodynia in chronic central pain following spinal cord injury. *Pain* 1996; 68:97–107.

Coderre TJ. Contribution of protein kinase C to central sensitization and persistent pain following tissue injury. *Neurosci Lett* 1992; 140:181–184.

Davidoff G, Roth EJ. Clinical characteristics of central (dysesthetic) pain in spinal cord injury patients. In: Casey KL (Ed). *Pain and Central Nervous System Disease: The Central Pain Syndromes*. New York: Raven Press, 1991, pp 77–83.

Dougherty PM, Staats PS. Intrathecal drug therapy for chronic pain: from basic science to clinical practice. *Anesthesiology* 1999; 9:1891.

Faden AI, Simon RP. A potential role for excitotoxins in the pathophysiology of spinal cord injury. *Ann Neurol* 1988; 23:623–626.

Hains BC, Chastain KM, Everhart AW, McAdoo DJ, Hulsebosch CE. Transplants of adrenal medullary chromaffin cells reduce forelimb and hindlimb allodynia in a rodent model of chronic central pain after spinal cord hemisection injury. *Exp Neurol* 2000a; 164:426–437.

Hains BC, Johnson KA, Eaton MJ, Hulsebosch CE. Transplantation of immortalized serotonergic neurons attenuates chronic central pain after spinal hemisection injury in rat. *Neurosci Abstracts* 2000b; 26:2303.

Hains BC, Johnson KM, McAdoo DJ, Eaton MJ, Hulsebosch CE. Engraftment of immortalized serotonergic neurons enhances locomotion function and attenuates chronic central pain following spinal hemisection injury in the rat. *Exp Neurol* 2001; 171:361–378.

Hao JX, Xu XJ, Aldskogious H, Seiger A, Wiesenfeld-Hallin Z. Allodynia-like effects in rat after ischemic spinal cord injury photochemically induced by laser irradiation. *Pain* 1991; 45:175–185.

Head H, Holmes G. Sensory disturbances from cerebral lesions. *Brain* 1911; 34:102–254.

Hulsebosch CE, Hains BC, Waldrep K, Young W. Bridging the gap: from discovery to clinical trials in spinal cord injury. *J Neurotrauma* 2000a; 17:1117–1128.

Hulsebosch CE, Taylor CP, Everhart A, Gonzalez FP. Gabapentin alleviates spontaneous measures of chronic central pain after spinal cord injury. *Neurosci Abstracts* 2000b; 26:1216.

Hulsebosch CE, Xu G-Y, Perez-Polo JR, et al. Rodent model of chronic central pain after spinal cord contusion injury and effects of gabapentin. *J Neurotrauma* 2000c; 17:1205–1217.

Koh JY, Goldberg MP, Hartley DM, Choi DW. Non-NMDA receptor-mediated neurotoxicity in cortical cultures. *J Neurosci* 1990; 10:693–705.

Lenz FA, Kwan HC, Martin R, et al. Characteristics of somatotopic organization and spontaneous neuronal activity in the region of the thalamic principal sensory nucleus in patients with spinal cord transection. *J Neurophysiol* 1994; 72:1570–1587.

Liu D, Thangnipon W, McAdoo DJ. Excitatory amino acids rise to toxic levels upon impact injury to the rat spinal cord. *Brain Res* 1991; 547:344–348.

Liu S, Ruenes GL, Yezierski RP. NMDA and non-NMDA receptor antagonists protect against excitotoxic injury in the rat spinal cord. *Brain Res* 1997; 756:160–167.

Loeser JD, Ward AA Jr, White LE Jr. Chronic deafferentation of human spinal cord neurons. *J Neurosurg* 1968; 29:48–50.

Ma Q-P, Woolf CJ. Noxious stimuli induce an *N*-methyl-D-aspartate receptor-dependent hypersensitivity of the flexion withdrawal reflex to touch: implications for the treatment of mechanical allodynia. *Pain* 1995; 61:383–390.

Mayer ML, Miller RJ. Excitatory amino acid receptors, second messengers and regulation of intracellular Ca^{2+} in mammalian neurons. *TIPS* 1990; 11:254–260.

McDonald JW, Schoepp DD. The metabotropic excitatory amino acid receptor agonist 1S, 3R-ACPD selectively potentiates *N*-methyl-D-aspartate-induced brain injury. *Eur J Pharmacol* 1992; 215:353–354.

Melzack R, Loeser JD. Phantom body pain in paraplegics: evidence for a central "pattern generating mechanism" for pain. *Pain* 1978; 4:195–210.

Merskey H, Bogduk (Eds). *Classification of Chronic Pain: Descriptions of Chronic Pain Syndromes and Definitions of Pain Terms*, 2nd ed. Seattle: IASP Press, 1994.

Mills CD, Hulsebosch CE. Changes in exploratory behavior as a measure of chronic central pain following spinal cord injury. *J Neurotrauma* 2001; 18:1091–1105.

Mills CD, Xu GY, Johnson KM, McAdoo DJ, Hulsebosch CE. AIDA reduces glutamate release and attenuates mechanical allodynia after spinal cord injury. *Neuroreport* 2000; 11:3067–3070.

Mills CD, Hains BC, Johnson KM, Hulsebosch CE. Strain and model differences in behavioral outcomes following spinal cord injury in rat. *J Neurotrauma* 2001; 18:743–756.

Mills CD, Johnson KM, Unabia GC, Hulsebosch CE. Group I metabotropic glutamate receptors in spinal cord injury: roles in neuroprotection and the development of chronic central pain. *J Neurotrauma* 2002; 19:23–42.

Monaghan DT, Bridges RJ, Cotman CW. The excitatory amino acid receptors: their classes, pharmacology and distinct properties in the function of the central nervous systems. *Annu Rev Pharmacol* 1989; 29:365–402.

Muir KW, Lees KR. Clinical experience with excitatory amino acid antagonist drugs. *Stroke* 1995; 26:503–513.

Ovelmen-Levitt J, Gorecki J, Nguyen K, Iskandar B, Nashold B. Spontaneous and evoked dysesthesias observed in the rat after spinal cordotomies. *Sterotact Funct Neurosurg* 1995; 65:157–160.

Richards JS, Meredith RL, Nepomuceno C, Fine PR, Bennett G. Psycho-social aspects of chronic pain in spinal cord injury. *Pain* 1980; 8:355–366.

Riddoch G. The clinical features of central pain. *Lancet* 1938; 34:1093–1098, 1150–1156, 1205–1209.

Rintala DH, Loubser PG, Castro J, Hart KA, Fuhrer MJ. Chronic pain in a community-based sample of men with spinal cord injury: prevalence, severity, and relationship with impairment, disability, handicap, and subjective well-being. *Arch Phys Med Rehabil* 1998; 79:604–614.

Rokkas CK, Helfrich LR, Lobner DC, Choi DW, Kouchoukos NT. Dextrorphan inhibits the release of excitatory amino acids during spinal cord ischemia. *Ann Thorac Surg* 1994; 58: 312–320.

Schoepp D, Bockaert J, Sladeczek F. Pharmacological and functional characteristics of metabotropic excitatory amino acid receptors. *TIPS* 1990; 11:508–515.

Siddall P, Xu CL, Cousins M. Allodynia following traumatic spinal cord injury in the rat. *Neuroreport* 1995; 6:1241–1244.

Siddall P, Yezierski R, Loeser J. Pain following spinal cord injury: clinical features, prevalence, and taxonomy. *IASP Newsletter* 2000; 3:3–7.

Tator CH, Fehlings MG. Review of the secondary injury theory of acute spinal cord trauma with emphasis on vascular mechanisms. *J Neurosurg* 1991; 75:15–26.

Vierck CJ Jr. Can mechanisms of central pain syndromes be investigated in animal models? In: Casey KL (Ed). *Pain and Central Nervous System Disease: The Central Pain Syndromes.* New York: Raven Press, 1991, pp 129–141.

Vierck CJ Jr, Light AR. Allodynia and hyperalgesia within dermatomes caudal to a spinal cord injury in primates and rodents. In: Sandkühler J, Bromm B, Gebhart G (Eds). *Nervous System Plasticity and Chronic Pain,* Vol. 129. Amsterdam: Elsevier, 2000, pp 411–428.

Vincler M, Maixner W, Vierck Jr CJ, Light AR. Effects of systemic morphine on escape latency and a hindlimb reflex response in the rat. *J Pain* 2001; 2:83–90.

Willis WD Jr. Central sensitization and plasticity following intense noxious stimulation. In: Moyer EA, Raybould HE (Eds.). *Basic and Clinical Aspects of Chronic Abdominal Pain.* Amsterdam: Elsevier Science, 1993, pp 201–217.

Woolf CJ. Long term alterations in the excitability of the flexion reflex produced by peripheral tissue injury in the chronic decerebrate rat. *Pain* 1984; 18:325–343.

Wrathall JR, Choinière D, Teng YD. Dose-dependent reduction of tissue loss and functional impairment after spinal cord trauma with the AMPA/kainate antagonist NBQX. *J Neurosci* 1994; 14:6598–6607.

Wrathall JR, Teng YD, Choinière D. Amelioration of functional deficits from spinal cord trauma with systemically administered NBQX, an antagonist of non-*N*-methyl-D-aspartate receptors. *Exp Neurol* 1996; 137:119–126.

Xu X-J, Hao J-X, Aldskogious H, Seiger A, Wiesenfeld-Hallin Z. Chronic pain-related syndrome in rats after ischemic spinal cord lesion: a possible animal model for pain in patients with spinal cord injury. *Pain* 1992; 48:279–290.

Yezierski RP, Liu S, Ruenes GL, Kajander KJ, Brewer KL. Excitotoxic spinal cord injury–behavioral and morphological characteristics of a central pain model. *Pain* 1998; 75:141–155.

Correspondence to: Claire E. Hulsebosch, PhD, Department of Anatomy and Neurosciences, University of Texas Medical Branch at Galveston, 301 University Boulevard, Galveston, TX 77555-1043, USA. Tel: 409-772-2939; Fax: 409-772-3222; email: cehulseb@utmb.edu.

Spinal Cord Injury Pain: Assessment, Mechanisms, Management. Progress in Pain Research and Management, Vol. 23, edited by Robert P. Yezierski and Kim J. Burchiel, IASP Press, Seattle, © 2002.

12

Plasticity in Supraspinal Viscerosomatic Convergent Neurons following Chronic Spinal Cord Injury

Richard D. Johnson and Charles H. Hubscher

Department of Physiological Sciences and the McKnight Brain Institute, University of Florida, Gainesville, Florida, USA

Chronic spinal cord injury (SCI) results in a number of sensory disturbances at or below the level of the lesion. Disturbances at the transitional zone between intact and anesthetic or dysesthetic dermatomes often leads to tactile allodynia in humans (Boivie 1992; Eide et al. 1996; Beric 1997; Defrin et al. 2001; Chapter 4, this volume). Such allodynia is usually associated with an incomplete cord injury (Boivie 1992; Chapter 2, this volume). Several studies in rats have demonstrated, using a variety of incomplete chronic lesions, that allodynia-like pain behavior is correlated with electrophysiological evidence of abnormal responses in spinal dorsal horn neurons near the lesion site (Xu et al 1992; Yezierski and Park 1993, 1996; Christensen and Hulsebosch 1997).

We have recently developed an electrophysiological animal model for investigating the effects of chronic SCI on responses in supraspinal neurons (Hubscher and Johnson 1999a,b). In rats, this model combines single-unit recording of medullary viscerosomatic convergent neurons in the anesthetized animal with assessment of functional behavior in the same animal. The neurons we studied are in the medullary reticular formation (MRF), specifically within a stereotactically identified portion of the nucleus reticularis gigantocellularis (Gi) and the pars alpha subregion (GiA). These neurons normally respond to high-threshold stimulation of discrete yet segmentally separated visceral and somatic regions. In contrast to dorsal horn neurons, the convergence of multiple inputs on these MRF neurons allows for the investigation of receptive fields with three different relationships to a midthoracic (T8) SCI (above-level, at-level, and below-level). Our interest here is the input from the skin of the lesion-level dorsal trunk. As reviewed in this chapter, chronic severe contusion injury can produce a situation where gentle low-threshold stroking of the dorsal trunk activates MRF convergent neurons and elicits allodynic-like pain behavior (Hubscher and Johnson 1999a). Neither of these responses are seen in uninjured animals. The inherently variable nature of a spinal cord contusion injury has, however, resulted in some animals that do not develop tactile allodynia and the concomitant high degree of low-threshold trunk neuronal responses in the MRF. In the discussion below, we suggest several central and peripheral mechanisms that may account for the development of SCI-induced plasticity in MRF neurons following specific types of incomplete SCI.

ANIMAL MODEL

Our animal model was originally developed for the electrophysiological study of MRF neurons receiving ascending sensory input from the male urogenital tract (Hubscher and Johnson 1996). We also studied the descending MRF modulation of perineal/sphincter motoneuron reflex circuits (Johnson and Hubscher 1998, 2000) and the effects of chronic midthoracic SCI on this spinobulbospinal coordinating center for male sexual function (Hubscher and Johnson 1999b, 2000). An unexpected finding was the development of novel low-threshold cutaneous receptive fields at the level of the lesion. The brief description of the methodology that follows is fully described elsewhere (Hubscher and Johnson 1996, 1999a,b).

Electrophysiological recordings. Urethane-anesthetized mature male rats were intubated for vital signs and stabilized with hip pins and a stereotactic head holder. Specially fabricated bipolar silicon-cuff microelectrodes were placed bilaterally around the dorsal nerve of the penis (DNP), the pelvic nerve (PN), and the motor branch of the pudendal nerve (Fig. 1). Two glass-coated platinum-plated tungsten microelectrodes with a 20-μm exposed tip attached to a stepping microdrive were configured for bilateral penetration of the MRF, in the same anterior/posterior plane (3400 μm rostral to obex) and equidistant from the midline. Two bilateral tracks (400 and 800 μm lateral to the midline) were made in the Gi and GiA, determined in our initial report (Hubscher and Johnson 1996) to contain the greatest number of viscerosomatic convergent neurons responsive to DNP/PN stimulation with convergent input from the ears, face, dorsal trunk, hindpaws, and forepaws (Fig. 1). Simultaneous-single neuron recordings were made extracellularly from both sides of the MRF. A hand-held pair of serrated forceps was used to determine the characteristics of cutaneous receptive fields and the

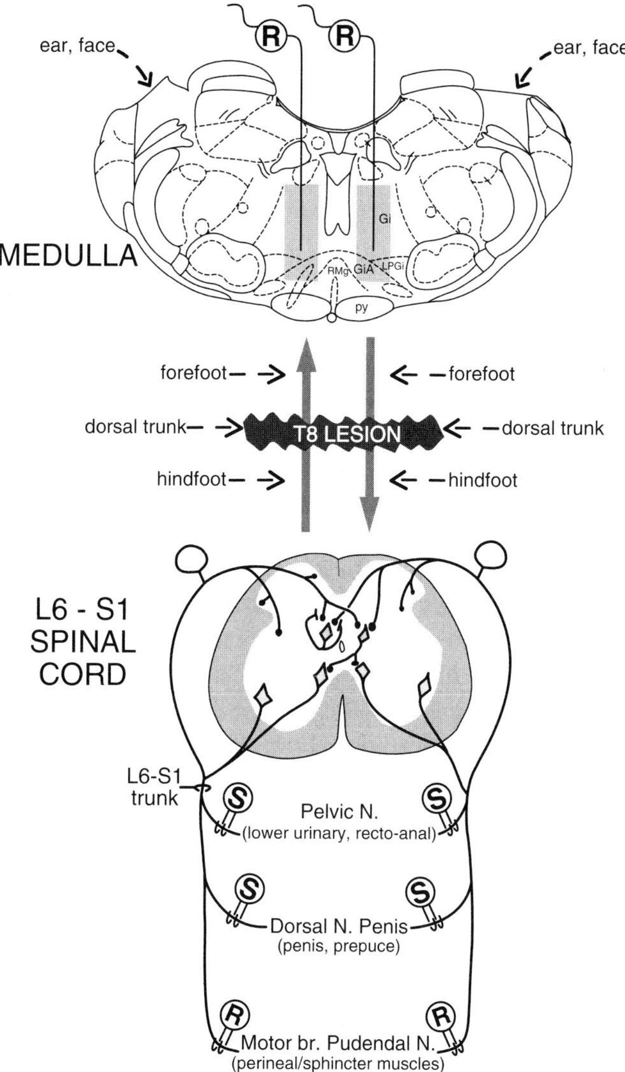

Fig. 1. Schematic diagram illustrating the experimental setup for bilateral electrical nerve stimulation (S) and recordings from the medullary reticular formation (MRF) and pudendal nerve (R). The shaded region in the MRF indicates the search region in all animals and postmortem location of all neurons. Gi = nucleus reticularis gigantocellularis; GiA = Gi pars alpha; LPGi = lateral paragigantocellularis nucleus; RMg = nucleus raphe magnus; py = medullary pyramidal tract.

mechanical threshold of the neuron. For low-threshold (LT) stimulation we used gentle non-noxious skin stroking; for high-threshold (HT) stimulation, we used gentle pressure/pinch, moderate pinch, and strong pinch (which left a temporary mark and indentation on the skin). To maintain consistency in stimulus intensity levels, the same experimenter stimulated all groups of animals and was blinded to the animals' behavioral status. A neuronal response was counted if the number of spikes firing was at least two times (excitation) or one-half (inhibition) that of background levels.

Chronic spinal cord lesions. To study the effects of chronic SCI, we made hemisections (lateral or dorsal) or contusions aseptically at spinal level T8 (full surgical and postoperative recovery details appear in Hubscher and Johnson 1999a). Lateral and dorsal hemisections were made through a longitudinal dural incision using a pair of microdissecting scissors. The dura was closed with a pair of 10–0 monofilament sutures. Severe contusion injuries were made using a rapid compression of the T8 spinal cord with a concave probe having a radius and size matching the overlying T7 vertebral lamina. The probe was attached to a displacement-controlled device driven with a trapezoid waveform using parameters (2.0 mm for 5 seconds) modified from previously described protocols (Bresnahan et al 1987; Theriault and Tator 1994). All surgical procedures except the lesion were also performed on sham surgical controls. The animals recovered for 30 days as previously described (Hubscher and Johnson 1999a), at which time the terminal electrophysiological experiment was performed.

Behavioral assessment of tactile allodynia. Qualitative assessments of sensitivity to gentle stroking stimulation of the skin on the dorsal trunk were made periodically throughout the recovery period using blunt forceps. This method of assessing skin surface sensitivity is similar to the touch-evoked agitation measure of behavioral response employed by Yaksh (1989), where vocalization in response to a probe (stroke) and efforts to escape it are taken as evidence of tactile allodynia.

Postmortem histology. At the end of the terminal experiment, animals were euthanized and perfused transcardially with saline and paraformaldehyde. The block of brainstem tissue containing the recording sites was removed and stored overnight in a 10% formalin/30% sucrose solution. The dorsal cutaneous nerves innervating the marked territory of hypersensitivity were anatomically traced to the spinal cord to determine the spinal segmental level receiving input from this area of skin. Recording sites were visualized in 50-μm vibratome sections stained with cresyl violet and reconstructed under light and dark field illumination (Paxinos and Watson 1986) as previously described (Johnson and Hubscher 1998). The perfused spinal cord was analyzed histologically (10-μm paraffin sections) to confirm the extent of the chronic lesion. Spinal cord tissue sections in and adjacent to the lesion epicenter were stained with both luxol fast blue and cresyl violet (Kluver-Barrera stain). In a subset of animals with contusion lesions, a 1-mm block of tissue at the lesion epicenter was postfixed in glutaraldehyde, osmicated, embedded in plastic, sectioned at 1 μm, and stained with toluidine blue using our existing protocols (Johnson and Halata 1991). Under high-power light microscopy, the number of surviving myelinated fibers passing through the epicenter was determined as described below. We combined ~50 digitized images of the stained sections at a magnification of 250× to produce a complete photomontage of the epicenter. We determined the total number of surviving myelinated axons (fiber diameter of 2 μm and above) in the core and perimeter of each epicenter. All the morphological analysis was performed by the same investigator, who was blinded to the behavioral status of the animal.

DEVELOPMENT OF NOVEL LOW-THRESHOLD LESION-LEVEL RECEPTIVE FIELDS

In unoperated and sham-operated control animals, bilaterally isolated MRF neurons had convergent inputs from mucocutaneous (penis, prepuce, anus), cutaneous (ears, face, forepaws, hindpaws, dorsal trunk), and visceral (urethra, colorectum) receptive fields (Hubscher and Johnson 1996, 1999a; unpublished observations). Regardless of whether the peripheral target was paired (e.g., paws, ears) or unpaired (e.g., urogenital tract), MRF neurons always responded to bilateral stimulation. With few exceptions, neurons responsive to stimulation of the ear also responded to urogenital stimulation, and vice versa. Therefore, both sites were used as search stimuli in animals with chronic SCI. As illustrated in Fig. 2, MRF neurons in this region of the gigantocellularis nuclear complex normally responded (often with an afterdischarge) only to high-threshold pinch stimuli. However, low-threshold stroking of the glans penis was often an effective stimulus, particularly following wind-up (Fig. 2). Receptive fields in the skin of the dorsal trunk all required moderate to strong pinching in unoperated and surgical sham control animals (Fig. 3). Subsequent to chronic T8 SCI, a strip of skin in the T6–T7 dermatomes (at the level of the lesion) exhibited novel low-threshold receptive fields that could be activated by a slow, gentle stroking of the dorsal trunk skin. Although some novel low-threshold lesion level fields were found in animals with dorsal and lateral hemisection injuries, a significantly greater number was found in animals with severe contusion injuries (Table I, Fig. 3; see Hubscher and Johnson 1999a). Low-threshold lesion level fields were not observed after acute (1–2-hour) partial or complete midthoracic transections (Hubscher and Johnson 1999b), but sometimes were observed following chronic transection (Fig. 3; R.D. Johnson and C.H. Hubscher, unpublished observations), suggesting that plasticity in MRF

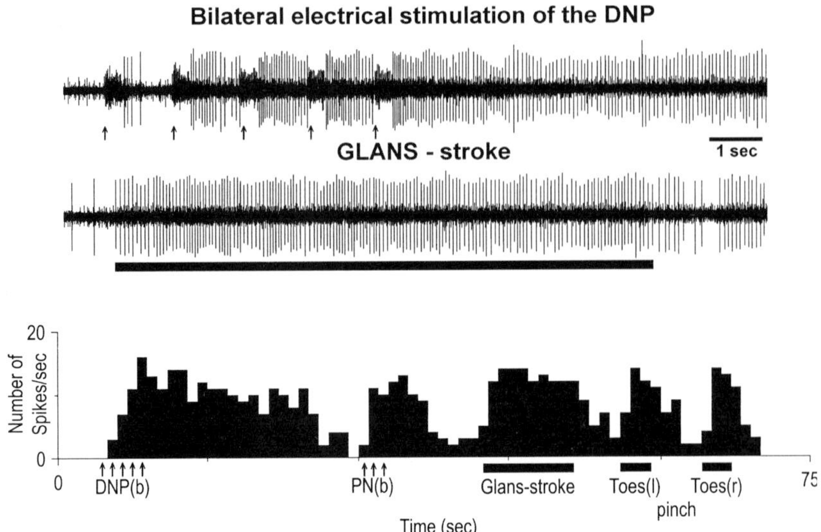

Fig. 2. Example of excitatory responses of a single neuron located in the right GiA to bilateral (b) electrical stimulation of the dorsal nerve of the penis (DNP) and pelvic nerve (PN), and natural stimulation of the glans penis and toes of the hindfoot. The same neuron also had excitatory responses to bilateral stimulation of the scrotum, anus, toes of the forefoot, ears, and urethra (none of which are shown). The upper two traces are raw spike records taken from the 75-second stimulation sequence shown as a peristimulus histogram in the bottom panel. The wind-up from electrical stimulation produced long afterdischarges. In the top trace, a responsive background unit (smallest deflection) as well as the electrical stimulus train artifact (medium-sized deflection) can be seen following the stimulus train onset arrows; neither was counted in the histogram below. Modified from Hubscher and Johnson (1996).

neuronal response requires a chronic injury. In some animals with contusion injury, however, low-threshold trunk fields did not develop.

In contrast to inputs from the level of the lesion, novel receptive fields activated by low-threshold stroking were not found in regions below the lesion (hindpaws) in any of the chronic injury groups, despite the survival of some of the ascending pathways. However, in most of the animals with lateral hemisections, increased response magnitude to pinch stimulation (relative to control) was observed in the lesion-side hindpaw (C.H. Hubscher and R.D. Johnson, unpublished observations).

DEVELOPMENT OF LESION-LEVEL ALLODYNIA

Qualitative behavioral testing for regions of skin sensitivity during the 30-day recovery period revealed tactile allodynia-like responses to stroking

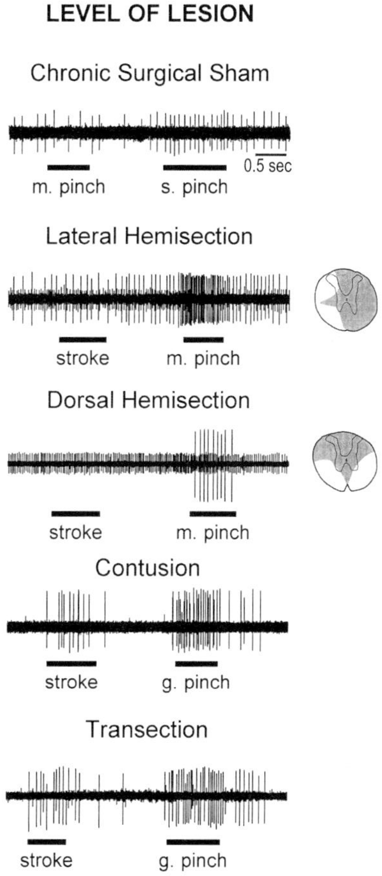

Fig. 3. Typical examples of excitatory responses of single medullary reticular formation (MRF) neurons to lesion-level (dorsolateral trunk) stimulation 30 days after a midthoracic chronic SCI or a sham injury. The intensity of the pinch stimulus was either gentle (g), moderate (m), or strong (s). Traces are raw 5-second spike records. Modified from Hubscher and Johnson (1999a).

in most of the animals with severe contusion injuries (Hubscher and Johnson 1999a). The response was elicited by gentle stroking of the dermatomal zone (T6–T7) just rostral to the T8 injury. The hypersensitive response was manifested by one or more of the following: obvious vocalization, a substantial increase in respiration and heart rate, or vigorous head-turning toward the stimulus. These responses were unusual in these tame animals, who were accustomed to daily handling for postoperative care and cleaning. Punctate low-threshold tactile stimulation did not produce an allodynia-like response. The onset of signs occurred between 2 and 3 weeks after surgery

Table I
Summary of neuronal responses (mean ± SEM) to stimulation at the lesion level in rats with SCI and control rats

Treatment	A	B	C
Control	27 ± 8* (68)	0/5*	0
Contusion	84 ± 4 (134)	11/15*	29 ± 6*
Dorsal hemisection	77 ± 8 (85)	2/7	10 ± 7
Lateral hemisection	57 ± 12* (53)	1/4	3 ± 3

Source: Modified from Hubscher and Johnson (1999a).
Note: A = percentage of medullary reticular formation neurons with receptive fields on the dorsal trunk (with total number of neurons in parentheses); B = number of animals with low-threshold dorsal trunk receptive fields; C = percentage of neurons in A with low-threshold dorsal trunk receptive fields.
* Significantly different from all other groups (χ^2, $P < 0.01$).

and continued throughout the recovery period. The behavioral responses were not observed in animals with chronic hemisection or transection injury (or in sham-operated and unoperated controls). In some animals with contusion injury, tactile allodynia was not observed, while in others it was only observed after “wind-up” (from repetitive stroking of the dorsal trunk or pinching the ear). At-level tactile allodynia also has been reported in other rat models of chronic contusion injury (Siddall et al. 1995; Lindsey et al. 2000), although the time course and symptomatology differ somewhat, presumably due to differences in contusion method, spinal level of injury, and behavioral paradigm.

SCI-INDUCED PLASTICITY IN MRF VISCEROSOMATIC NEURONS

As has been found for spinal dorsal horn neurons (Xu et al 1992; Yezierski and Park 1993; Christensen and Hulsebosch 1997; Chapter 10, this volume), our electrophysiological studies have demonstrated that chronic SCI changes the response characteristics of supraspinal neurons. The reorganization of viscerosomatic inputs and enhanced responses to regions associated with tactile allodynia and/or hyperalgesia are most likely due to a combination of central and peripheral events. We attribute much of this reorganization to the removal of convergent inputs from below the lesion, which has the effect of strengthening the remaining inputs. The lack of novel low-threshold receptive fields in skin at the lesion level after acute lesions suggests that this reorganization occurs over time (Hubscher and Johnson 1999b).

The strong correlation between a high percentage of stroke-sensitive trunk receptive fields and allodynia-like behavior suggests that this subregion of the MRF has a role in the perception of SCI pain. Somal lesion of this MRF subregion attenuates allodynia and hyperalgesia, possibly by eliminating a descending nociceptive facilitatory projection (Zhuo and Gebhart 1991; Pertovaara et al. 1996; Wei et al. 1999). Alternatively, we have reported that microstimulation of bulbospinal axons originating from this region produces presynaptic inhibition of primary afferents (Johnson and Hubscher 1998), which would contribute to disinhibition after chronic SCI (Hubscher and Johnson 2000). Ascending MRF projections may affect pain relay centers in the thalamus. In a pilot study, we have demonstrated that low-threshold receptive fields at the lesion level develop in neurons located in medial thalamic nuclei (Fig. 4; Hubscher and Johnson 1999c) following a chronic contusion injury that correlates with allodynia-like behavior.

CENTRAL MECHANISMS

Several physiological and anatomical characteristics of the spinal cord lesion area may contribute to the development of lesion-level sensitivity in MRF neurons and the concomitant behavioral signs of tactile allodynia. Lowered sensitivity of wide-dynamic-range (WDR) dorsal horn neurons to tactile stimulation of the dorsal trunk, including increased afterdischarge (Chapter 10), could contribute to changes in MRF neuronal responses.

Interruption or sparing of specific midthoracic spinal pathways may be a factor in determining whether or not tactile allodynia develops. For example, spinothalamic tract (STT) axons project through the midthoracic

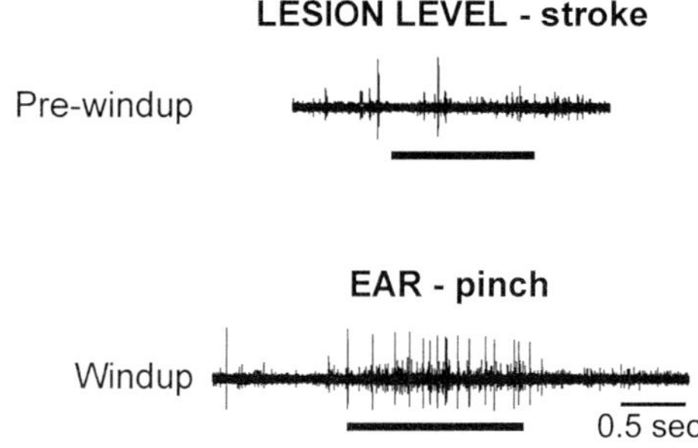

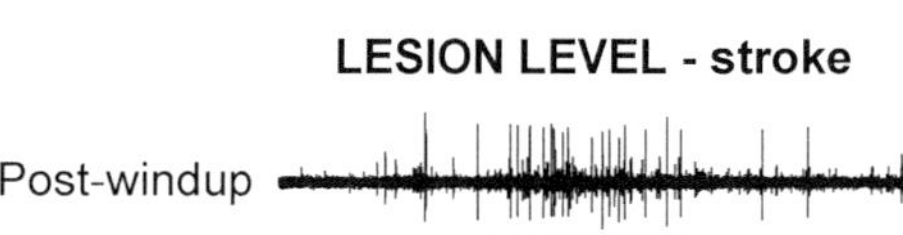

Fig. 4. Example of excitatory responses of a single viscerosomatic neuron from the medial thalamus to lesion-level stimulation 30 days after a midthoracic chronic contusion injury that produced wind-up-dependent tactile allodynia. Wind-up from a remote site (the ear) elicited a low-threshold stroke response from the lesion-level skin.

lateral funiculus (Zhang et al. 2000) and have collaterals ending on neurons in the MRF (Geisler et al. 1981; Kevetter and Willis 1982). Based on SCI data in humans and animals, damage to the STT is probably required for the development of tactile allodynia (Boivie 1992; Weng et al. 2000; Defrin et al. 2001). Data obtained in our model, in combination with other data from human and animal studies, provide evidence that in addition to STT damage, some sparing of the dorsal column is required for the expression of tactile allodynia below the lesion. In rats, thoracic lateral hemisection that severed the STT but spared the dorsal columns (Berkley and Hubscher 1995; Al-Chaer et al. 1997) led to tactile allodynia in the lesion-side hindpaw (Christensen and Hulsebosch 1996). In contrast, our lateral hemisections that did not spare the dorsal columns led only to the development of lesion-side hyperalgesic MRF responses from the hindpaw (C.H. Hubscher and R.D. Johnson, unpublished observations).

Relative to lesion-level effects in our animals with contusion injuries, sparing of myelinated axons in the core region of the epicenter may be important for the development of tactile allodynia and MRF plasticity (Fig. 5). Some animals exhibited an allodynia-like response only after wind-up pinch stimuli to above-level (Fig. 4) or below-level territories. With the latter, urogenital stimulation often was an effective wind-up stimulation for

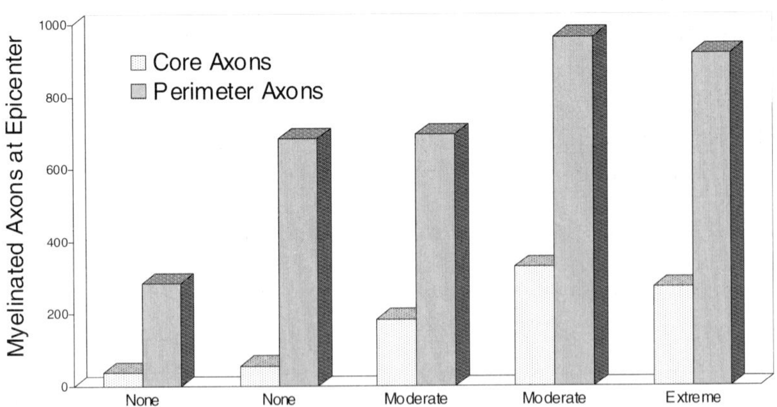

Fig. 5. Number of spared myelinated axons passing through the contusion injury epicenter in five animals. Behavioral assessment of lesion-level tactile allodynia for each animal is expressed as None (no evidence of sensitivity), Moderate (wind-up-dependent allodynia), or Extreme (strong reactions to stroking the allodynic area). Axonal profiles were counted for the perimeter and core regions of the epicenter section. Note the correlation between behavioral status and number of spared myelinated axons in the core.

contusion-induced lesion-level tactile allodynia (and for wind-up of low-threshold MRF responses), despite the lack of any conscious perception of the penile stimulus or of stimulation of any other below-level region. Clinically, tactile allodynia is frequently associated with distension of the bladder and colon, despite the lack of sensation from the viscera (Defrin et al. 2001). As such, the efficacy of the below-level stimulus in winding up the lesion-level response (electrophysiological and behavioral) may depend on some of the spared interior axons.

PERIPHERAL MECHANISMS

Events in the primary afferents may contribute to the development of contusion-induced MRF neuronal plasticity and allodynia to skin stroking. Central sensitization probably occurs, caused by ectopic discharges in dorsal root ganglion (DRG) neurons or by sprouting of myelinated afferents into lamina II of the spinal cord (reviewed by Woolf and Salter 2000). The development of novel stroke-activated receptive fields may be due to increased activity or sprouting of unmyelinated C-fiber afferents. In humans, tactile allodynia is almost always elicited by a repetitive moving (stroking) stimulus over the skin surface (Boivie 1992; Defrin et al. 2001; Chapter 4, this volume) similar to the stimulus required to activate C-mechanoreceptors. We have shown that viscerosomatic MRF neurons in the Gi have a large input from C-fiber afferents (Petruska et al. 1998), which are common in the glans penis (Johnson and Halata 1991). Compression of the dorsal roots, which occurs in our contusion injuries (but not with partial or complete transection lesions), can lead to cutaneous hyperalgesia (Song et al. 1999) and close-proximity DRG cell loss (R.D. Johnson and C.H. Hubscher, unpublished observations). The latter leads to collateral sprouting of unmyelinated afferents from the uninjured dermatome (reviewed in Petruska 2000).

ACKNOWLEDGMENTS

The authors wish to thank V. Dugan, J. Levinson, O. Bertozzi, R. Odama, and M. Seplow for excellent technical assistance. Studies were supported by NIH, the American Paralysis Association, the Paralyzed Veterans of America, and the Brain and Spinal Cord Rehabilitation Trust Fund of Florida.

REFERENCES

Al-Chaer ED, Westlund KN, Willis WD. Nucleus gracilis: an integrator for visceral and somatic information. *J Neurophysiol* 1997; 78:521–527.

Beric A. Post-spinal cord injury pain states. In: Wallace M, Dunn J, Yaksh T (Eds). *Anesthesiology Clinics of North America—Pain: Nociceptive and Neuropathic Mechanisms*. Philadelphia: W.B. Saunders, 1997, pp 445–463.

Berkley KJ, Hubscher CH. Are there separate central nervous system pathways for touch and pain? *Nat Med* 1995; 1:766–773.

Boivie J. Central pain. In: Wall PD, Melzack R (Eds). *Textbook of Pain*. Churchill Livingstone, 1992, pp 871–902.

Bresnahan JC, Beattie MS, Todd FD, et al. A behavioral and anatomical analysis of spinal cord injury produced by a feedback-controlled impaction device. *Exp Neurol* 1987; 95:548–570.

Christensen MD, Hulsebosch CE. Chronic central pain after spinal cord injury. *J Neurotrauma* 1997; 14:517–537.

Defrin R, Ohry A, Blumen N, et al. Characterization of chronic pain and somatosensory function in spinal cord injury subjects. *Pain* 2001; 89:253–263.

Eide PK, Jørum E, Stenehjem AE. Somatosensory findings in patients with spinal cord injury and central dysaethesia pain. *J Neurol Neurosurg Psychiatry* 1997; 60:411–415.

Geisler Jr GJ, Spiel HR, Willis WD. Organization of spinothalamic tract axons within the rat spinal cord. *J Comp Neurol* 1981; 195:243–252.

Hubscher CH, Johnson RD. Responses of medullary reticular formation neurons to input from the male genitalia. *J Neurophysiol* 1996; 76:2474–2482.

Hubscher CH, Johnson RD. Changes in neuronal receptive field characteristics in caudal brain stem following chronic spinal cord injury. *J Neurotrauma* 1999a; 16:533–541.

Hubscher CH, Johnson RD. Effects of acute and chronic midthoracic spinal cord injury on neural circuits for male sexual function. I. Ascending pathways. *J Neurophysiol* 1999b; 82:1381–1389.

Hubscher CH, Johnson RD. Changes in neuronal receptive field characteristics in thalamus following chronic contusion injury. *Soc Neurosci Abstracts* 1999c; 22:1843.

Hubscher CH, Johnson RD. Effects of acute and chronic midthoracic spinal cord injury on neural circuits for male sexual function. II. Descending pathways. *J Neurophysiol* 2000; 83:2508–2518.

Johnson RD, Halata Z. Topography and ultrastructure of sensory nerve endings in the glans penis of the rat. *J Comp Neurol* 1991; 312:229–310.

Johnson RD, Hubscher CH. Brainstem microstimulation differentially inhibits pudendal motoneuron reflex inputs. *Neuroreport* 1998; 9:341–345.

Johnson RD, Hubscher CH. Brainstem microstimulation activates sympathetic fibers in pudendal nerve motor branch. *Neuroreport* 2000; 11:379–382.

Kevetter GA, Willis WD. Spinothalamic cells in the rat lumbar cord with collaterals to the medullary reticular formation. *Brain Res* 1982; 238:181–185.

Lindsey AE, LoVerso RL, Tovar CA, et al. An analysis of changes in sensory thresholds to mild tactile and cold stimuli after experimental spinal cord injury in the rat. *Neurorehabil Neural Repair* 2000: 14:287–300.

Paxinos G, Watson C. *The Rat Brain in Stereotaxic Coordinates*, 2nd ed. San Diego: Academic Press, 1986.

Pertovaara A, Wei H, Hämäläinen MM. Lidocaine in the rostroventromedial medulla and the periaqueductal gray attenuates allodynia in neuropathic rats. *Neurosci Lett* 1996; 218:127–130.

Petruska JC. Collateral sprouting of unmyelinated primary afferents lacking receptors for nerve growth factor. University of Florida: Dissertation, 2000.

Petruska JC, Hubscher CH, Johnson RD. Anodally-focussed polarization of peripheral nerve allows discrimination of myelinated and unmyelinated fiber input to brainstem nuclei. *Exp Brain Res* 1998; 121:379–390.

Siddall P, Xu CL, Cousins M. Allodynia following traumatic spinal cord injury in the rat. *Neuroreport* 1995; 6:1241–1244.

Song XJ, Hu SJ, et al. Mechanical and thermal hyperalgesia and ectopic neuronal discharge after chronic compression of dorsal root ganglia. *J Neurophysiol* 1999; 82:3347–3358.

Theriault E, Tator CH. Persistence of rubrospinal projections following spinal cord injury in the rat. *J Comp Neurol* 1994; 342:249–258.

Wei F, Dubner R, Ren K. Nucleus reticularis gigantocellularis and nucleus raphe magnus in the brainstem exert opposite effects on behavioral hyperalgesia and spinal Fos protein expression after peripheral inflammation. *Pain* 1999; 80:127–141.

Weng H-R, Lee JI, Lenz FA, et al. Functional plasticity in primate somatosensory thalamus following chronic lesion of the ventral lateral spinal cord. *Neuroscience* 2000; 101:393–401.

Woolf CJ, Salter MW. Neuronal plasticity: increasing the gain in pain. *Science* 2000; 288:1765–1768.

Xu X-J, Hao J-X, Aldskogius H, et al. Chronic pain-related syndrome in rats after ischemic spinal cord lesion: a possible animal model for pain in patients with spinal cord injury. *Pain* 1992; 48:279–290.

Yaksh TL. Behavioral and autonomic correlates of the tactile evoked allodynia produced by spinal glycine inhibition: effects of modulatory receptor systems and excitatory amino acid antagonists. *Pain* 1989; 37:111–123.

Yezierski RP. Pain following spinal cord injury: the clinical problem and experimental studies. *Pain* 1996; 68:185–194.

Yezierski RP, Park SH. The mechanosensitivity of spinal sensory neurons following intraspinal injections of quisqualic acid in the rat. *Neurosci Lett* 1993; 157:115–119.

Zhang X, Honda CN, Geisler GJ. Position of spinothalamic tract axons in upper cervical spinal cord of monkeys. *J Neurophysiol* 2000; 84:1180–1185.

Zhuo M, Gebhart GF. Spinal serotonin receptors mediate descending facilitation of a nociceptive reflex from nuclei reticularis gigantocellularis and gigantocellularis pars alpha in the rat. *Brain Res* 1991; 550:35–48.

Correspondence to: Richard D. Johnson, PhD, Department of Physiological Sciences, University of Florida, Box 100144, Gainesville, FL 32610-0144, USA. Tel: 352-392-4700 ext. 3834; Fax: 352-392-5145; email: johnson@ufbi.ufl.edu.

Spinal Cord Injury Pain: Assessment, Mechanisms, Management. Progress in Pain Research and Management, Vol. 23, edited by Robert P. Yezierski and Kim J. Burchiel, IASP Press, Seattle, © 2002.

13

Microelectrode Studies of the Thalamus in Patients with Central Pain and in Control Patients with Movement Disorders

Shinji Ohara, Ira Garonzik, Sherwin Hua, and Frederick A. Lenz

Department of Neurosurgery, Johns Hopkins Hospital, Baltimore, Maryland, USA

In order to understand the organization of the region of the principal somatic sensory nucleus of the thalamus in patients with central pain secondary to spinal cord injury (SCI), it is essential to understand the normal organization of this area in primates without abnormalities of the somatic sensory system. Fortunately, this region has been well studied in primates. The human principal sensory nucleus is known as the ventral caudal nucleus (Vc) in Hassler's (1959) atlas, which corresponds in monkeys (Hirai and Jones 1989) to the ventral posterior (VP) nucleus, as defined in Olszewski's (1952) atlas.

NORMAL ORGANIZATION OF THE HUMAN PRINCIPAL SOMATIC SENSORY NUCLEUS

This chapter describes studies in the region of the ventral caudal portion of the human principal sensory nucleus (Vc). Human studies cannot obtain histological verification of nuclear location, so we must identify the Vc region based on physiological criteria. We can divide the Vc region into a cutaneous core area and a posterior-inferior area. The core is defined as the area where the majority of cells respond to innocuous, mechanical, and cutaneous stimuli, and probably corresponds to the Vc (Lenz et al. 1993a, 1994a, 1998a), the human equivalent of the monkey VP (Hirai and Jones 1989). The posterior inferior area is the cellular area below and behind the core and probably corresponds to the posterior subnucleus of Vc (nucleus ventral caudal portae, Vcpor), the inferior subnucleus of Vc (ventral caudal parvocellular nucleus, Vcpc), the posterior nucleus, the magnocellular medial geniculate (Mehler 1962, 1966; Lenz et al. 1993a), and the ventral medial posterior nucleus (Vmpo) of Craig et al. (1994).

In the core region, receptive field (RF) locations for the cells responding to nonpainful stimuli remain unchanged over distances of several millimeters in the anterior-posterior and superior-inferior directions. However, RFs do change markedly over similar distances in the mediolateral direction (see Fig. 1). Observations of this kind have established that parts of the body are represented within the Vc in parasagittal planes or lamellae. The sequence of neuronal, cutaneous RFs indicates that lamellae, from medial to lateral, represent intraoral structures, the face, thumb, fingers (radial to ulnar), and toes (Lenz et al. 1988a). Proximal parts of the limbs are represented dorsal to the corresponding digits. This medial-lateral somatotopy is consistent with some (Cohen and Grundfest 1953; Albé-Fessard et al. 1963; McComas et al. 1970; Bates 1972; Guiot et al. 1973), but not all, studies of the human thalamus (Ohye 1982).

Characteristic shifts in RFs are observed on microelectrode trajectories in the parasagittal plane through the region of Vc from anterior-dorsal to posterior-ventral. Specifically, cells with RFs on parts of the body that are represented laterally in the Vc are found along any trajectory both anterior-superior and posterior-inferior to cells with RFs on parts of the body that are represented medially in the thalamus (see Figs. 7 and 8 of Lenz et al. 1988a).

Fig. 1. Map of receptive fields for trajectories in the region of Vc in a patient with Parkinsonian tremor. Receptive field (RF) mapping is shown along two trajectories within the parasagittal planes at 16 mm (A) and 18 mm (B) lateral to the midline. The stereotactically predicted course of each trajectory is drawn on the appropriate sagittal map of the thalamus and the AC–PC line is indicated (top). Directly beneath, these same trajectories are redrawn. Lines at right angles to each trajectory indicate the positions at which single units were recorded. The response pattern of each cell is indicated by symbols at the end of each line. Filled circles = deep lemniscal; open squares = light touch; filled squares = cutaneous pressure. The cutaneous responses were sometimes classified as slowly adapting (filled triangle) or rapidly adapting (open triangle). Lines without symbols indicate cells without RFs. The arrow at the end of each trajectory indicates the position of the last cell recorded. Letters to the upper left indicate the left (side) of the brain and the number of millimeters lateral (16 or 18 mm). In the lower panels, graphics indicating the size and location of RFs for each neuron are numbered to correspond to the numbers shown in the middle panel. NR indicates a recorded cell for which no RF was found. Abbreviations: Vc = ventralis caudalis; Vcpor = ventralis caudalis portae; Vcpc = ventralis caudalis parvocellularis; Lim = limitans; MG = medial geniculate; ML = medial lemniscus; WM = white matter below the ventral nuclear group; PC = posterior commissure. Reproduced from Lenz et al. (1988a), with permission. →

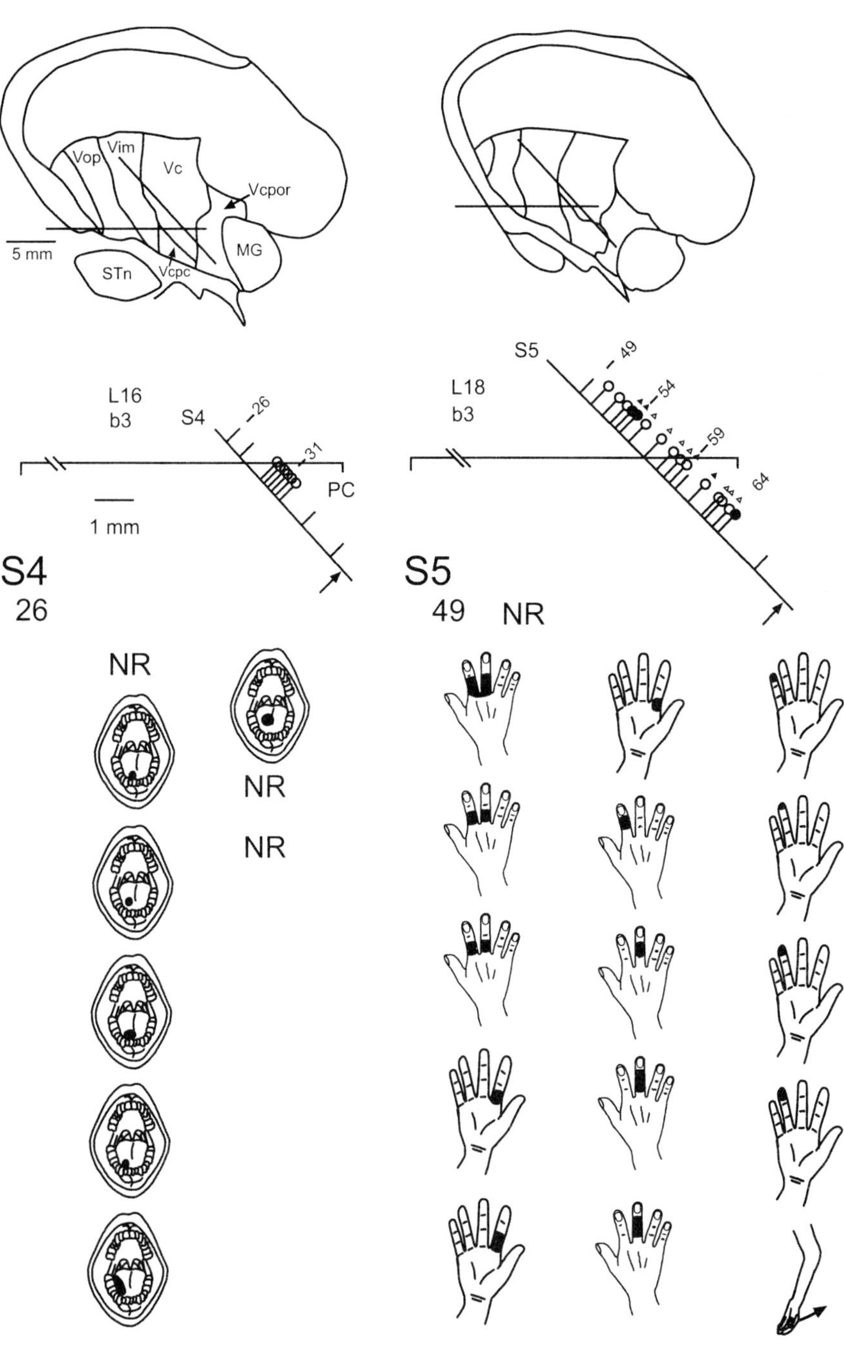
Vop
Vim
Vc
Vcpor
5 mm
MG
STn
Vcpc
L16
b3
S4
26
31
PC
1 mm
S4
26
NR
NR
NR
L18
b3
S5
49
54
59
64
S5
49
NR

Another example is shown in Fig. 1B, where the RFs change from the second and third digit to the fourth digit and then to the fifth digit (represented lateral to all digits) and then back to the fourth digit (represented medial to the fifth digit). This organization suggests that lamellae representing different parts of the body are concave medially, consistent with studies in nonhuman primates (Mountcastle and Henneman 1952; Jones et al. 1982).

IS THE REGION OF VC INVOLVED IN PAIN PROCESSING?

Several lines of evidence demonstrate that the region of Vc is important in human pain-signaling pathways. Studies of patients at autopsy following lesions of the spinothalamic tract (STT) show the most dense STT termination in the Vc (Walker 1943; Bowsher 1957; Mehler et al. 1960, 1962, 1966). Additionally, terminations are observed posterior to the Vc in the magnocellular medial geniculate (Mehler 1962, 1969), and in the limitans, the Vc portae nuclei, and inferior to the Vc in the Vcpc (Mehler 1966). In monkeys, STT terminations are found in the Vmpo, which appears, by immunohistochemistry and physiology, to have a human analogue (Craig et al. 1994; Davis et al. 1999).

Two groups of cells have been identified in the Vc: one with a differential response to painful thermal and mechanical stimuli (Lenz et al. 1994b; Lee et al. 1999), and another with a response to innocuous cool and mechanical stimuli (Lenz and Dougherty 1998). Cells in the posterior-inferior region have a significant selective response to noxious heat stimuli (Lenz et al. 1993b). These reports extend to humans the results of numerous monkey studies in which cells within the VP (Casey 1966; Kenshalo et al. 1980; Gautron and Guilbaud 1982; Casey and Morrow 1983; Chung et al. 1986; Bushnell and Duncan 1987; Bushnell et al. 1993; Apkarian and Shi 1994) and posterior and inferior to the VP respond to noxious stimuli (Casey 1966; Apkarian and Shi 1994; Craig et al. 1994).

Lesioning and stimulation studies suggest that cells in the region of the human Vc and monkey VP that respond to noxious stimuli probably signal pain. Blockade of the activity in this region by injection of local anesthetic into the monkey VP significantly interferes with the monkey's ability to discriminate temperature in both the innocuous and noxious ranges (Duncan et al. 1993). Stimulation within the Vc and posterior-inferior to it can evoke both pain (Hassler and Reichert 1959; Halliday and Logue 1972; Dostrovsky et al. 1991; Lenz et al. 1993a) and thermal sensations (Lenz et al. 1993a; Davis et al. 1999).

The Vc and the region posterior and inferior to it are likely to be involved in pain-signaling pathways because (1) this region receives input from pain-signaling pathways, (2) it contains cells that respond to noxious stimuli, (3) stimulation can evoke pain, and (4) temporary lesioning of the monkey VP disables the discrimination of pain and temperature. Thalamic sites that normally signal thermal sensations may signal pain in patients with chronic pain. Therefore, studies of this region are critical to understanding acute and chronic pain sensations.

SOMATOTOPIC REPRESENTATION IN THE REGION OF THE HUMAN PRINCIPAL SENSORY NUCLEUS IN PATIENTS WITH SPINAL TRANSECTION

We explored the region of the principal sensory nucleus of the thalamus (Vc) during stereotactic surgical procedures to treat patients with central pain after spinal cord transection (n = 5) and patients with movement disorders (n = 23) (Lenz et al. 1988a). Receptive fields (RFs) of thalamic single neurons and locations of sensations evoked by stimulation (projected fields, PFs) were determined by standard methods. For this analysis, the "region of Vc" was defined as the cellular thalamic region where sensations were evoked at less than 25 μA. The region of Vc in spinal patients was subdivided into different areas, according to RF and PF locations. Fig. 2 shows two trajectories through the thalamus of a patient with a complete spinal cord transection at the T8 level. Areas that were distant from the representation of the anesthetic part of the body were termed "spinal control" areas (Fig. 2A), while those that were adjacent to or included in the representation of the area of absolute sensory loss were classified in the "border zone anesthetic" area.

The next trajectory (Fig. 2B) was made in the 17-mm lateral plane where the representation of the leg should be located, given the representation of the hand on the first trajectory (Lenz et al. 1988a). Along the second trajectory many cells lacked RFs. Cells that did respond to sensory stimulation all had RFs on the chest wall just above the anesthetic level. Cells with RFs on the chest wall occurred over a distance of 1.5 mm along the trajectory. This is a large representation for the chest wall, which normally occupies a sliver dorsal to the representation of the digits and upper extremity in monkeys (Jones and Friedman 1982; Kaas et al. 1984; Jones 1985; see also Fig. 4 of Lenz et al. 1994c). Finally, the RFs are poorly matched with the PFs, which were located on the leg. In border zone anesthetic areas, RFs were often located on the border of the anesthetic part of the body, whereas PFs were

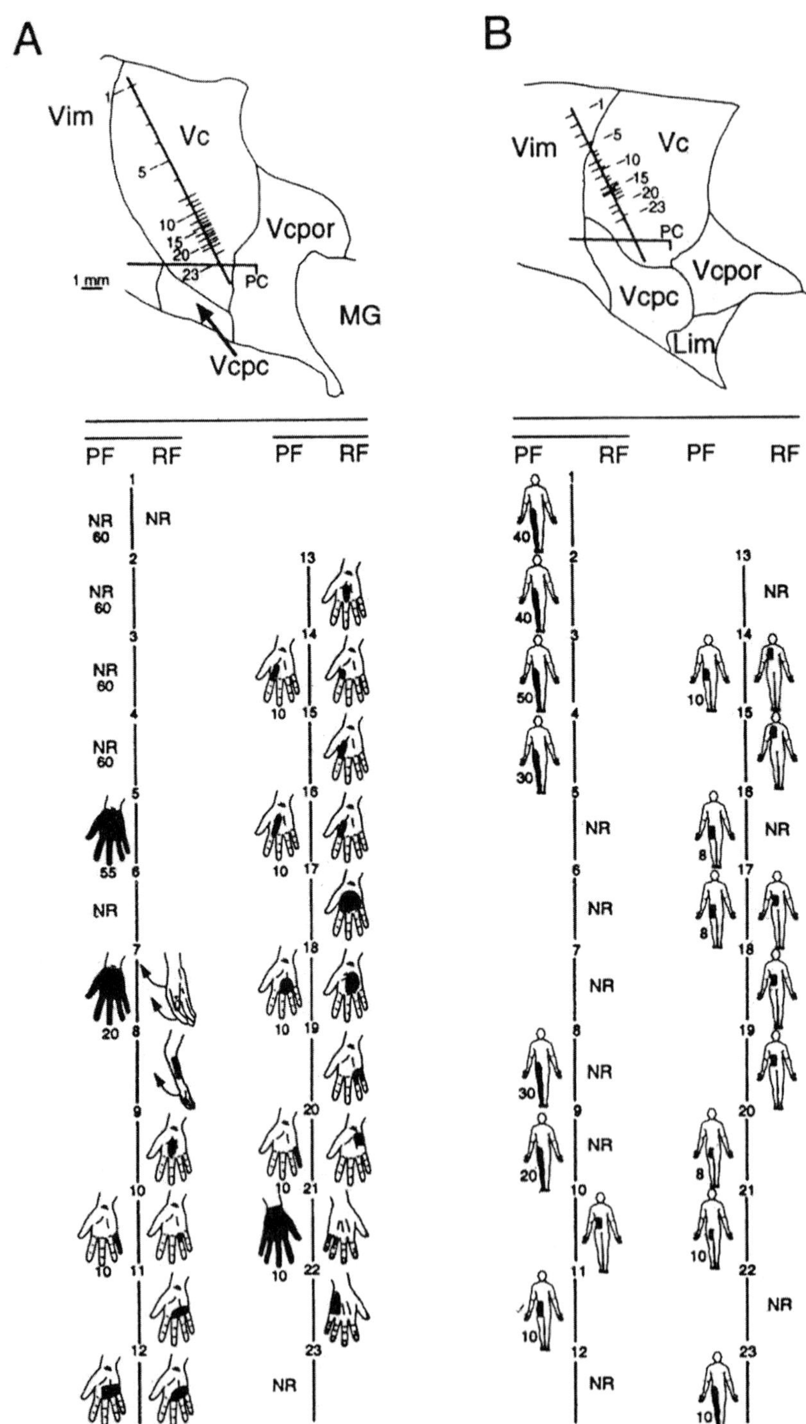
A
Vim
Vc
Vcpor
MG
Vcpc
PC
1 mm
B
Vim
Vc
PC
Vcpor
Vcpc
Lim
PF
RF
PF
RF
NR

referred to anesthetic parts of the body. The anesthetic part of the body was normally represented in these areas, which the PFs continued to represent, whereas the RFs had changed to represent the border zone of the anesthetic part of the body. Similar changes are seen in patients with amputations (Lenz et al. 1998b).

In summary, in patients with spinal cord transection, the region of Vc that represents the border zone anesthetic part of the body is characterized by an increase in the representation of the border zone part of the body, an increase in the number of cells without RFs, and a mismatch between RFs and PFs, so that RFs represent the border zone, whereas PFs are referred to the anesthetic part of the body. Therefore, the activity of cells in the border zone anesthetic part of the thalamus may be responsible for sensations that are felt in these areas.

IS THALAMIC FUNCTIONAL MODE ALTERED IN CHRONIC PAIN STATES?

Spontaneous thalamic activity is often discussed in terms of thalamic functional mode, which refers to the firing of thalamic cells either in bursts (spike-bursts, bursting mode) or as tonic firing (tonic mode) (Steriade et al. 1990). Many studies have suggested that increased spike-bursting occurs in the thalamus of patients with chronic pain (Albé-Fessard and Lombard 1983; Lenz et al. 1989; Rinaldi et al. 1991; Jeanmonod et al. 1993; Jeanmonod et al. 1994; Lenz et al. 1994c, 1998b; compare Radhakrishnan et al. 1999). This kind of spike-bursting has a particular pattern of interspike intervals (ISIs) within intervals so that a spike-burst occurs after a relatively long ISI and

---

← **Fig. 2.** Map of receptive and projected fields for trajectories in the region of Vc in a patient with spinal cord transection at T8. Panel A shows a trajectory in the 15-mm lateral parasagittal plane (Lat 15 mm) through the region of Vc that represents the arm. Panel B shows a trajectory 2 mm lateral to the first (Lat 17 mm). The AC–PC line is indicated by the horizontal line in the panel, while the trajectories are shown by the oblique lines in the posterior commissure as labeled. The locations of cells are indicated by tick marks to the right of the trajectory. Cells with RFs are indicated by long ticks; those without are indicated by short ticks. Stimulation sites are shown to the left of the trajectory. Long ticks indicate a somatosensory response to stimulation, while short ticks indicate no response to microstimulation. Based upon evoked sensations at ≤25 μA the region of Vc includes sites 7 to 23 in A and sites 9 to 23 in B. The graphic to the right of the trajectory indicates the RF; NR indicates that the cell had no RF. The graphic to the left of the trajectory indicates the PF for threshold microstimulation at that site, while the number below the graphic indicates the threshold in microamperes. At all sites along both trajectories where sensations were evoked, that sensation was described as tingling. Other conventions are as described in the legend for Fig. 1; Vim = ventral intermediate nucleus.

starts with a short ISI (typically <6 ms). Thereafter, the ISIs progressively lengthen so that the cell's firing decelerates throughout the spike-burst (see Fig. 3).

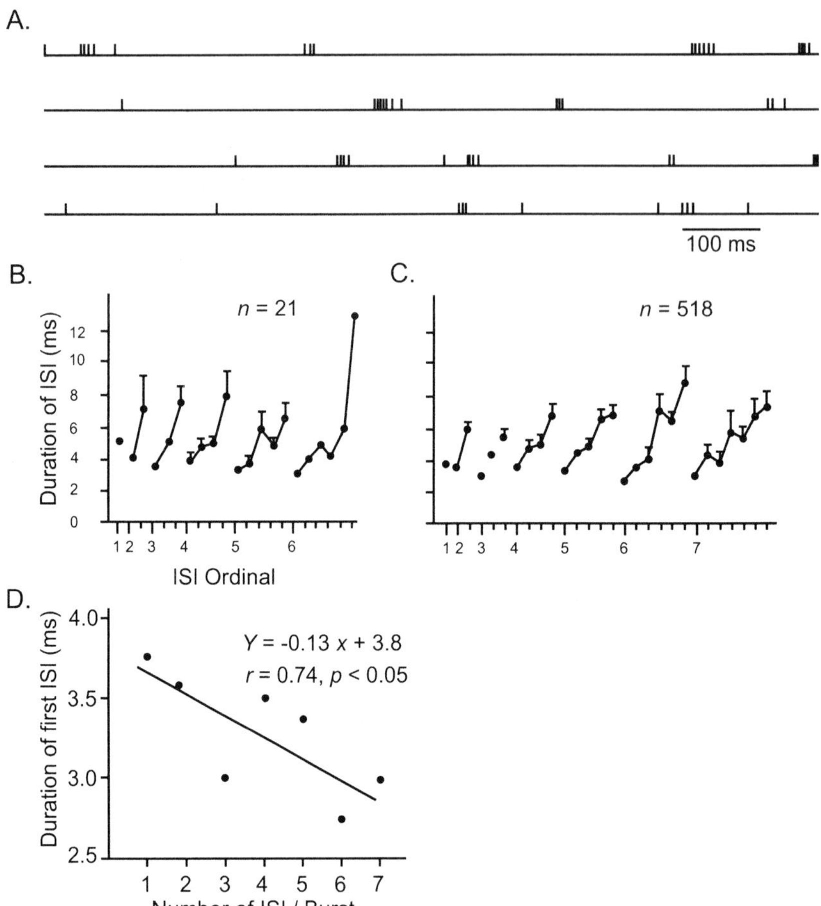

Fig. 3. Interspike interval (ISI) characteristics of bursts recorded in patients with central pain secondary to spinal cord transection. Panel A shows the digitized spike train from a cell recorded in a patient with central pain. Time scale is as indicated. Panel B plots the average ISI duration (mean and SEM) as a function of the ordinal number of the ISI within the burst for the 21 bursts recorded for that cell. For example, the three points located above and to the right of the number 3 show results for bursts composed of three ISIs and four action potentials. The three points represent from left the right the durations of the first, second, and third ISIs in bursts of three ISIs. Panel C demonstrates the same analysis for 22 cells (518 bursts) located in the border zone anesthetic region in two patients. Panel D shows the decrease in first ISI duration as the number of spikes increases. This pattern is typical of spike-bursts. Reproduced from Lenz et al. (1989), with permission.

We divided the region of Vc in patients with spinal transection into regions representing body parts adjacent to the anesthetic part of the body (Fig. 2B, border zone/anesthetic region) and those representing body parts distant from the representation of the anesthetic part of the body (Fig. 2A, spinal control). In patients with spinal transection, the highest rate of bursting occurs in cells that do not have RFs and that are located in the representation of the anesthetic part of the body (see Table I). These cells also have the lowest firing rates between spike-bursts (principal event rate, Table I) (Lenz et al. 1994c). The low firing rates suggest that these cells have decreased tonic excitatory drive and are hyperpolarized, perhaps due to loss of excitatory input from the STT (Eaton and Salt 1990; Young 1990; Ericson et al. 1993; Dougherty et al. 1996). Therefore, the available evidence suggests that affected thalamic cells in patients with spinal transection were dominated by spike-bursting consistent with membrane hyperpolarization (Steriade and Deschenes 1984; Steriade and Llinas 1988; Steriade et al. 1990; Davis et al. 1998; Lenz et al. 1998a).

In patients with SCI, spike-bursting activity was maximal in the region posterior and inferior to the core (Table IV in Lenz et al. 1994c). This posterior-inferior region is strongly related to pain by several lines of evidence (Lenz and Dougherty 1997). Neurons in this region respond preferentially to pain-producing stimuli (Lenz et al. 1993b). Stimulation evokes the sensation of pain more frequently in this area than in the core of the Vc (Hassler and Reichert 1959; Hassler 1970; Halliday and Logue 1972; Dostrovsky et al. 1991; Lenz et al. 1993a). Thus, increased spike-bursting activity might be correlated with some aspects of the abnormal sensations (e.g., dysesthesia or pain) that these patients experience. However, in patients with spinal transection the painful area overlaps with the area of sensory loss (Lenz et al. 1994c). Therefore, the bursting might be related to sensory loss, rather than to pain.

Our findings about spike-bursting activity in spinal patients have been called into question by a recent study in patients with chronic pain (Radhakrishnan et al. 1999). This report found the same number of bursting cells per trajectory in patients with movement disorders and in patients with chronic pain. The study grouped results in all pain patients; the only diagnoses that were considered separately were anesthesia dolorosa and phantom pain. The subset of patients with central pain secondary to SCI was not studied. In both studies (Lenz et al. 1994c; Radhakrishnan et al. 1999), results in patients with movement disorders served as controls for those in patients with pain. Cells studied by Radhakrishnan and colleagues were largely located anterior-superior or posterior-ventral to the Vc so that "very few cells in either group (pain or nonpain patients) were within Vc"

Table I
Indexes of burst firing (e.g. bursts with >3 ISIs/burst) and associated ISI indexes in patients with central pain secondary to spinal cord transection and control patients with movement disorders

	Control		Spinal Control		Border/Anesthetic	
ISI Index	No RF ($n = 9$)	RF ($n = 31$)	No RF ($n = 2$)	RF ($n = 27$)	No RF ($n = 16$)	RF ($n = 12$)
2nd-order ISI <10 ms (%)	**0.115**	**0.399**	6.05	**0.59**	**<u>9.78</u>**	0.6
Bursts/second	1.12	**1.03**	36.6	2.68	**<u>11.9</u>**	1.78
(Bursts ≥4 ISIs)/second	**0.0037**	0.0033	1.32	0.0153	**<u>0.98</u>**	0.0185
Preburst interval (ms)	62.2	120	66.2	102.5	**<u>146.9</u>**	**60.9**
Principal events/second	11.5	7.8	23.9	9.76	**<u>7.39</u>**	**19.7**

Note: ISI = interspike interval; RF = receptive field. Numbers in boldface type indicate categories in which post hoc testing of means (Bonferroni correction) revealed significant differences from the border zone anesthetic, no RF category (numbers in bold and underlined).

(Radhakrishnan et al. 1999). In contrast, we examined cells only within or posterior-inferior to the Vc. Finally, Radhakrishnan and coworkers studied the burst index (the number of bursting cells per track), whereas we studied cellular bursting rates, rates of bursts with more than three ISIs, and other measures of bursting (e.g., percentage of second-order ISIs of less than 11 ms) for all cells in the region of Vc. Thus, there are significant differences between the two studies in terms of the diagnoses of patients studied, the location of cells studied, and the analytical techniques. Clearly, the increase in bursting activity demonstrated by Lenz and coworkers is more applicable to the region of the principal somatic sensory nucleus of patients with central pain secondary to spinal cord transection.

Further support for increased spike-bursts occurring in patients with spinal cord transection is found in thalamic recordings from monkeys with thoracic, anterolateral cordotomies (Weng et al. 2000). Some of these animals showed increased responsiveness to electrocutaneous stimuli and thus the study may represent a model of central pain (Vierck 1991). The most pronounced changes in firing were found in thalamic multireceptive cells, which respond to both cutaneous brushing and compressive stimuli with activity that is not graded into the noxious range. In comparison with normal controls, multireceptive cells in the monkeys with cordotomies showed significant increases in the number of bursts occurring spontaneously or in response to brushing or compressive stimuli. The changes in bursting behavior were widespread, occurring in the thalamic representation of the upper and lower extremities, both ipsilateral and contralateral to the cordotomy. The studies of this monkey model of central pain strengthen the case that spike-bursting rates are higher in patients with central pain secondary to SCI than in patients without any abnormality of the somatic sensory system (movement disorder patients).

Clearly, there is no direct relationship between spike-burst firing and pain. Spike-bursts are found in the thalamic representation of the monkey upper extremity and in the thalamic representation of the arm and leg ipsilateral to the cordotomy. Typically, pain is not experienced in these parts of the body in patients with thoracic spinal cord transection or cordotomy (Beric et al. 1988). Spike-bursts are increased in frequency during slow-wave sleep in all mammals studied (Steriade et al. 1990), including humans (Zirh et al. 1997). However, such bursting could cause pain if stimulation in the vicinity of the bursting cell produced the sensation of pain. This finding has been reported in two recent studies of sensations evoked by stimulation of the region of Vc in patients with chronic pain secondary to neural injury (Davis et al. 1996; Lenz et al. 1998a).

SENSATIONS EVOKED BY STIMULATION WITHIN THE REGION OF VC

Microstimulation studies suggest partitioning of thermal and pain sensations at different locations in the region of Vc in control patients without somatosensory abnormality. Patients were trained preoperatively to use a standard questionnaire to describe the location (projected field) and quality of sensations evoked by threshold microstimulation intraoperatively. Thermal and pain sensations were evoked by stimulation over a relatively large area extending up to 4 mm posterior to the core and up to 4 mm below the anterior-posterior commissure (AC–PC) line (see Fig. 3 in Lenz et al. 1993a). Within the core of the Vc, sites where stimulation evoked thermal or pain sensations were located near the border with the posterior-inferior area. Thermal pain sensations were evoked at a significantly greater percentage of sites located in the posterior-inferior area (30%) than of sites in the core area (5%). The threshold of current for evoking a sensation did not vary with location of the stimulation site (core versus posterior-inferior) or with quality of sensation (paresthesia or thermal/pain sensations). Other reports have identified the presence of sites where pain, but not thermal sensations, were evoked posterior and inferior to the core of the Vc (Hassler and Reichert 1959; Halliday and Logue 1972; Dostrovsky et al. 1991).

There is also anatomical organization based on the modality of the thermal or pain sensations and the part of the body where a sensation was evoked. For example, the sensation of warmth was evoked by stimulation at sites that were located significantly posterior to sites where pain or cool sensations were evoked. The sensation of paresthesia was more likely to be evoked in a large PF by stimulation in the posterior-inferior area (11%) than by stimulation in the core (3%). Differences in the size of the PFs were related to the quality of the sensation within the thermal/pain category. The sensation of cool was usually evoked in small PFs located on the lips. The sensation of warmth or pain was evoked in PFs that were larger than those where cool sensations were evoked on the same part of the body (Lenz et al. 1993a). Locations of projected fields in terms of depth relative to the skin also varied relative to the location of the stimulation site. Evoked sensations were more likely to be referred to deep structures at stimulation sites in the posterior-inferior (50%) than in the core area (28%).

MODALITY REPRESENTATION IN THE REGION OF VC IN PATIENTS WITH CHRONIC PAIN AND CENTRAL PAIN

In patients with chronic pain, the incidence of thalamic stimulation-evoked pain both in the Vc and posterior-inferior to the Vc is significantly higher than in control patients (Levin 1966; Obrador and Dierssen 1966; Dierssen et al. 1969; Mazars et al. 1974; Lenz et al. 1988b; Davis et al. 1996). A more recent study also suggests changes in the incidence of sites where stimulation evokes nonpainful thermal sensations (Lenz et al. 1998a). In this study, stimulation of the region of Vc was more likely to evoke pain in patients with chronic neuropathic pain (n = 12) after nervous system injury than in control patients without somatosensory abnormalities (patients with movement disorders, n = 10) (Lenz et al. 1998a).

On the basis of PFs, the region of Vc was divided into areas representing the part of the body where the patients experienced chronic pain (pain-affected), where the patients did not experience chronic pain (pain-unaffected), and into a control area located in the thalamus of patients with movement disorders with no experience of chronic pain. The region of Vc was also divided into a core region, where the majority of cells responded to innocuous cutaneous stimulation, and a region posterior-inferior to the core.

In both the core and posterior-inferior regions of patients with chronic neuropathic pain, the proportion of sites where threshold microstimulation evoked pain was larger in pain-affected and pain-unaffected areas than in control areas (see Fig. 4). The number of sites where thermal (warm or cold) sensations were evoked was correspondingly smaller, so that the total of pain sites plus thermal sites was not significantly different across all areas (see Fig. 4) (Lenz et al. 1998a). Therefore, sites where stimulation evoked pain in patients with neuropathic pain may correspond to sites where stimulation evoked thermal sensations in patients without somatosensory abnormality.

The same kind of change was found in patients with central pain. In these patients the number of sites where cold was evoked was significantly lower than in controls, whereas the number of sites where warmth was evoked was not different from controls (Lenz et al. 1994c). In these patients there

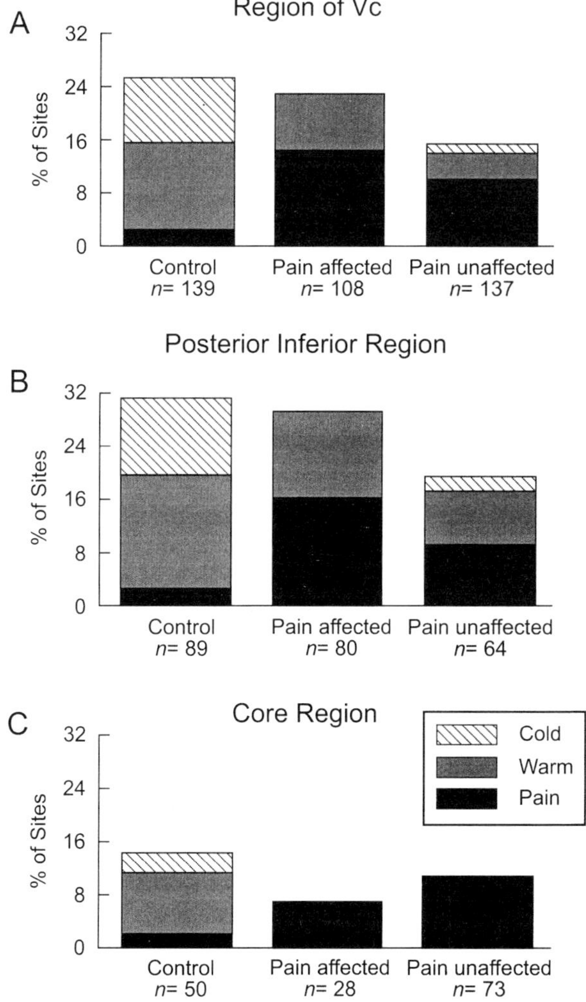

Fig. 4. Percentages of sites where pain, cold, and warm sensations were evoked by stimulation in the core (panel C), in the posterior-inferior areas (panel B) and combined (panel A). These percentages are shown for movement disorder patients (control) and for areas of the thalamus representing the part of the body where the chronic pain patients did (pain affected) or did not experience pain (pain unaffected).

was a significant increase in the number of sites where pain was evoked, but no significant difference from controls in the number of pain sites plus thermal sites. Stimulation of the STT in the cervical spine produces both pain and thermal sensations (Tasker and Organ 1973; Mayer et al. 1975). Therefore, the results of Lenz et al. (1994c) suggest that the terminus of the STT may have been relabeled to signal pain rather than cold in patients with central pain. This finding could account for the occurrence of cold hyperalgesia in patients with central pain.

The changes in modality representation suggest that pain is evoked in patients with neuropathic pain by stimulation at sites where thermal sensations would normally be evoked. Therefore, our data suggest that the STT, or elements to which the STT projects, signal pain rather than thermal sensations in patients with neuropathic pain. This suggestion is consistent with the finding that stimulation of the STT at the craniospinal junction evokes pain in patients with neuropathic pain (Tasker 1982), but evokes nonpainful thermal sensations in patients who do not have neuropathic pain (Tasker 1988). Anterolateral cordotomy relieves pain in a much greater proportion of patients with somatic pain than it does in patients with neuropathic pain (Tasker et al. 1980; Sweet et al. 1994). The failure of cordotomy to relieve neuropathic pain might be anticipated from the occurrence of central pain in patients with impaired function of the STT (Cassinari and Pagni 1969; Beric et al. 1988; Boivie et al. 1989; Andersen et al. 1995). These results suggest that the generator for pain in patients with central pain is the terminus of the STT.

In patients with central pain, anatomical evidence of damage to STT is a common finding (Cassinari and Pagni 1969), and loss of STT function, indicated by impaired thermal and pain sensibility, is a uniform finding (Beric et al. 1988; Boivie et al. 1989; Andersen et al. 1995). Stimulation-evoked pain is more common in patients with central pain than in controls, while stimulation-evoked cold sensations are correspondingly less common. These findings suggest a reorganization of the termination of the STT such that cold modalities are relabeled to signal pain in the thalamus of patients with central pain. Such reorganization might occur in response to STT injury because dramatic changes in thalamic anatomy can result from interruption of sensory input (Rausell et al. 1992; Ralston et al. 1996). The relationship between thalamic stimulation-evoked cold and pain in patients with central pain may explain the perception of cold as pain (cold hyperalgesia or allodynia) that can occur in these patients (Boivie et al. 1989).

In summary, the studies reviewed here show that after SCI there is an increase in the size of the thalamic representation of parts of the body adjacent to the anesthetic area. Cells in this area are much less likely to have RFs than are cells in normal controls. Additionally, there is a mismatch between the RFs and PFs, which suggests that the representation of sensory input (RFs) is much more plastic than the central representation of the part of the body (PFs). In the region of Vc, where RFs and PFs confirm the representation of the border zone anesthetic region, cells are more likely to fire with a spike-bursting pattern, and firing between bursts is likely to be decreased. Finally, thalamic stimulation in these regions is more likely to evoke sensations of pain and correspondingly less likely to evoke thermal sensations, suggesting that the STT terminations in the region of Vc now signal pain more than innocuous thermal sensations. In combination with the increased spike-burst rate described above, the increase in stimulation-evoked pain could explain the ongoing pain of central pain states.

ACKNOWLEDGMENTS

Supported by grants to F.A. Lenz from the NIH: NS39498 and NS40059.

REFERENCES

Albé-Fessard DG, Lombard MC. Use of an animal model to evaluate the origin of and protection against deafferentation pain. *Adv Pain Res Ther* 1983; 5:691–700.

Albé-Fessard DG, Arfel G, Guiot G. Activités electriques characteristiques de quelques structures cerebrales chez l'homme. *Ann Chir* 1963; 17:1185–1214.

Andersen P, Vestergaard K, Ingeman-Nielsen M, Jensen TS. Incidence of post-stroke central pain. *Pain* 1995; 61:187–193.

Apkarian AV, Shi T. Squirrel monkey lateral thalamus. I. somatic nociresponsive neurons and their relation to spinothalamic terminals. *J Neurosci* 1994; 14:6779–6795.

Bates JAV. Electrical recording from the thalamus in human subjects. In: Iggo A (Ed). *Handbook of Sensory Physiology: Somatosensory System*. Berlin: Springer Verlag, 1972, pp 561–578.

Beric A, Dimitrijevic MR, Lindblom U. Central dysesthesia syndrome in spinal cord injury patients. *Pain* 1988; 34:109–116.

Boivie J, Leijon G, Johansson I. Central post-stroke pain-a study of the mechanisms through analyses of the sensory abnormalities. *Pain* 1989; 37:173–185.

Bowsher D. Termination of the central pain pathway in man: the conscious appreciation of pain. *Brain* 1957; 80:606–620.

Bushnell MC, Duncan GH. Mechanical response properties of ventroposterior medial thalamic neurons in the alert monkey. *Exp Brain Res* 1987; 67:603–614.

Bushnell MC, Duncan GH, Tremblay N. Thalamic VPM nucleus in the behaving monkey. I. Multimodal and discriminative properties of thermosensitive neurons. *J Neurophysiol* 1993; 69:739–752.

Casey KL. Unit analysis of nociceptive mechanisms in the thalamus of the awake squirrel monkey. *J Neurophysiol* 1966; 29:727–750.

Casey KL, Morrow TJ. Ventral posterior thalamic neurons differentially responsive to noxious stimulation of the awake monkey. *Science* 1983; 221:675–677.

Cassinari V, Pagni CA (Eds). *Central Pain. A Neurosurgical Survey*. Cambridge, Massachusetts: Harvard University Press, 1969.

Chung JM, Lee KH, Surmeier DJ, et al. Response characteristics of neurons in the ventral posterior lateral nucleus of the monkey thalamus. *J Neurophysiol* 1986; 56:370–390.

Cohen SM, Grundfest H. Thalamic loci of electrical activity initiated by afferent impulses in the cat. *J Neurophysiol* 1953; 17:193–207.

Craig AD, Bushnell MC, Zhang ET, Blomqvist A. A specific thalamic nucleus for pain and temperature sensation in macaques and humans. *Nature* 1994; 372:770–773.

Davis KD, Kiss ZHT, Tasker RR, Dostrovsky JO. Thalamic stimulation-evoked sensations in chronic pain patients and nonpain (movement disorder) patients. *J Neurophysiol* 1996; 75:1026–1037.

Davis KD, Kiss ZHT, Luo L, et al. Phantom sensations generated by thalamic microstimulation. *Nature* 1998; 391:385–387.

Davis KD, Lozano AM, Manduch M, et al. Thalamic relay site for cold perception in humans. *J Neurophysiol* 1999; 81:1970–1973.

Dierssen G, Odoriz B, Hernando C. Sensory and motor responses to stimulation of the posterior cingulate cortex in man. *J Neurosurg* 1969; 31:435–440.

Dostrovsky JO, Wells FEB, Tasker RR. Pain evoked by stimulation in human thalamus. In: Sjigenaga Y (Ed). *International Symposium on Processing Nociceptive Information.* Amsterdam: Elsevier, 1991, pp 115–120.

Dougherty PM, Li Y-J, Lenz FA, Rowland LH, Mittman S. Evidence that excitatory amino acids mediate afferent input to the primate somatosensory thalamus. *Brain Res* 1996; 278:267–273.

Duncan GH, Bushnell MC, Oliveras JL, Bastrash N, Tremblay N. Thalamic VPM nucleus in the behaving monkey. III. Effects of reversible inactivation by lidocaine on thermal and mechanical discrimination. *J Neurophysiol* 1993; 70:2086–2096.

Eaton SA, Salt TE. Thalamic NMDA receptors and nociceptive sensory synaptic transmission. *Neurosci Lett* 1990; 110:297–302.

Ericson AC, Blomqvist A, Craig AD, Ottersen OP, Broman J. Enrichment of Glutamate-like immunoreactivity in spinothalamic tract terminals in the nucleus submedius of cat. *Soc Neurosci Abstracts* 1993; 18:832.

Gautron M, Guilbaud G. Somatic responses of ventrobasal thalamic neurones in polyarthritic rats. *Brain Res* 1982; 237:459–471.

Guiot G, Derome P, Arfel G, Walter SG. Electrophysiological recordings in stereotaxic thalamotomy for parkinsonism. In: Krayenbuehl H, Maspes PE, Sweet WH (Eds). In: *Progress in Neurological Surgery.* Basel: Karger, 1973, pp 189–221.

Halliday AM, Logue V. Painful sensations evoked by electrical stimulation in the thalamus. In: Somjen GG (Ed). *Neurophysiology Studied in Man.* Amsterdam: Excerpta Medica, 1972, pp 221–230.

Hassler R. Anatomy of the thalamus. In: Schaltenbrand G, Bailey P (Eds). *Introduction to Stereotaxis with an Atlas of the Human Brain.* Stuttgart: Thieme, 1959, pp 230–290.

Hassler R. Dichotomy of facial pain conduction in the diencephalon. In: Hassler R, Walker AE (Eds). *Trigeminal Neuralgia: Pathogenesis and Pathophysiology.* Stuttgart: Thieme, 1970, pp 123–138.

Hassler R, Reichert T. Klinische und anatomische Befunde bei stereotaktischen Schmerzoperationen im Thalamus. *Arch Psychiat Nerverkr* 1959; 200:93–122.

Hirai T, Jones EG. A new parcellation of the human thalamus on the basis of histochemical staining. *Brain Res Rev* 1989; 14:1–34.

Jeanmonod D, Magnin M, Morel A. Thalamus and neurogenic pain: physiological, anatomical and clinical data. *Neuroreport* 1993; 4:475–478.

Jeanmonod D, Magnin M, Morel A. A thalamic concept of neurogenic pain. In: Gebhart GF, Hammond DL, Jensen TS (Eds). *Proceedings of the 7th World Congress on Pain,* Progress in Pain Research and Management, Vol. 2. Seattle: IASP Press, 1994, pp 767–787.

Jones EG (Ed). *The Thalamus.* New York: Plenum, 1985.

Jones EG, Friedman DP. Projection pattern of functional components of thalamic ventrobasal complex on monkey somatosensory cortex. *J Neurophysiol* 1982; 48:521–544.

Jones EG, Friedman DP, Hendry SHC. Thalamic basis of place and modality-specific columns in monkey somatosensory cortex: a correlative anatomical and physiological study. *J Neurophysiol* 1982; 48:545–568.

Kaas JH, Nelson RJ, Sur M, Dykes RW, Merzenich MM. The somatotopic organization of the ventroposterior thalamus of the squirrel monkey, *Saimiri sciureus. J Comp Neurol* 1984; 226:111–140.

Kenshalo DR, Giesler GJ, Leonard RB, Willis WD. Responses of neurons in primate ventral posterior lateral nucleus to noxious stimuli. *J Neurophysiol* 1980; 43:1594–1614.

Lee J-I, Antezanna D, Dougherty PM, Lenz FA. Responses of neurons in the region of the thalamic somatosensory nucleus to mechanical and thermal stimuli graded into the painful range. *J Comp Neurol* 1999; 410:541–555.

Lenz FA, Dougherty PM. Pain processing in the human thalamus. In: Steriade M, Jones EG, McCormick DA (Eds). *Thalamus,* Vol. II. Oxford: Elsevier, 1997, pp 617–651.

Lenz FA, Dougherty PM. Cells in the human principal thalamic sensory nucleus (ventralis caudalis—Vc) respond to innocuous mechanical and cool stimuli. *J Neurophysiol* 1998; 79:2227–2230.

Lenz FA, Dostrovsky JO, Tasker RR, et al. Single-unit analysis of the human ventral thalamic nuclear group: somatosensory responses. *J Neurophysiol* 1988a; 59:299–316.

Lenz FA, Tasker RR, Dostrovsky JO, et al. Abnormal single-unit activity and responses to stimulation in the presumed ventrocaudal nucleus of patients with central pain. *Pain Res Clin Manage* 1988b; 3:157–164.

Lenz FA, Kwan HC, Dostrovsky JO, Tasker RR. Characteristics of the bursting pattern of action potentials that occur in the thalamus of patients with central pain. *Brain Res* 1989; 496:357–360.

Lenz FA, Seike M, Lin YC, et al. Thermal and pain sensations evoked by microstimulation in the area of the human ventrocaudal nucleus (Vc). *J Neurophysiol* 1993a; 70:200–212.

Lenz FA, Seike M, Lin YC, et al. Neurons in the area of human thalamic nucleus ventralis caudalis respond to painful heat stimuli. *Brain Res* 1993b; 623:235–240.

Lenz FA, Gracely RH, Hope EJ, et al. The sensation of angina can be evoked by stimulation of the human thalamus. *Pain* 1994a; 59:119–125.

Lenz FA, Gracely RH, Rowland LH, Dougherty PM. A population of cells in the human principal sensory nucleus respond to painful mechanical stimuli. *Neurosci Lett* 1994b; 180:46–50.

Lenz FA, Kwan HC, Martin R, et al. Characteristics of somatotopic organization and spontaneous neuronal activity in the region of the thalamic principal sensory nucleus in patients with spinal cord transection. *J Neurophysiol* 1994c; 72:1570–1587.

Lenz FA, Gracely RH, Baker FH, Richardson RT, Dougherty PM. Reorganization of sensory modalities evoked by stimulation in the region of the principal sensory nucleus (ventral caudal—Vc) in patients with pain secondary to neural injury. *J Comp Neurol* 1998a; 399:125–138.

Lenz FA, Zirh AT, Garonzik IM, Dougherty PM. Neuronal activity in the region of the principle sensory nucleus of human thalamus (ventralis caudalis) in patients with pain following amputations. *Neurosci* 1998b; 86:1065–1081.

Levin G. Electrical stimulation of the globus pallidus and thalamus. *J Neurosurg* 1966; 24:415.

Mayer DJ, Price DD, Becker DP. Neurophysiological characterization of the anterolateral spinal cord neurons contributing to pain perception in man. *Pain* 1975; 1:59–72.

Mazars G, Merienne L, Cioloca C. Traitement de certains types de douleurs par des stimulateurs thalamiques implantables. *Neurochirurgie* 1974; 20:117–124.

McComas AJ, Wilson P, Martin-Rodriguez J, Wallace C, Hankinson J. Properties of somatosensory neurons in the human thalamus. *J Neurol Neurosurg Psychiatry* 1970; 33:716–717.

Mehler WR. The anatomy of the so-called "pain tract" in man: an analysis of the course and distribution of the ascending fibers of the fasciculus anterolateralis. In: French JD, Porter RW (Eds). *Basic Research in Paraplegia.* Springfield: Thomas, 1962, pp 26–55.

Mehler WR. The posterior thalamic region in man. *Confin Neurol* 1966; 27:18–29.

Mehler WR. Some neurological species differences—a posteriori. *Ann N Y Acad Sci* 1969; 167:424–468.

Mehler WR, Feferman ME, Nauta WHJ. Ascending axon degeneration following anterolateral cordotomy. An experimental study in the monkey. *Brain* 1960; 83:718–750.

Mountcastle VB, Henneman E. The representation of tactile sensibility in the thalamus of the monkey. *J Comp Neurol* 1952; 97:409–440.

Obrador S, Dierssen G. Sensory responses to subcortical stimulation and management of pain disorders by stereotactic methods. *Confin Neurol* 1966; 27:45–52.

Ohye C. Depth microelectrode recordings. In: Schaltenbrand G, Walker AE (Eds). *Stereotaxy of the Human Brain.* Stuttgart: Thieme, 1982, pp 372–389.

Olszewski J (Ed). *The Thalamus of Maccaca Mulatta.* New York: Karger, 1952.

Radhakrishnan V, Tsoukatos J, Davis KD, et al. A comparison of the burst activity of lateral thalamic neurons in chronic pain and non-pain patients. *Pain* 1999; 80:567–575.

Ralston HJ, Ohara PT, Meng XW, Wells J, Ralston DD. Transneuronal changes in the inhibitory circuitry of the macaque somatosensory thalamus following lesions of the dorsal column nuclei. *J Comp Neurol* 1996; 371:325–335.

Rausell E, Cusick CG, Taub E, Jones EG. Chronic Deafferentation in monkeys differentially affects nociceptive and non-nociceptive pathway distinguished by specific calcium-binding proteins and down-regulates gamma-aminobutyric acid type A receptors at thalamic levels. *Proc Natl Acad Sci USA* 1992; 89:2571–2575.

Rinaldi PC, Young RF, Albé-Fessard DG, Chodakiewitz J. Spontaneous neuronal hyperactivity in the medial and intralaminar thalamic nuclei in patients with deafferentation pain. *J Neurosurg* 1991; 74:415–421.

Steriade M, Deschenes M. The thalamus as a neuronal oscillator. *Brain Res Rev* 1984; 8:1–63.

Steriade M, Llinas RR. The functional states of the thalamus and the associated neuronal interplay. *Physiol Rev* 1988; 68:649–742.

Steriade M, Jones EG, Llinas RR (Eds). *Thalamic Oscillations and Signaling.* New York: Wiley, John & Sons, 1990.

Sweet WH, Poletti CE, Gybels GM. Operations in the brainstem and spinal canal with an appendix on the relationship of open and percutaneous cordotomy. In: Wall PD, Melzack R (Eds). *Textbook of Pain.* New York: Churchill Livingstone, 1994, pp 1113–1136.

Tasker RR. Identification of pain processing systems by electrical stimulation of the brain. *Hum Neurobiol* 1982; 1:261–272.

Tasker RR. Percutaneous cordotomy: the lateral high cervical technique. In: Schmidek HH, Sweet WH (Eds). *Operative Neurosurgical Techniques: Indications, Methods, and Results.* Philadelphia: Saunders, 1988, pp 1191–1205.

Tasker RR, Organ LW. Percutaneous cordotomy: physiological identification of target site. *Confin Neurol* 1973; 35:110–117.

Tasker RR, Organ LW, Hawrylyshyn P. Deafferentation and causalgia. In: Bonica JJ (Ed). *Pain.* New York: Raven Press, 1980, pp 305–329.

Vierck CJ. Can mechanisms of central pain syndromes be investigated in animal models? In: Casey KL (Ed). *Pain and Central Nervous System Disease: The Central Pain Syndromes.* New York: Raven Press, 1991, pp 129–141.

Walker AE. Central representation of pain. *Res Publ Assoc Res Nerv Ment Dis* 1943; 23:63–85.

Weng HR, Lee JL, Lenz FA, et al. Functional plasticity in primate somatosensory thalamus following chronic lesion of the ventral lateral spinal cord. *Neuroscience* 2000; 101:393–401.

Young RF. Brain stimulation. *Neurosurg Clin N Am* 1990; 1:865–879.

Zirh AT, Lenz FA, Reich SG, Dougherty PM. Patterns of bursting occurring in thalamic cells during parkinsonian tremor. *Neuroscience* 1997; 83:107–121.

Correspondence to: Frederick A. Lenz, MD, PhD, FRCS(C), Department of Neurosurgery, Meyer Building 7-113, Johns Hopkins Hospital, 600 North Wolfe Street, Baltimore, MD 21287-7713, USA. Tel: 410-955-2257; Fax: 410-614-9877; email: fal@pallidum.med.jhu.edu.

Spinal Cord Injury Pain: Assessment, Mechanisms, Management. Progress in Pain Research and Management, Vol. 23, edited by Robert P. Yezierski and Kim J. Burchiel, IASP Press, Seattle, © 2002.

14

New and Old Thoughts on the Mechanisms of Spinal Cord Injury Pain

Arthur D. (Bud) Craig

Atkinson Pain Research Laboratory, Division of Neurosurgery, Barrow Neurological Institute, Phoenix, Arizona, USA

This chapter addresses the fundamental mechanisms that generate intractable pain in many patients subsequent to spinal cord injury (SCI). The two sensory levels of the nervous system that can be affected by damage to the spinal cord are the segmental level, i.e., the dorsal horn of the spinal cord at or near the site of injury, and the suprasegmental or forebrain level. The former must be responsible for *at-level* pain, and the latter must be responsible for *below-level* pain, identical to the central pain syndrome. Several reviews of SCI pain and central pain have appeared recently (Boivie 1994; Pagni 1998; Craig 2000; Yezierski 2000), and Chapters 6 and 15 address the central neural bases of SCI pain. This chapter provides a brief review of important old ideas along with a deeper synopsis of attractive new ideas, with particular emphasis on a new hypothesis for central pain.

FUNDAMENTAL MECHANISMS OF ABNORMAL ACTIVITY

Whether at the site of spinal damage or at more rostral levels, there are three fundamental mechanisms for intractable pain. The abnormal neural activity that must underlie generation of SCI pain could occur due to *disinhibition, sensitization,* or *plasticity.*

Disinhibition. The concept of disinhibition (or "release") postulates that abnormal activity occurs because of a loss of inhibition that results in a release of activity, whether due to a direct loss of the action of local inhibitory interneurons or to the loss of an inhibitory interaction between converging systems. Thus, activity in particular neurons may appear that is normally damped or masked by ongoing inhibitory processes. This concept can easily explain the appearance of novel sensory phenomena, such as allodynia, in which a normally non-noxious stimulus such as cold or touch produces pain. This phenomenon would be consistent with a fairly abrupt post-traumatic appearance of pain.

Sensitization. The concept of sensitization suggests that abnormal activity occurs because of an unusual increase of activity or responsiveness in particular neurons. Such increases could be due to the development of a hyperactive focus of neural discharge (also referred to as ectopic activity or an irritable focus), or they could result from increased sensitivity to a normally occurring source of input. In general, physiological sensitization must result from biochemical changes, whether in the levels of released transmitters or modulators, the levels of circulating paracrine agents, or the levels and availability of receptors and intracellular messengers. Adaptation to changing conditions is a fundamental feature of biology, and pathological sensitization to pain must be a dysfunctional epiphenomenon of an adaptive process. This concept can easily explain the symptom of hyperalgesia, in which a stimulus that is normally only mildly painful causes unbearable pain. This phenomenon would require some time to develop, ranging from hours to weeks.

Plasticity. The concept of plasticity refers to abnormal activity due to a change in anatomical or functional connections. Anatomical changes ("sprouting") could produce abnormal connections that result in terminations on inappropriate neurons. Functional changes could occur, such as imbalanced modulation or the unmasking of latent inputs, that result in a reorganization of functional activity within a region and a change in the effects of its output activity. This concept could easily explain the slow (weeks to years) post-traumatic development of unusual cross-modal or nontopographic symptoms, including late-developing mechanical (touch-evoked) allodynia or the illusory sensations that can occur in a phantom limb after stimulation of the face (Ramachandran et al. 1995).

These mechanisms are certainly not exclusive, and each probably occurs to some degree following any damage to the spinal cord or central nervous system. Nonetheless, separating these concepts provides useful avenues for mechanism-based analyses of the causes of SCI pain.

SEGMENTAL MECHANISMS OF SCI PAIN

Several lines of current research are addressing segmental mechanisms for the generation of abnormal activity that could result in chronic pain. Such investigations are examining possibilities based on all three of the fundamental mechanisms described above. Contributors to this volume include several of the primary investigators active in this area, and Chapters 6, 7, 10, and 11 describe the use of different animal models of SCI to examine possible causes of segmental disinhibition and sensitization. Additional possibilities are being actively pursued in other laboratories that are examining neuropathic pain resulting from damage to a peripheral nerve rather than to the spinal cord, and similar segmental mechanisms could be involved in the at-level pain of SCI.

One possibility considered in many studies is degeneration of the local inhibitory interneurons in the spinal dorsal horn after injury to a peripheral nerve or to the spinal cord itself (Sugimoto et al. 1990; Eaton et al. 1998). These neurons may be particularly sensitive to the acute rise in excitatory amino acids following injury. Such interneurons are concentrated in the substantia gelatinosa (lamina II) of the superficial dorsal horn, where C fibers from the skin terminate. This loss of inhibitory interneurons could directly disinhibit neurons in the spinal dorsal horn that produce an ascending message of pain. Recent data from Yezierski's laboratory (Chapter 7) indicate that such neurons with ascending projections are probably located in the superficial dorsal horn, because pain behavior in this SCI model is observed only if this region remains intact.

Another possibility being considered is disinhibition due to the loss of descending inhibitory modulation. Some studies show that neuropathic pain behavior in rats can be reduced by lesions of the ascending fibers in the dorsal columns or in the midline medullary reticular formation (Bian et al 1998; Maier and Watkins 1998; Ossipov et al. 2000). Such lesions are thought to decrease descending inhibitory actions in the spinal dorsal horn (Urban and Gebhart 1999).

Both local and descending modulation of activity may affect the level of dynorphin in the superficial dorsal horn, which has recently been recognized as an important mediator of chronic neuropathic pain. Wang et al. (2001) showed, using dynorphin-knockout mice, that the upregulation of dynorphin is critical for maintained pain behavior days to weeks following peripheral nerve damage. Fig. 1 shows data from their study indicating that the enhanced dynorphin immunoreactivity seen in the superficial dorsal horn of the wild-type mouse does not appear in the knockout model and also that the late phase of allodynia-like pain behavior is reversed (after 8 days in their model). This evidence indicates that the upregulation of this neuromodulator in the superficial dorsal horn is critical for sensitized pain behavior.

Sensitization of ascending spinal nociceptive neurons after peripheral nerve injury in the primate was directly examined in a physiological study by Palecek et al. (1992). The authors recorded spinothalamic tract (STT)

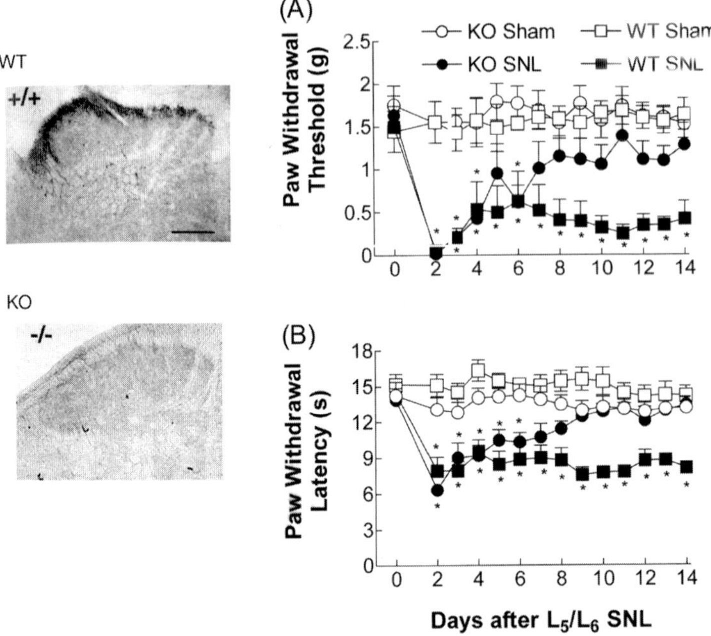

Fig. 1. Left: The immunohistochemical demonstration of dynorphin in the superficial dorsal horn of the wild-type (WT) mouse and the dynorphin-knockout (KO) mouse. Right: Behavioral data indicating allodynia-like pain behavior in mice with sciatic nerve ligation (SNL) was maintained in WT but not in KO mice. Reproduced from Wang et al. (2001), with permission.

neurons in the primate deep dorsal horn at the segment innervated by the damaged nerve and found them to be unresponsive, but they showed that such neurons in the immediately rostral segments were hyper-responsive to low-threshold somatic stimulation and were sensitized to thermal stimuli to which they would not normally respond. For further details on their work, see Chapter 6 by Willis, whose laboratory has examined many possible biochemical mechanisms for the sensitization of deep dorsal horn neurons. The deep neurons this group studied seem to integrate much of the activity of the more superficial layers of the dorsal horn, and thus they provide a representative indication of the segmental changes that occur following injury.

A critical role for the superficial dorsal horn in neuropathic pain is indicated by the recent study of Bester et al. (2000), who used the activation of neuronal *c-fos* as a measure to determine which neurons in the dorsal horn could explain mechanical allodynia-like activity. They found that low-threshold stimulation (brushing) that produced pain behavior in rats with sciatic nerve (crush) lesions produced correlative *c-fos* expression in laminae I–II neurons (Fig. 2), as well as in the major lamina I projection target in rats, the midbrain parabrachial nucleus. Because such neurons are normally activated only by noxious stimulation, their data directly reveal abnormal activity that could be the basis for allodynia-like pain behavior. Their data corroborate the evidence cited above, indicating that hyper-responsiveness and sensitization in the superficial dorsal horn is critical for neuropathic pain and segmental SCI pain. The clinical findings of Edgar et al. (1993) support this view, as do recent comparative studies showing that abolition of substance P-responsive lamina I neurons reduces pain behavior in rats (Mantyh et al. 1997; Cao et al. 1998). Nociceptive lamina I projection neurons can be sensitized to low-threshold mechanical and innocuous thermal stimulation, which could provide the basis for the mechanical and thermal allodynia that can appear in neuropathic and at-level SCI pain (see Craig 2000). However, Bester et al. (2000) found that the abnormally activated laminae I–II neurons were distributed only within the terminal territory of the intact saphenous nerve, which they interpreted to indicate that the activation of lamina I nociceptive projection neurons by low-threshold stimulation was due not to sensitization, but rather to abnormal anatomical sprouting of large-diameter mechanoreceptor terminals into the superficial dorsal horn (Woolf et al. 1992). This important result indicates the possible role of anatomical plasticity in segmental pain, although several major issues remain to be clarified regarding their interpretation (Blomqvist and Craig 2000).

Finally, a startling new direction to consider is the possibility that neuronal sensitization at the segmental level may be caused by an inflammatory

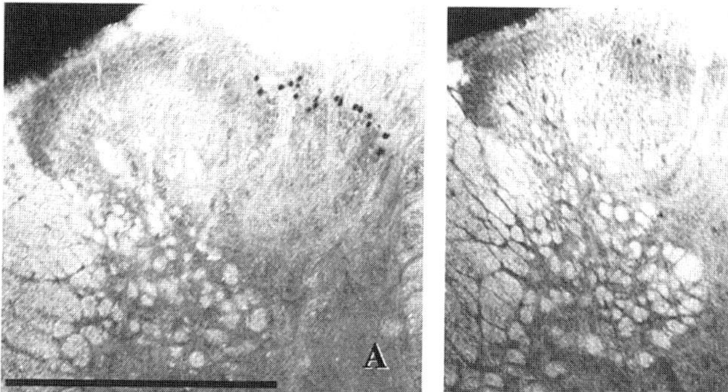

Fig. 2. Photomicrographs showing brush-evoked *c-fos* expression in superficial dorsal horn (laminae I–II) neurons in a rat with a sciatic nerve lesion (A) but not in a rat with a sham control operation (B). Scale bar = 500 μm. Reproduced from Bester et al. (2000), with permission.

glial response. Both microglia and astrocytes within the spinal cord can be activated by peripheral nerve or spinal damage, and they release a cascade of cytokines and eicosanoids (prostaglandins) that directly affect excitatory amino acid release and local neuronal activity (DeLeo and Yezierski 2001; Watkins 2001). This enhanced glutamate release may be responsible for neuronal death and hyperactivity, and the cytokines may act on second-messenger systems in spinal neurons (Bezzi et al. 2001; Samad et al. 2001). Intrathecal administration of antagonists to cytokines and prostaglandins (e.g., IL-1 receptor antagonist, IL-10, and acetaminophen) can reduce neuropathic and SCI pain behavior. The role of cytokines and glia in clinical SCI pain at the segmental level is an exciting prospect that requires immediate investigation.

THE ROLE OF LAMINA I PROJECTION NEURONS IN SEGMENTAL SCI PAIN

Considerable evidence indicates that ascending projection neurons in the superficial dorsal horn are important for segmental pain. Such neurons are located almost entirely in lamina I, the thin marginal zone at the top of the dorsal horn. The functional anatomy of lamina I has recently been reviewed (Craig 2000). Briefly, lamina I receives monosynaptic input from Aδ and C fibers from all tissues of the body. This zone contains modality-selective nociceptive, thermoreceptive, and chemoreceptive neurons that are functionally and morphologically distinct. It projects to spinal and brainstem autonomic and homeostatic sites, as well as to the thalamus, and it receives descending controls from brainstem pre-autonomic regions and the hypothalamus. It is the source of the lateral spinothalamic tract (STT), which is critical for the sensations of pain, temperature, itch and other feelings from the body that represent its physiological condition. The available evidence supports the concept that lamina I is the source of ascending activity important for homeostasis, and that the lamina I STT projection comprises discrete sensory channels that provide the basis for distinct sensations, or "labeled lines" (Craig et al. 2001). The recent identification of histamine-(itch)-selective lamina I STT cells in our laboratory demonstrates the selectivity inherent in the lamina I projection system (Andrew and Craig 2001): such cells receive input only from a specific subset of very slowly conducting C fibers that are selectively responsive to histamine, and they are distinct with respect to their ongoing activity, central conduction velocities, and thalamic projections. Their temporal response profile mirrors itch sensation in humans, and clinical evidence indicates that their axons in the lateral STT are critical for the sensation of itch. Recent analyses indicate that thermoreceptive-specific (COOL and WARM) lamina I STT cells in the cat are similarly unique in their functional and anatomical characteristics and can also be directly associated with human thermal sensations (Craig et al. 2001).

There are two major classes of nociceptive lamina I STT neurons, and our most recent findings indicate that they constitute discrete channels for distinct aspects of pain. The nociceptive-specific (NS) lamina I STT neurons, which are dominated by input from Aδ nociceptors, show responses that parallel the human sensations of "first" pain and "sharpness," whereas the polymodal nociceptive lamina I neurons (termed HPC cells, because they respond to noxious heat, noxious pinch, and noxious cold) show responses that parallel the human sensation of "second" (burning) pain (Andrew and Craig 1999; Craig and Andrew 1999). Like second pain, which is dependent on C-nociceptor input, HPC cells are dominated by monosynaptic input from polymodal C-fiber nociceptors.

Fig. 3 documents the association of HPC lamina I STT activity with human second pain sensation. The upper left panels show the psychophysical reports by human volunteers of the augmenting second pain sensation elicited by a repeated brief contact heat stimulus (Vierck et al. 1997). In this paradigm, a painfully hot stimulus is used that is perceived only as warm if contacted very briefly (0.7 seconds). Repeated brief contacts at short intervals (<3 seconds) reliably elicit a strongly augmenting second (burning) pain sensation, but only a weak first (sharp) pain sensation. This phenomenon is characterized by its direct dependence on the stimulus temperature and its inverse dependence on the interstimulus interval (ISI), as shown in the upper left panels. The upper right panels in Fig. 3 show that lamina I HPC cells display the same response patterns with the same dependencies and the same rate of augmentation (temporal summation). The original records at the bottom of Fig. 3 document the rapid temporal summation in the responses of a single HPC lamina I STT neuron to repeated brief contact heat stimulation at shorter ISIs. In contrast, NS lamina I STT neurons do not show such temporal summation, and their responses parallel the human reports of first pain in response to repeated heat as well as to mechanical stimulation. The activity of STT neurons in the deep dorsal horn similarly does not parallel the human report of second pain in response to repeated heat stimulation.

As discussed further by Vierck (Chapters 8, 9), this temporal summation phenomenon could be a very important segmental mechanism for neuropathic and SCI pain. Temporal summation with repeated noxious stimuli is a cardinal characteristic of SCI and central pain (sometimes called "wind-up" pain; see Chapters 4, 15, and 20). Most strikingly, Vierck et al. (1997) showed

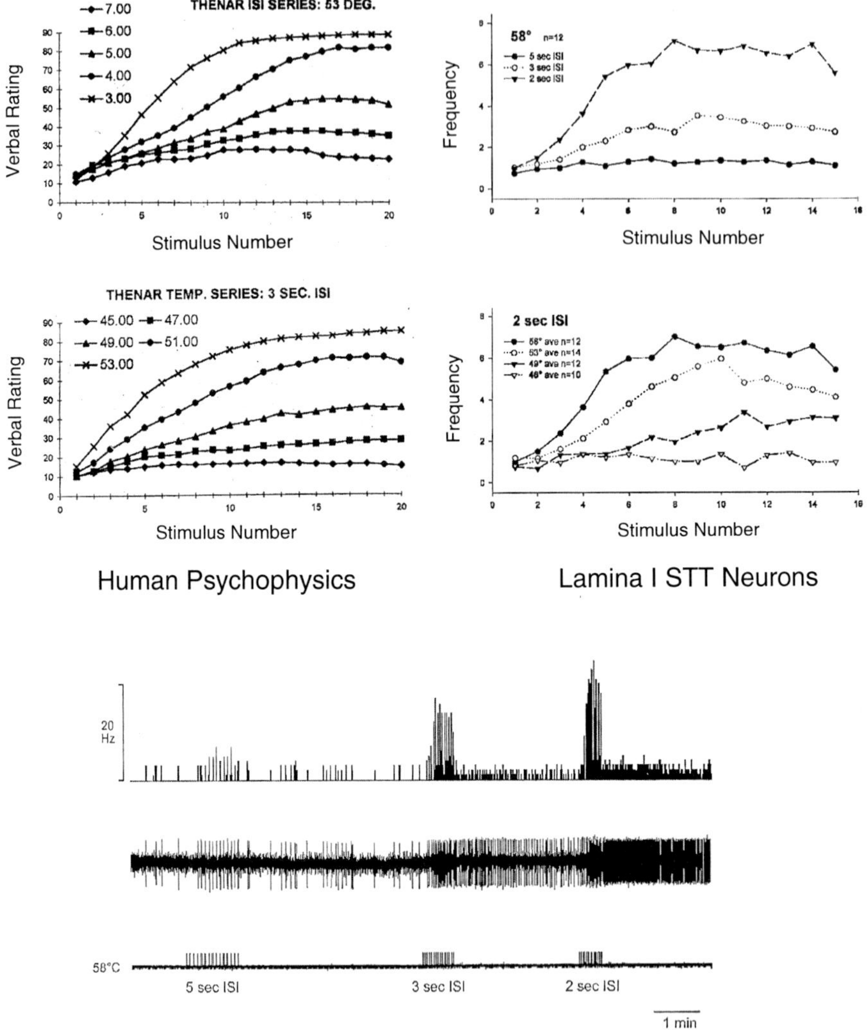

Fig. 3. Upper left: Psychophysical data showing that the augmenting second pain response of human volunteers to repeated brief contact heat stimulation is dependent on the stimulus temperature and inversely dependent on the interstimulus interval (ISI). Reprinted from Vierck et al. (1997), with permission. Upper right: The average responses of HPC lamina I spinothalamic tract (STT) neurons in the anesthetized cat show the same response augmentation and the same dependence on temperature and ISI. Bottom: Original data showing the augmenting responses in the histogrammed (1-second bins) record (upper trace) and the action potential (middle trace) record evoked from a single HPC lamina I STT neuron by the repeated brief contact heat stimuli at the times indicated in the lower trace (unpublished data from A.D. Craig and D. Andrew).

that this augmenting second pain sensation displays a rapid "re-set" phenomenon in normal human subjects, in which the temporal summation begins again from baseline following very short intertrial intervals. Although direct investigation is still needed, this re-set seems to be lacking in hyperpathic SCI and central pain patients. The HPC lamina I STT neurons show the same re-set phenomenon, exactly in parallel with the reported psychophysics, and thus the role of these neurons in the abnormal temporal summation of neuropathic and SCI pain must be further examined. For example, identification of the gene expression profile of HPC (multipolar) lamina I cells could be revealing, because such a profile must be unique for this particular cell type, and it may be quite different in chronic pain conditions. Further, it seems quite possible that the re-set observed in normal human volunteers and in HPC neurons represents the rapid restoration of an inhibitory process that is released by the repeated stimulation (i.e., disinhibited). The abnormal temporal summation of pain in SCI might represent the loss of this (descending?) inhibitory mechanism. Thus, identification of the source of this inhibitory deficiency might be critical. These considerations indicate several areas that could be important to study.

FOREBRAIN MECHANISMS OF SCI PAIN

Damage to the central nervous system at any level can result in ongoing pain, and this condition is known generically as *central pain*. Below-level SCI pain can be considered central pain. Several reviews of central pain have appeared in recent years (Boivie 1994; Bowsher 1996; Pagni 1998; Craig 2000). Such pain is characteristically described as burning and hyperpathic (augmenting), and it is often (although not necessarily) accompanied by mechanical or thermal (cold) allodynia. It is always referred to deep and cutaneous tissues where a paradoxical loss of acute pain (pinprick and heat) and thermal (cool and warm) sensation can be demonstrated (Bowsher et al. 1998), whereas there is no consistent correlation with the presence or absence of mechanical sensation. Thus, central pain is considered to result from damage to the spinothalamic tract at any level. Histological and imaging observations indicate that lesions of the dorsal horn, the contralateral spinal anterolateral funiculus, the path of the STT in the medulla and midbrain, the posterolateral thalamus, and the parieto-insular region of cortex can cause central pain. Central pain is not produced by lesions of the spinal dorsal columns, the medial thalamus, or parietal somatosensory cortices.

Several hypotheses for the basis of central pain build upon the three fundamental mechanisms of abnormal neural activity described above (Craig

2000). The oldest is a disinhibition hypothesis suggesting that a medial thalamic substrate for the emotional aspect of pain is released by the loss of a lateral thalamic substrate for discriminative pain sensation (Head and Holmes 1911). Head and Holmes deduced that the infarct in the posterolateral thalamus that was characteristic of the thalamic pain syndrome (the first recognized type of central pain) destroyed a specific sensory substrate for pain and temperature. They presumed that this insult released essential activity in the medial thalamus responsible for the emotional aspect of pain, which they thought was manifested by the hyperpathic response evoked by repeated noxious stimulation, in contrast to the lack of perception of single acute noxious stimuli. The specific pain and temperature relay nucleus that Head and Holmes envisioned has been identified as the posterior part of the ventral medial nucleus (VMpo), but their hypothesis left several gaps, one of which was the means by which medial thalamus was still activated following loss of the lateral pain and temperature pathway.

Melzack and Casey (1968) subsequently formalized the hypothesis that spinoreticulothalamic activity was responsible for this activation. They followed Riddoch's (1938) and Bishop's (1959) conjecture that such a multisynaptic pathway exists as a phylogenetically old substrate for forebrain integration. The existence of such a pathway is still uncertain, although new data suggest an important possibility (the spino-parabrachial projection). Thus, Melzack and Casey suggested a disinhibition phenomenon similar to that of Head and Holmes whereby central pain results from the release of the so-called paleospinothalamic (medial) projections from the inhibition normally imposed by neospinothalamic (lateral) projections.

Two hypotheses based on sensitization have been proposed. One idea is that hyperactive thalamic bursting develops in the medial thalamus due to excessive inhibition by the reticular thalamic nucleus, in turn caused by the deafferentation of the posterolateral thalamus (Jeanmonod et al. 1994). Inhibitory GABAergic reticular neurons can cause a characteristic periodic bursting discharge in thalamic cells, which is called "low-threshold calcium spiking (LTS)," as occurs in synchronized sleep activity or barbiturate spindling or epileptic discharges. This hypothesis presumes bidirectional reticular nucleus interconnections between pain-related cells in the medial and lateral thalamus, which is an unlikely anatomical arrangement because the thalamic reticular nucleus is topographically related to the various nuclei of the thalamus. A related hypothesis is that LTS bursting within deafferented regions of lateral thalamus could itself be associated with chronic pain, because such activity can be recorded in human neuropathic pain patients (Lenz and Dougherty 1997). Such bursting might also be due to changes in thalamic neurotransmitter regulation (Bowsher et al. 1998), to differences in

GABAergic modulation of STT terminations within VP (Ralston and Ralston 1994), or to anatomical plasticity in the deafferented thalamus (Woods et al. 2000), although a directly comparable study in the primate found physiological changes throughout the somatosensory thalamus, not only in the deafferented region (Weng et al. 2000). These two sensitization hypotheses would be consistent with the delay (months to years) in the onset of central pain observed in some patients following stroke or SCI, but they are not compatible with most cases, in which the onset of central pain immediately follows the damage. Furthermore, both of these sensitization hypotheses presume that bursting thalamic activity is abnormal and generates pain, but such bursting occurs normally during sleep and also in the thalamus of awake patients who do not have pain (Radhakrishnan et al. 1999).

Foerster (1927) suggested that loss of the dorsal column pathway was responsible for pain, but his considerations probably confounded burning central pain with the dysesthesia of lemniscal deafferentation (Boivie 1994). On the other hand, Beric (1997) suggested that below-level SCI pain occurs only if damage to the lateral STT is coupled with spared dorsal column function, resulting in dissociated sensory loss and a sensory imbalance. This idea is consonant with the notion that imbalanced integration between lemniscal activity in area 3b and STT-related activity in area 3a can occur following spinal lesions (Tommerdahl et al. 1996). However, central pain can occur following complete spinal transection or following supratentorial lesions that affect both spinothalamic and lemniscal sensibilities.

The possibility of plastic reorganization of the lateral thalamus in central pain is suggested by the observations of Dostrovsky and colleagues (Davis et al 1998; Dostrovsky 2000). They found that electrical stimulation with a microelectrode in the deafferented region of VP can occasionally elicit phantom pain in amputees with chronic pain or can lead to reports of pain in central (post-stroke) pain patients. This finding contrasts with the repeated observations by Dostrovsky and others that VP stimulation in nonpain patients almost never causes pain. This difference indicates that the output of the deafferented region of VP in amputees is still connected to sites that generate a sensation in the phantom limb, but that this output is somehow misrouted or aberrantly integrated to generate a sensation of pain. However, when the stimulation in chronic pain patients produced pain, it was topographically inappropriate, suggesting that either disordered anatomical rewiring had occurred in their VP projections to the cortex, or more likely, that ascending thalamocortical fibers of passage from the VMpo were activated. This possibility is supported by the observation that the incidence of pain reports from stimulation in the posterior thalamus was also greatly increased in these patients. The incidence of evoked thermal sensations, however, was reduced. Nevertheless, these observations contrast with the clinically useful finding that such stimulation in chronic pain patients is usually therapeutic (Gybels and Sweet 1989). The basis for these observations remains to be established, because the VP thalamus is primarily the thalamic relay for the lemniscal (mechanoreceptive) system, which is critical for fine tactual discrimination.

THE THERMOSENSORY DISINHIBITION HYPOTHESIS OF CENTRAL PAIN

I have proposed a new hypothesis for central pain that is based on the original disinhibition hypothesis of Head and Holmes, but updated by several new findings (Craig 1998, 2000). This thermosensory disinhibition hypothesis proposes that central pain results from the disinhibition of pain by release from ongoing thermosensory activity, or in other words, from imbalanced integration caused by the loss of temperature sensation (rather than by the loss of discriminative pain sensation; see also Kendall 1939). In essence, I suggest that central pain is a thermoregulatory disorder that produces an ongoing thermal distress signal that is modulated by homeostatic processing. My proposal also updates the ideas of Melzack and Casey (1968) by suggesting that the loss of the lateral thalamic spinothalamic pathway unmasks a homeostatic spinobulbothalamic pathway to the medial thalamus that is responsible for the pain. Specifically, the thermosensory disinhibition hypothesis states that a lesion that interferes with the output of the thermosensory area in the insula disinhibits a limbic network involving brainstem homeostatic sites, the medial thalamus, and the anterior cingulate cortex (ACC) that engenders affect (burning pain) associated with thermoregulatory motivation.

The thermosensory disinhibition hypothesis is based on several clinical characteristics of central pain. First and foremost, virtually all central pain patients have a thermosensory deficit in the region where the ongoing pain is perceived (Boivie 1994; Andersen et al. 1995; Bowsher 1996; Pagni 1998). At the least, they have elevated warming/cooling thresholds, and most have a complete regional loss of innocuous temperature sensation, or thermanesthesia, whereas many, but not all, also have a paradoxical reduction in acute pain sensation, or hypoalgesia. This consistent correlation suggests a causal role for the loss of thermal sensation. Second, at least half of central pain patients experience the onset of ongoing pain immediately after the precipitating incident, whether a cerebrovascular event or spinal trauma. This time frame is consistent with the mechanism of disinhibition. Third, most central pain patients describe the ongoing pain as burning, and many have cold allodynia (pain caused by a cool stimulus). This description is consistent with the burning sensation of deep cold pain, a distinct thermoregulatory signal. Incidentally, Head and Holmes (1911) noted that many thalamic pain patients felt better in a warm room, also an indication of a thermoregulatory dysfunction. Fourth, most have vague autonomic dysfunction (inappropriate flushing, sweating, and regional vasoconstriction), and nearly all show signs of an emotional dependence in their pain (hyperpathia). This phenomenon is also consistent with the concept of a homeostatic disorder. Last, the lesions associated with central pain nearly always destroy the lateral spinothalamocortical pathway of lamina I neurons. This pathway incorporates the ascending thermosensory pathway.

Fig. 4 summarizes the projections of lamina I neurons, which as noted above have an integral role in pain and temperature sensations. Their ascending projections define the lateral spinothalamic tract in the middle of the lateral funiculus in the contralateral spinal cord. They project to a number of spinal and brainstem sites associated with autonomic function; in the upper brainstem they project to two particular sites that are important for whole-body homeostasis, the parabrachial nucleus (PB) and the periaqueductal gray (PAG). These are the primary sensory and motoric homeostatic (limbic) sites of the brainstem, respectively. Most importantly, our anatomical and physiological work has shown that there is a direct lamina I spinothalamocortical pathway that is unique to primates conveyed by a specific lateral thalamic relay nucleus within the posterolateral thalamus, i.e., the VMpo. Fig. 5 shows that the human VMpo nucleus, distinguished by its cytoarchitecture, its immunohistochemical labeling, and its dense STT input, is a very large structure (Blomqvist et al. 2000). This topographic pathway courses to the dorsal margin of the mid/posterior insular cortex. This cortical area forms, in conjunction with the (similarly unique) direct vagal/solitarius representation that in primates is relayed by the adjacent VMb to a contiguous cortical field, a complete first-order (interoceptive) representation of the physiological condition of the body. In addition, a medial lamina I spinothalamocortical pathway passes through the ventrocaudal portion of the medial dorsal nucleus (MDvc) to reach the ACC.

Functional imaging data confirm that the interoceptive representation in the insular cortex is activated specifically by stimuli associated with feelings from the body, including pain, temperature, itch, hunger, thirst, taste, exercise, cardiovascular activity, inspiration, and air hunger (for references see Craig 2000; Drzezga et al. 2001). In particular, this region is the only cortical field activated in a graded fashion by contralateral thermal stimuli (Fig. 6; Craig et al. 2000), and therefore this cortical field includes the

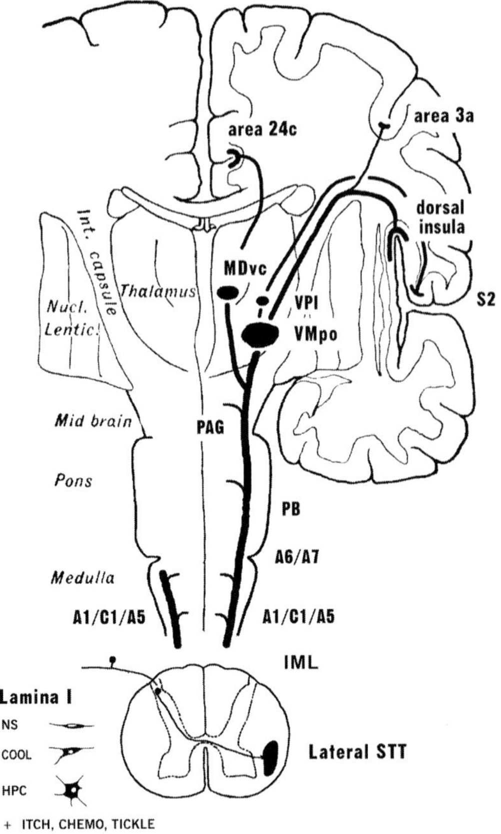

Fig. 4. Diagram summarizing the projections of lamina I neurons in the primate, based on anterograde tracing following precise injections into lamina I at different spinal levels (see Craig 2000). A1/C1/A5 and A6/A7 = catecholaminergic cell groups; IML = intermediolateral cell column in the thoracolumbar spinal cord; MDvc = ventrocaudal portion of the medial dorsal nucleus; PAG = periaqueductal gray; PB = parabrachial nucleus; VMpo = posterior part of the ventral medial nucleus; VPI = ventral posterior inferior nucleus; S2 = secondary somatosensory cortex.

discriminative thermosensory cortex of humans, consistent with clinical studies of cortical lesions that produce thermanesthesia (Greenspan et al. 1999). This evidence manifests the concept described above that temperature is an emergent aspect of interoceptive sensation, rather than an exteroceptive sensation associated with touch (and so are pain and other bodily feelings), which is contrary to long-held beliefs. The homeostatic nature of this cortical field is supported by its delineation by labeling for receptors for corticotropin-releasing factor, as shown in Fig. 7.

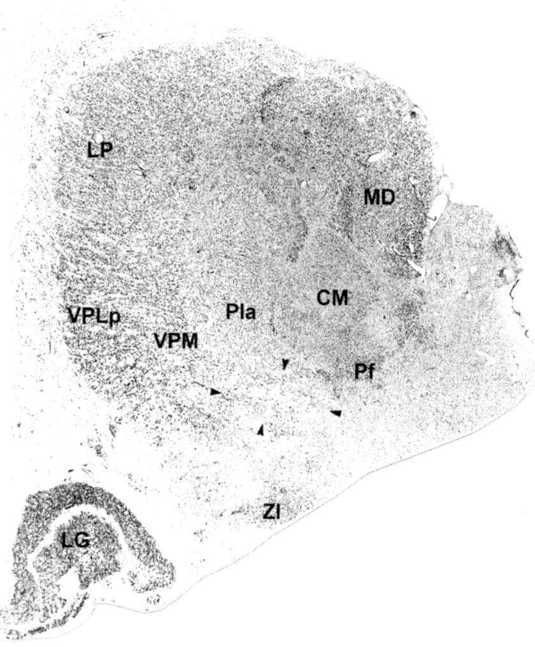

Fig. 5. Photomicrograph illustrating the location and size of the posterior part of the ventral medial nucleus (VMpo) in the human thalamus (arrows). CM = center median nucleus; LG = lateral geniculate nucleus; LP = lateral posterior nucleus; MD = mediodorsal nucleus; Pf = parafascicular nucleus; Pla = anterior pulvinar nucleus; VPLp = ventral posterior lateral nucleus; VPM = ventral posterior medial nucleus; ZI = zona incerta. Adapted from Blomqvist et al. (2000).

Most significantly, this region of cortex exactly matches the cortical site that is damaged in patients with central pain, shown in Fig. 8 (Schmahmann and Leifer 1992). Similarly, lesions at spinal, bulbar, and thalamic levels that are associated with central pain are all located such that they would interfere with the rostrad transmission in the lamina I spinothalamocortical pathway. Thus, the loss of function of this thermosensory cortical region occurs in central pain, consistent with the finding that all central pain patients have a thermosensory deficit. This finding strongly suggests that it is the loss of this thermosensory cortical activity that disinhibits central pain.

In fact, it is well known that thermal stimuli normally inhibit pain; this phenomenon is used every day therapeutically. It is not well recognized that this phenomenon has a central as well as a peripheral basis. Cold can block activity in peripheral nerve terminals and reduce peripheral inflammation, but it also reduces the pain caused by electrical stimulation of a peripheral

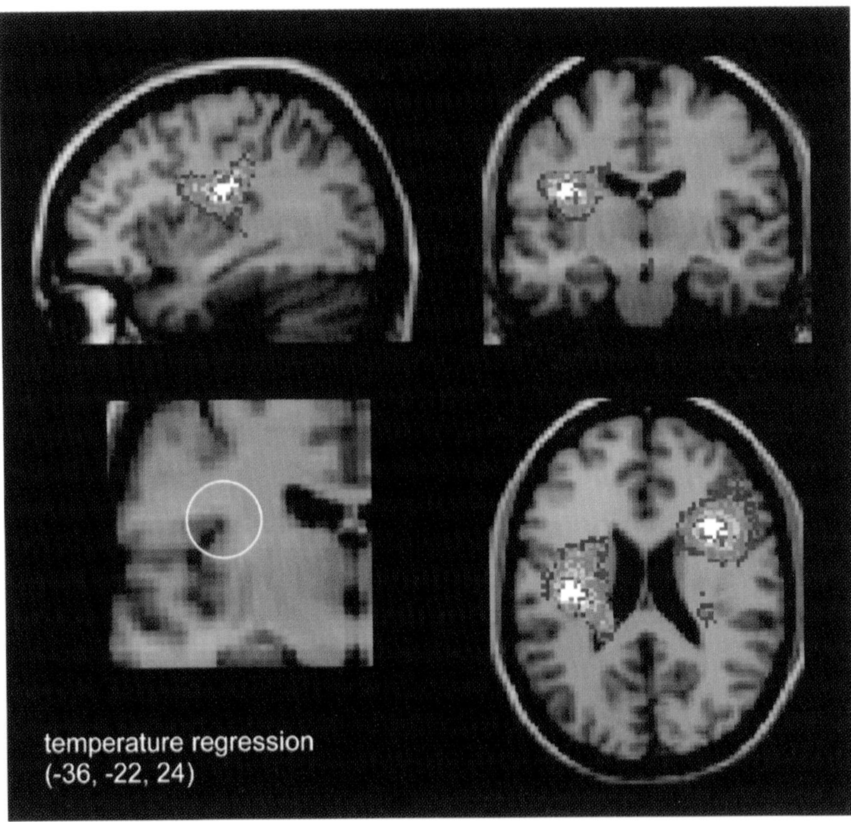

Fig. 6. PET data indicating the location of discriminative thermosensory human cortex in the fundus of the superior limiting (circular) sulcus at the dorsal margin of the mid/posterior insula (coordinates –36, –22, 24), identified by regression analysis of regional cerebral blood flow against stimulus temperatures between 20° and 34°C applied tonically to the hand. From Craig et al. (2000).

nerve (Bini et al. 1984). A pressure block of A-fiber conduction in a peripheral nerve that eliminates both touch and cooling sensations will enable a cool stimulus to elicit a painful burning sensation, just like the burning pain normally associated with noxious cold (see, e.g., Yarnitsky and Ochoa 1990). In other words, the burning pain sensation caused by polymodal C nociceptors (which are sensitive both to cool and to noxious cold) is normally masked centrally by the activity of the specific cutaneous Aδ-fiber thermoreceptors that are responsible for the sensation of cooling. When the activity of cooling receptors is reduced, then the C-fiber activity evoked by cooling is disinhibited centrally and causes a burning sensation at both cool and cold temperatures.

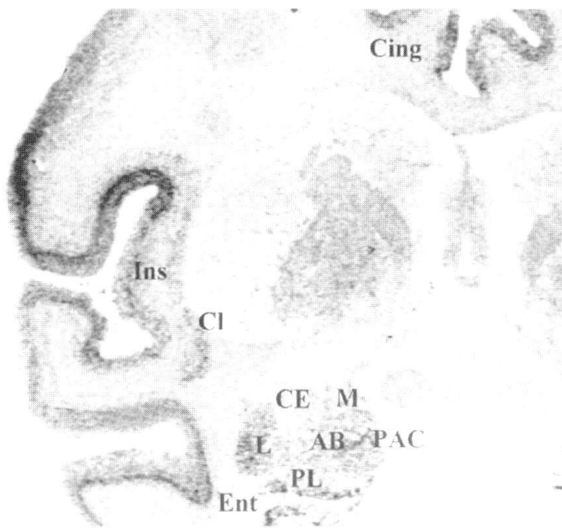

Fig. 7. Photomicrograph identifying the location of mRNA binding for corticotropin-releasing factor receptor in the fundus of the superior limiting sulcus. From Sanchez et al. (1997), with permission; see this reference for abbreviations.

Thermal disinhibition of burning pain is demonstrable without a nerve block by the thermal grill illusion (Thunberg 1896), in which a sensation of burning, ice-like pain is generated by innocuous cool (20°C) and warm (40°C) stimuli presented together in a spatially unusual fashion. Just as for the peripheral nerve block, this illusion can be explained physiologically by an unmasking of the activity of cold-evoked polymodal C-nociceptor activation (of HPC lamina I STT cells) due to a (warm-induced) reduction in the activity of specific Aδ thermoreceptors and thermosensory lamina I cells (Craig and Bushnell 1994). The grill effectively produces a relative balance of polymodal and thermosensory activity like that caused by noxious cold. This phenomenon demonstrates that the thermoreceptive-specific sensory channel inhibits the polymodal nociceptive channel at thalamocortical levels, and that a reduction in this inhibition releases or unmasks a burning pain sensation. A similar intense, painful burning sensation is perceived if warm water is applied to a foot that is numbed by cold, which is an unmistakable thermoregulatory distress signal. The mechanism is just like that of the thermal grill, because the warm water inhibits the cutaneous thermosensory receptors and the lamina I STT thermosensory cells but not the deep polymodal C fibers and the lamina I STT polymodal nociceptive HPC cells.

Functional imaging has confirmed that the thermal grill produces a pattern of activity in the cortex identical to the activation produced by noxious

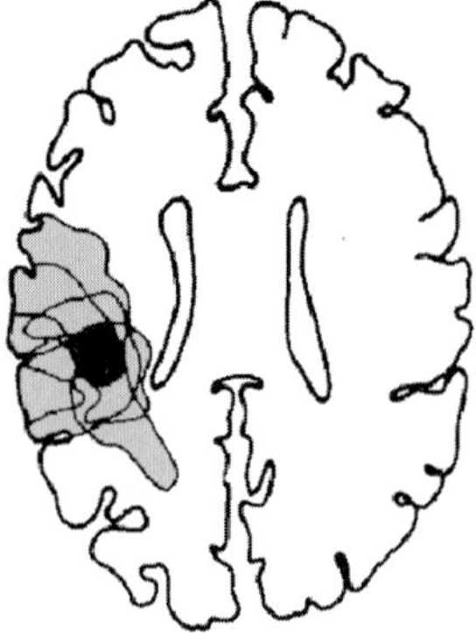

Fig. 8. Summary diagram of the locations of cortical lesions in six central pain patients, showing that the common site of damage is in the dorsal margin of the mid/posterior insular cortex. Compare with the axial projection in Fig. 6. Redrawn from Schmahmann and Leifer (1992).

cold (Craig et al. 1996). The cortical activation unmasked by the grill is in the ACC, indicating that anterior cingulate activation is selectively associated with the perception of thermal pain, or the affect that signals thermoregulatory distress. Therefore, a reduction of thermosensory activity in the lateral lamina I spinothalamocortical pathway to the insular cortex unmasks activity in the medial lamina I pathway that activates the ACC and is associated with burning pain. Thus the medial thalamic lamina I STT target MDvc may be the critical site for the inhibition of thermal pain by cold; preliminary physiological recordings in the MDvc support that conjecture (Craig 1997).

Thus, the thermosensory disinhibition hypothesis for central pain proposes that loss of activity in the thermosensory (interoceptive) cortex in the dorsal mid/posterior insula disinhibits polymodal activation of the MDvc and the ACC, which engenders burning pain. The descending outputs from the insular cortex include the brainstem PB and PAG, as well as lamina I (Yasui et al. 1991), and so the effects of deactivating the thermosensory cortex may be to release these brainstem sites from descending control. Recent anatomical findings indicate that these brainstem structures project to the posteromedial thalamus (Krout and Loewy 2000a,b), and preliminary data in my laboratory indicate that their projections include the MDvc. The PB in particular receives a strong lamina I input that is integrated with vagal inputs, and it is crucial for cardiovascular and thermoregulatory homeostatic control; thus, our current hypothesis is that the loss of activity in the insular thermosensory cortex disinhibits the integration of lamina I and PB inputs in the MDvc, as illustrated in Fig. 9. The resemblance of this concrete anatomical hypothesis to the earlier heuristic proposals by Head and Holmes (1911) and Melzack and Casey (1968) is remarkable.

It remains to be determined whether activity in the ACC can be observed in central pain patients. Functional imaging studies averaged across chronic pain patients have produced inconsistent results (see Craig 2000). One PET study reported that therapeutic stimulation in the lateral thalamus for chronic pain activated the insular cortex and caused thermal sensations (Duncan et al. 1998). A PET study of patients with Wallenberg's syndrome (a form of central pain) reported that allodynic cold stimuli produced activation in the insular cortex, but activity was not observed in the ACC during allodynic or control stimulation, perhaps for methodological reasons (Peyron et al. 1998). A similar PET study of a single central pain patient showed anomalous allodynic activation of the ipsilateral insular cortex (Peyron et al. 2000), and imbalanced activity was observed in the dorsal margin of the insular cortex in another patient with ongoing pain (Kupers et al. 2000). However, novel short-latency laser-evoked activation of the ACC was recorded in one central pain patient (Lorenz et al. 1998). We are performing functional magnetic resonance imaging (fMRI) studies of activation by noxious cold and the thermal grill in anesthetized monkeys (Fig. 10) in order to obtain comparable data in the experimental primate. Similarly, there is a need for single-subject imaging analyses of central pain patients and SCI patients.

Finally, as noted above, the lamina I projection system may be viewed as the source of sensory input to a hierarchical network involved in homeostasis and in the behavioral maintenance of the integrity and well-being of the body. The unique lateral (insular) pathway in humans provides a first-order interoceptive representation of the condition of the body, including the specific sensations of pain, temperature, and itch, while the medial (cingulate) pathway provides an integrative substrate for emotional affect, or motivation. One function of the thermosensory inhibition of the integration of brainstem homeostatic and polymodal nociceptive activity in the medial thalamus may be to generate a graded sensation of burning pain that differentiates noxious cold from innocuous cool, and thereby to motivate appropriate integrative homeostatic responses to different levels of thermoregulatory distress that require appropriately different protective behaviors. Thus, the deep, burning ache experienced by many central pain patients may be related to dysfunctional regional thermoregulation. This suggestion is consistent with the essential role of behavioral motivation in thermoregulation in primates and with its hierarchical evolutionary refinement (Satinoff 1978; Blatteis 1998). Thermoregulation is known to interact with many aspects of homeostasis, e.g., food, energy, fat and salt balance, and cardiovascular control, and to be an adaptive (acclimating) system, which could account for the delayed onset in some patients and the emotional dependency of central pain. Notably, the pleasantness or unpleasantness of a thermal stimulus depends directly on core temperature, whereas the discriminative percept does not (Mower 1976); that is, a cold stimulus may feel pleasant if the body is

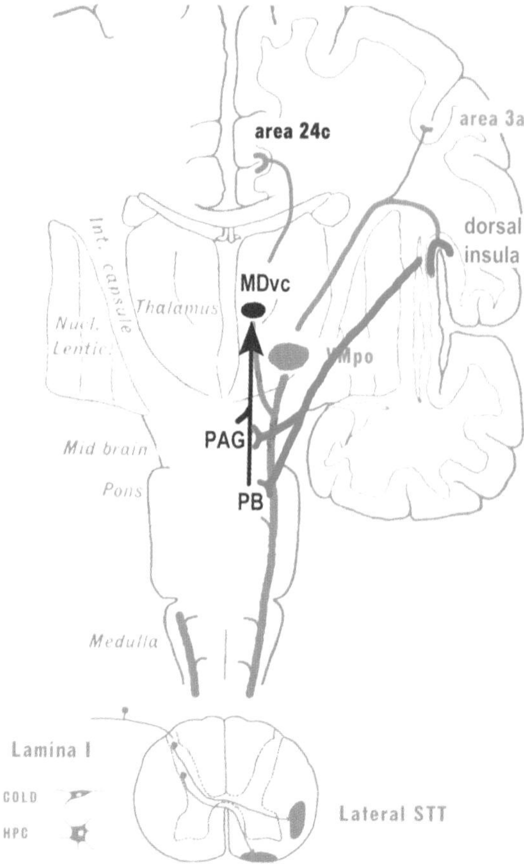

Fig. 9. Diagram summarizing the thermosensory disinhibition hypothesis for central pain, indicating the proposal that damage to the interoceptive lamina I/ posterior part of the ventral medial nucleus (VMpo) projection cortical field in the dorsal mid/posterior insula interrupts its descending inhibitory control of homeostatic integration in the parabrachial nucleus (PB) and periaqueductal gray (PAG). The disinhibited activity in these brainstem nuclei is integrated in the ventrocaudal portion of the medial dorsal nucleus (MDvc) to produce homeostatic activation in area 24c of the anterior cingulate cortex that engenders thermoregulatory motivation, or pain.

overly warm (and needs cooling), but the same stimulus feels unpleasant if the body is cold (and needs warming). In other words, the affect (or motivation) generated by a thermal stimulus is governed by the needs of thermoregulatory integration, independent of the sensory perception of cool or warm. Similarly, some patients have lost the ability to perceive cold and warm due to spinal or thalamocortical lesions, but they can distinguish warm or cool objects by the distinctly different "feelings" they evoke, and cats with thalamic lesions seem to do the same (Norrsell and Craig 1999). This finding is consistent with the idea that central pain is due to imbalanced (disinhibited) integration of ascending thermosensory lamina I activity in brainstem and forebrain homeostatic centers. This imbalance produces a dysfunctional thermoregulatory drive. Furthermore, this imbalance would explain the occurrence of central pain in a patient with a hemi-thalamus (Parrent et al. 1992) and would account for the correlation of central pain in Wallenberg's patients with unilateral but not bilateral thermosensory loss (MacGowan et al. 1997).

These considerations suggest that central pain and below-level SCI pain might be alleviated by altering homeostatic conditions in the body, for example

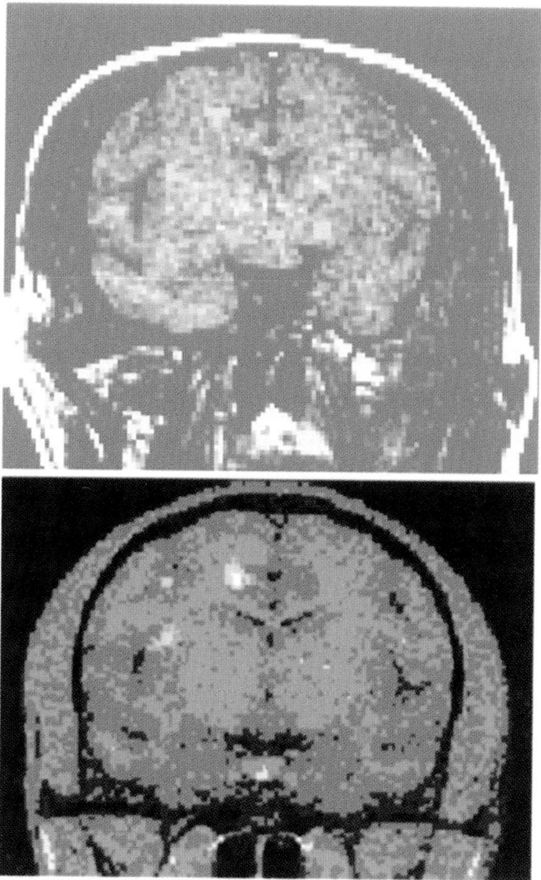

Fig. 10. Preliminary fMRI data indicating activation of the posterior part of the ventral medial nucleus (VMpo) and anterior cingulate cortex (and also area 3a) by noxious cold in two anesthetized monkeys.

by increasing peripheral tissue perfusion or core temperature, which would diminish thermoregulatory drive. Perhaps this is why amitriptyline works to alleviate central pain in many patients. These considerations certainly indicate that pain can be viewed as an aspect of homeostasis, and they provide a sound scientific foundation for the view that chronic pain should be treated with an integrative, holistic approach.

CONCLUSION

Modern studies based on the fundamental mechanisms of disinhibition, sensitization, and plasticity are providing new insights into the possible causes of SCI pain. Exciting new findings and important directions for future studies discussed in this chapter could generate new therapeutic avenues for both segmental, at-level pain and suprasegmental, below-level (or central) pain. In particular, the functional anatomical identification of the lamina I spinothalamocortical pathway as a critical substrate for pain, temperature, and other feelings from the body has generated new concepts that should help guide future studies of pain.

ACKNOWLEDGMENTS

The research in this laboratory was supported by NIH grant NS 25616 and by the Atkinson Pain Research Fund administered by the Barrow Neurological Foundation.

REFERENCES

Andersen G, Vestergaard K, Ingeman-Nielsen M, Jensen TS. Incidence of central post-stroke pain. *Pain* 1995; 61:187–193.

Andrew D, Craig AD. Responses of lamina I spinothalamic tract (STT) cells to tonic noxious mechanical stimuli. *Proceedings of the 9th World Congress on Pain,* Progress in Pain Research and Management, Vol. 16. Seattle: IASP Press, 1999.

Andrew D, Craig AD. Spinothalamic lamina I neurons selectively sensitive to histamine: a central neural pathway for itch. *Nat Neurosci* 2001; 4:72–77.

Beric A. Post-spinal cord injury pain states. *Pain* 1997; 72:295–298.

Bester H, Beggs S, Woolf CJ. Changes in tactile stimuli-induced behavior and c-Fos expression in the superficial dorsal horn and in parabrachial nuclei after sciatic nerve crush. *J Comp Neurol* 2000; 428:45–61.

Bezzi P, Domercq M, Brambilla L, et al. CXCR4-activated astrocyte glutamate release via TNFalpha: amplification by microglia triggers neurotoxicity. *Nat Neurosci* 2001; 4:702–710.

Bian D, Ossipov MH, Zhong C, et al. Tactile allodynia, but not thermal hyperalgesia, of the hindlimbs is blocked by spinal transection in rats with nerve injury. *Neurosci Lett* 1998; 241:79–82.

Bini G, Cruccu G, Hagbarth K-E, et al. Analgesic effect of vibration and cooling on pain induced by intraneural electrical stimulation. *Pain* 1984; 18:239–248.

Bishop GH. The relation between nerve fiber size and sensory modality: phylogenetic implications of the afferent innervation of cortex. *J Nerv Ment Dis* 1959; 128:89–114.

Blatteis CM. *Physiology and Pathophysiology of Temperature Regulation.* Singapore: World Scientific, 1998.

Blomqvist A, Craig AD. Is neuropathic pain caused by the activation of nociceptive-specific neurons due to anatomic sprouting in the dorsal horn? *J Comp Neurol* 2000; 428:1–4.

Blomqvist A, Zhang ET, Craig AD. Cytoarchitectonic and immunohistochemical characterization of a specific pain and temperature relay, the posterior portion of the ventral medial nucleus, in the human thalamus. *Brain* 2000; 123:601–619.

Boivie J. Central pain. In: Wall PD, Melzack R (Eds). *Textbook of Pain.* Edinburgh: Churchill Livingstone, 1994, pp 871–902.

Bowsher D. Central pain: clinical and physiological characteristics. *J Neurol Neurosurg Psychiatry* 1996; 61:62–69.

Bowsher D, Leijon G, Thoumas KA. Central poststroke pain—correlation of MRI with clinical pain characteristics and sensory abnormalities. *Neurology* 1998; 51:1352–1358.

Cao YQ, Mantyh PW, Carlson EJ, et al. Primary afferent tachykinins are required to experience moderate to intense pain. *Nature* 1998; 392:390–394.

Craig AD. The primate MDvc contains nociceptive neurons. *Soc Neurosci Abstr* 1997; 23:1012.

Craig AD. A new version of the thalamic disinhibition hypothesis of central pain. *Pain Forum* 1998; 7:1–14.

Craig AD. The functional anatomy of lamina I and its role in post-stroke central pain. In: Sandkühler J, Bromm B, Gebhart GF (Eds). *Nervous System Plasticity and Chronic Pain.* Amsterdam: Elsevier, 2000, pp 137–151.

Craig AD, Andrew D. Lamina I spinothalamic neurons display temporal summation to repeated brief contact heat stimuli. *Soc Neurosci Abstracts* 1999; 25:148.

Craig AD, Bushnell MC. The thermal grill illusion: unmasking the burn of cold pain. *Science* 1994; 265:252–255.

Craig AD, Reiman EM, Evans A, Bushnell MC. Functional imaging of an illusion of pain. *Nature* 1996; 384:258–260.

Craig AD, Chen K, Bandy D, Reiman EM. Thermosensory activation of insular cortex. *Nat Neurosci* 2000; 3:184–190.

Craig AD, Krout K, Andrew D. Quantitative response characteristics of thermoreceptive and nociceptive lamina I spinothalamic neurons in the cat. *J Neurophysiol* 2001; 86:1459–1480.

Davis KD, Kiss ZHT, Luo L, et al. Phantom sensations generated by thalamic microstimulation. *Nature* 1998; 391:385–387.

DeLeo JA, Yezierski RP. The role of neuroinflammation and neuroimmune activation in persistent pain. *Pain* 2001; 90:1–6.

Dostrovsky JO. Role of thalamus in pain. In: Sandkühler J, Bromm B, Gebhart GF (Eds). *Nervous System Plasticity and Chronic Pain.* Amsterdam: Elsevier, 2000, pp 245–258.

Drzezga A, Darsow U, Treede R, et al. Central activation by histamine-induced itch: analogies to pain processing: a correlational analysis of O-15 H(2)O positron emission tomography studies. *Pain* 2001; 92:295–305.

Duncan GH, Kupers RC, Marchand S, et al. Stimulation of human thalamus for pain relief: possible modulatory circuits revealed by positron emission tomography. *J Neurophysiol* 1998; 80:3326–3330.

Eaton MJ, Plunkett JA, Karmally S, et al. Changes in GAD- and GABA-immunoreactivity in the spinal dorsal horn after peripheral nerve injury and promotion of recovery by lumbar transplant of immortalized serotonergic precursors. *J Chem Neuroanat* 1998; 16:57–72.

Edgar RE, Best LG, Quail PA, Obert AD. Computer-assisted DREZ microcoagulation: posttraumatic spinal deafferentation pain. *J Spinal Disorders* 1993; 6:48–56.

Foerster O. *Die Leitungsbahnen des Schmerzgefühls und die chirurgische Behandlung der Schmerzzustände.* Berlin: Urban & Schwarzenberg, 1927, pp 1–307.

Greenspan JD, Lee RR, Lenz FA. Pain sensitivity alterations as a function of lesion location in the parasylvian cortex. *Pain* 1999; 81:273–282.

Gybels JM, Sweet WH. *Neurosurgical Treatment of Persistent Pain: Physiological and Pathological Mechanisms of Human Pain*, Pain and Headache, Vol. 11. Basel: Karger, 1989, pp 1–442.

Head H, Holmes G. Sensory disturbances from cerebral lesions. *Brain* 1911; 34:102–254.

Jeanmonod D, Magnin M, Morel A. A thalamic concept of neurogenic pain. *Proceedings of the 7th World Congress on Pain*, Progress in Pain Research and Management, Vol. 2. Seattle: IASP Press, 1994, pp 767–787.

Kendall D. Some observations on central pain. *Brain* 1939; 62:253–273.

Krout KE, Loewy AD. Parabrachial nucleus projections to midline and intralaminar thalamic nuclei of the rat. *J Comp Neurol* 2000a; 428:475–494.

Krout KE, Loewy AD. Periaqueductal gray matter projections to midline and intralaminar thalamic nuclei of the rat. *J Comp Neurol* 424:111–141, 2000b.

Kupers RC, Gybels JM, Gjedde A. Positron emission tomography study of a chronic pain patient successfully treated with somatosensory thalamic stimulation. *Pain* 2000; 87:295–302.

Lenz FA, Dougherty PM. Pain processing in the human thalamus. In: Steriade M, Jones EG, McCormick DA (Eds). *Experimental and Clinical Aspects*, Thalamus, Vol. II. Amsterdam: Elsevier, 1997, pp 617–652.

Lorenz J, Kohlhoff H, Hansen HC, et al. Aβ-fiber mediated activation of cingulate cortex as correlate of central post-stroke pain. *Neuroreport* 1998; 9:659–663.

MacGowan DJ, Janal MN, Clark MC, et al. Central poststroke pain and Wallenberg's lateral medullary infarction: frequency, character, and determinants in 63 patients. *Neurology* 1997; 49:120–125.

Maier SF, Watkins LR. Cytokines for psychologists: implications of bidirectional immune-to-brain communication for understanding behavior, mood, and cognition. *Psychol Rev* 1998; 105:83–107.

Mantyh PW, Rogers SD, Honoré P, et al. Inhibition of hyperalgesia by ablation of lamina I spinal neurons expressing the substance P receptor. *Science* 1997; 278:275–279.

Melzack R, Casey KL. Sensory, motivational, and central control determinants of pain. In: Kenshalo DR (Ed). *The Skin Senses*. Springfield: Thomas, 1968, pp 423–443.

Mower G. Perceived intensity of peripheral thermal stimuli is independent of internal body temperature. *J Comp Physiol Psychol* 1976; 90:1152–1155.

Norrsell U, Craig AD. Behavioral thermosensitivity after lesions of thalamic target areas of a thermosensory spinothalamic pathway in the cat. *J Neurophysiol* 1999; 82:611–625.

Ossipov MH, Lai J, Malan Jr P, Porreca F. Spinal and supraspinal mechanisms of neuropathic pain. *Ann NY Acad Sci* 2000; 909:12–24.

Pagni CA. *Central Pain: A Neurosurgical Challenge*. Turin: Ediziona Minerva Medica S.P.A., 1998.

Palecek J, Dougherty PM, Kim SH, et al. Responses of spinothalamic tract neurons to mechanical and thermal stimuli in an experimental model of peripheral neuropathy in primates. *J Neurophysiol* 1992; 68:1951–1966.

Parrent AG, Lozano AM, Dostrovsky JO, Tasker RR. Central pain in the absence of functional sensory thalamus. *Stereotact Funct Neurosurg* 1992; 59:9–14.

Peyron R, Garcéa-Larrea L, Gregoire MC, et al. Allodynia after lateral-medullary (Wallenberg) infarct—a PET study. *Brain* 1998; 121:345–356.

Peyron R, Garcéa-Larrea L, Gregoire MC, et al. Parietal and cingulate processes in central pain: a combined positron emission tomography (PET) and functional magnetic resonance imaging (fMRI) study of an unusual case. *Pain* 2000; 84:77–87.

Radhakrishnan V, Tsoukatos J, Davis KD, et al. A comparison of the burst activity of lateral thalamic neurons in chronic pain and non-pain patients. *Pain* 1999; 80:567–575.

Ralston III HJ, Ralston DD. Medial lemniscal and spinal projections to the macaque thalamus: an electron microscopic study of differing GABAergic circuitry serving thalamic somatosensory mechanisms. *J Neurosci* 1994; 14:2485–2502.

Ramachandran VS, Rogers-Ramachandran D, Cobb S. Touching the phantom limb. *Nature* 1995; 377:489–490.

Riddoch G. The clinical features of central pain. *Lancet* 1938; 1:1093–1156.

Samad TA, Moore KA, Sapirstein A, et al. Interleukin-1-beta-mediated induction of COX-2 in the CNS contributes to inflammatory pain hypersensitivity. *Nature* 2001; 410:471–475.

Sanchez MM, Young LJ, Plotsky PM, Insel TR. Autoradiographic and in situ hybridization localization of corticotropin-releasing factor 1 and 2 receptors in nonhuman primate brain. *J Comp Neurol* 1999; 408:365–377.

Satinoff E. Neural organization and evolution of thermal regulation in mammals. *Science* 1978; 201:16–22.

Schmahmann JD, Leifer D. Parietal pseudothalamic pain syndrome: clinical features and anatomic correlates. *Arch Neurol* 1992; 49:1032–1037.

Sugimoto T, Bennett GJ, Kajander KC. Transsynaptic degeneration in the superficial dorsal horn after sciatic nerve injury: effects of a chronic constriction injury, transection, and strychnine. *Pain* 1990; 42:205–213.

Thunberg T. Fornimmelserne vid till samma stelle lokaliserad, samtidigt pogoende kald-och Ermeretning. *Upsala Lokforen Forh* 1896; 2(1):489–495.

Tommerdahl M, Delemos KA, Vierck Jr CJ, et al. Anterior parietal cortical response to tactile and skin-heating stimuli applied to the same skin site. *J Neurophysiol* 1996; 75:2662–2670.

Urban MO, Gebhart GF. Central mechanisms in pain. *Med Clin North Am* 1999; 83:585–596.

Vierck CJ Jr, Cannon RL, Fry G, et al. Characteristics of temporal summation of second pain sensations elicited by brief contact of glabrous skin by a preheated thermode. *J Neurophysiol* 1997; 78:992–1002.

Wang ZJ, Gardell LR, Ossipov MH, et al. Pronociceptive actions of dynorphin maintain chronic neuropathic pain. *J Neurosci* 2001; 21:1779–1786.

Watkins LR, Milligan ED, Maier SF. Glial activation: a driving force for pathological pain. *Trends Neurosci* 2001; 24:450–455.

Weng HR, Lee JI, Lenz FA, et al. Functional plasticity in primate somatosensory thalamus following chronic lesion of the ventral lateral spinal cord. *Neuroscience* 2000; 101:393–401.

Woods TM, Cusick CG, Pons TP, et al. Progressive transneuronal changes in the brainstem and thalamus after long-term dorsal rhizotomies in adult macaque monkeys. *J Neurosci* 2000; 20:3884–3899.

Woolf CJ, Shortland P, Coggeshall RE. Peripheral nerve injury triggers central sprouting of myelinated afferents. *Nature* 1992; 355:75–78.

Yarnitsky D, Ochoa JL. Release of cold-induced burning pain by block of cold-specific afferent input. *Brain* 1990; 113:893–902.

Yasui Y, Breder CD, Saper CB Cechetto DF. Autonomic responses and efferent pathways from the insular cortex in the rat. *J Comp Neurol* 1991; 303:355–374.

Yezierski RP. Pain following spinal cord injury: pathophysiology and central mechanisms. In: Sandkühler J, Bromm B, Gebhart GF (Eds). *Nervous System Plasticity and Chronic Pain.* Amsterdam: Elsevier, 2000, pp 429–450.

Correspondence to: A.D. Craig, PhD, Division of Neurosurgery, Barrow Neurological Institute, 350 West Thomas Road, Phoenix, AZ 85013, USA. Tel: 602-406-3385; Fax: 602-406-4121; email: bcraig@mha.chw.edu.

Part III

Imaging

Spinal Cord Injury Pain: Assessment, Mechanisms, Management. Progress in Pain Research and Management, Vol. 23, edited by Robert P. Yezierski and Kim J. Burchiel, IASP Press, Seattle, © 2002.

15

Understanding Central Pain: New Insights from Forebrain Imaging Studies of Patients and of Animals with Central Lesions

Thomas J. Morrow and Kenneth L. Casey

Neurology Research Laboratories, Veterans Affairs Hospital, and Departments of Neurology and Physiology, University of Michigan, Ann Arbor, Michigan, USA

Functional imaging of pain-related central nervous system (CNS) activity provides a powerful method for exploring the complex neural mechanisms that support the pain experience. Over the last decade, major advances in brain imaging techniques in humans using positron emission tomography (PET) and functional magnetic resonance imaging (fMRI) have expanded our knowledge of the neurophysiology of pain and enhanced our understanding of the central mechanisms of pain processing far beyond the limits of traditional electrophysiological and lesion studies. Functional imaging, by allowing us to examine the responses of multiple CNS regions simultaneously in awake, behaving subjects during acute and chronic pain states, provides clear evidence that there is no common "center" or pathway for the generation of pain. Instead, the evidence points to a distributed parallel network or matrix of cortical and subcortical structures that receives afferent input via distinct anatomical pathways (see Apkarian 1995; Casey and Minoshima 1997).

Although most functional imaging studies of pain have used PET or fMRI to examine human subjects, the number of imaging studies performed on animal models of pain is increasing due to recent advances in methodology. Human studies have an obvious advantage in being able to simultaneously assess both experiential/cognitive aspects of pain and brain activation. However, both PET and fMRI have relatively limited spatial resolutions, whereas film-based animal imaging studies boast spatial resolutions on the order of 20–50 μm. This fine spatial resolution, coupled with the availability of tissue sections, allows us to correlate activation with very small, histologically defined CNS regions. Human functional imaging studies of chronic pain states are subject to significant variability arising from inter-individual differences in the chronic pain syndrome itself. In contrast, inter-individual variation in animal models of chronic pain is considerably reduced by the fact that the pain syndrome can be produced in a carefully controlled fashion. For these reasons our laboratory has employed regional cerebral blood flow (rCBF) imaging in animal models of chronic pain to complement our related human studies using PET. These imaging approaches combine to provide a powerful platform for the investigation of CNS mechanisms of pain. This chapter presents data from these complementary human and animal imaging studies.

STUDIES OF NORMAL HUMANS

We have just begun to identify the sources of variation in the normal pain activation of the human forebrain. However, the results reviewed elsewhere (Casey 1999; Derbyshire 1999) provide a background of information that is sufficiently consistent, even across genders (Paulson et al. 1998), to support studies of the physiological variables that determine the patterns of brain activation during normal pain. For example, Derbyshire and Coghill, with colleagues, used correlation analyses to investigate the inter-regional distribution of information about heat pain intensity (Derbyshire et al. 1997; Coghill et al. 1999). Both groups found that such information is widely distributed among pain-activated regions. In related investigations, Rainville and colleagues (1997) used hypnotic suggestion to uncouple the perception of heat pain unpleasantness from heat pain intensity in normal subjects. They were able to show a positive correlation of pain unpleasantness with the intensity of rCBF response in a far-anterior (dorsal perigenual) region of the anterior cingulate cortex; this correlation was not found in a specific examination of the primary somatosensory (S1) cortex. In differentiating the perception of pain from the anticipation of pain, Ploghaus and colleagues (1999) used fMRI to show that the activation of some regions, previously identified in PET studies of heat pain, is better correlated with the anticipation of pain than with pain perception. Thus, the anticipation of heat pain was related to activity in the far frontal cingulate cortex, anterior insula, and anterior cerebellar vermis, while the perception of pain was related to activity in adjacent regions (mid-anterior cingulate, mid-insula, and paravermian cerebellum). Finally, we have recently shown the importance of the duration of the heat pain experience in determining the pattern of forebrain activation (Casey et al. 2001). This PET study of normal subjects showed that the pattern of brain activation and the perception of heat pain both change during repetitive noxious heat stimulation. The perceived intensity and unpleasantness of pain both increase with greater duration of the repetitive stimulation. These psychophysical changes could be mediated by brain structures that show increased activity with longer periods of stimulation; these structures include the contralateral M1/S1 cortex, bilateral S2 and mid-insular cortex, contralateral ventral posterior thalamus, medial ipsilateral thalamus, and the vermis and paravermis of the cerebellum. Structures that are equally active throughout stimulation (the contralateral mid-anterior cingulate cortex and premotor cortex) are less likely to mediate these psychophysical changes. Structures showing significant or borderline activation only during the early scans (ipsilateral premotor cortex, contralateral perigenual anterior cingulate cortex, lateral prefrontal cortex, and anterior insular cortex) could mediate pain-related attentive or anticipatory functions, but this hypothesis remains to be tested.

Other forms of pain have been studied less intensively. We have compared the pattern of brain activation produced by cutaneous mechanical contact heat pain with the pain produced by infrared laser stimulation, by ice water immersion, and by deep electrical stimulation of muscle (Casey et al. 1996; Svensson et al. 1997). Cutaneous heat pain and deep immersion cold pain produce similar, but not identical, patterns of brain response. Five regions that are responsive during both heat and cold pain (the cerebellar vermis, ipsilateral thalamus, contralateral premotor cortex, contralateral anterior cingulate cortex, and the confluent activation of contralateral anterior insula and lenticular nucleus) each show a greater response during cold pain than during heat pain. However, the extensive spatial overlap of responses suggests a pattern common to these different types of pain (Casey et al. 1996). Similarly, when perceived pain intensity is similar, direct statistical comparisons between cutaneous laser and intramuscular stimulation show no reliable differences between these two forms of noxious stimulation, indicating a substantial overlap in the pattern of brain activation (Svensson et al. 1997).

Imaging studies of visceral pain are also at an early stage of development, but evidence indicates that these studies will reveal important CNS abnormalities in patients with myocardial and visceral disease (Rosen and Camici 2000). A review of imaging studies of normal visceral pain shows again that similar cerebral structures are activated during visceral and somatic pain (Ladabaum et al. 2000). We used voxelwise correlations with perceived pain to compare cutaneous heat pain with the pain produced with a gastric balloon (Cross et al. 1999). Although visceral pain preferentially activates structures in the left hemisphere and medial thalamus, both somatic and visceral pain activate the thalami, brainstem, cingulate cortex, premotor cortex, cerebellar hemispheres, caudate nucleus, and cerebellar vermis. There appears, then, to be a common activation of cerebral nociceptive pathways during somatic and visceral pain. In certain pathological conditions, however, there may be abnormalities of visceral nociceptive processing that have serious clinical consequences (Rosen and Camici 2000).

STUDIES OF PATIENTS WITH NEUROPATHIC PAIN

The few examples given above show that, although we are at an early stage in the investigation of the forebrain responses during some forms of normal pain, progress has been significant and is accelerating. However, the study of normal subjects has been largely restricted to subjects below the age of 40 years. To investigate the pathophysiology of central pain syndromes, it is necessary to establish a population of normal subjects within the age range of those most likely to develop central pain. In ongoing studies of patients with central neuropathic pain (Casey et al. 1999), we have compared the forebrain responses to contact heat stimuli in 17 normal men with that of 4 men with unilateral central pain following forebrain or spinal stroke (all aged 40–68 years). On average, the normal subjects identified 38.5°C as the level of heat detection (HD) and gave this intensity a rating of 2.3 out of 10 on a visual analogue scale (VAS). The average heat pain threshold (HPT) was 46.5°C (VAS 4.8), and 49.5°C (VAS 7.9) was the average highest level (near tolerance; HPTol) for 1 minute of repetitive 5-second heat contacts. All participants underwent 21 PET scans ($H_2{}^{15}O$, 3D), with three baseline scans (no stimulation) and three repetitions of each intensity on each forearm. Compared to baseline, normal subjects activated the contralateral insula and right inferior parietal lobule at HD and HPT, added the contralateral premotor cortex (B6) and cerebellum at HPT, and added the contralateral sensorimotor M1/S1, bilateral thalamus, and lenticular nucleus at HPTol.

All four central pain patients underwent PET scanning with the same protocol as the normal subjects. Each patient had clinically detectable impairment of heat and/or mechanical pain on the side of central pain. We used each patient's clinically normal side to establish the stimulus intensities (HD, HPT, and HPTol) for stimulation of the pathological side. For PET analysis, we measured the heat responsiveness of the thalamus and cortex at each stimulus temperature compared to the resting rCBF. Preliminary results show that each patient has abnormal thalamic and/or cortical asymmetry at rest and increased thalamic and/or cortical responsiveness to contralateral stimulation at HPT and above. At rest, three patients have hemithalamic hypoactivity, and one patient has hemithalamic hyperactivity in the hemisphere contralateral to the pathological pain. In contrast, a patient with global left arm hypoesthesia due to a nerve root lesion has contralateral resting hemithalamic hypoactivity but no evidence for thalamic hyper-responsiveness.

One advantage of PET, as compared with fMRI, for these studies is that it provides the opportunity to determine the excitability of cerebral structures as determined by the rCBF response compared to the resting (no stimulation) level. Fig. 1 shows an example taken from the analysis of a patient with a lacunar infarction adjacent to the right ventral posterior lateral thalamus (yellow arrow, left image, top panel). This patient, a hypertensive 67-year-old man, has painful dysesthesia of the left hemibody at rest, while his right thalamus is hypoactive compared to the left thalamus (Fig. 1, "rest" image). This patient has an elevated HPT (49°C) and high HPTol on both sides, so we tested his thalamic responses to contralateral stimulation at the three temperatures shown. As shown in the images and accompanying bar graph, his right hemithalamus, which is hypoactive at rest, is significantly more responsive to contralateral noxious heat than the left. Whether the left hemithalamus is also abnormally hyporesponsive remains to be determined in this sample case. It is clear, however, that in this patient, as in others we have studied thus far, the thalamus contralateral to the central pain may be hypoactive at rest but hyper-responsive during contralateral heat stimulation. This observation could not be made without information about regional activity during the resting, unstimulated state as determined by PET. In addition, both the psychophysical and cerebral responses in patients can be compared quantitatively with those of our sample of normal men in the same age range.

These results suggest that the pathological hypoactivity in the resting hemithalamus masks an underlying hyper-responsiveness to noxious stimulation. This phenomenon may be due to a loss of resting inhibitory activity within the thalamus, leading to bilateral and widespread cortical abnormalities. Other imaging studies have shown reduced thalamic activity during ongoing peripheral (Hsieh et al. 1995; Iadarola et al. 1995) or central (Pagni and Canavero 1995) neuropathic pain without stimulation. Cesaro and colleagues (1991) used single photon emission computed tomography (SPECT) to investigate the cerebral responses to pain in four patients with central post-stroke pain (CPSP). They found thalamic hyperactivity exclusively in

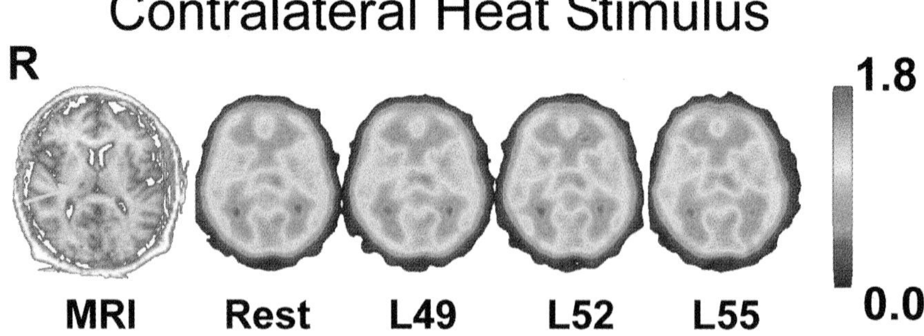

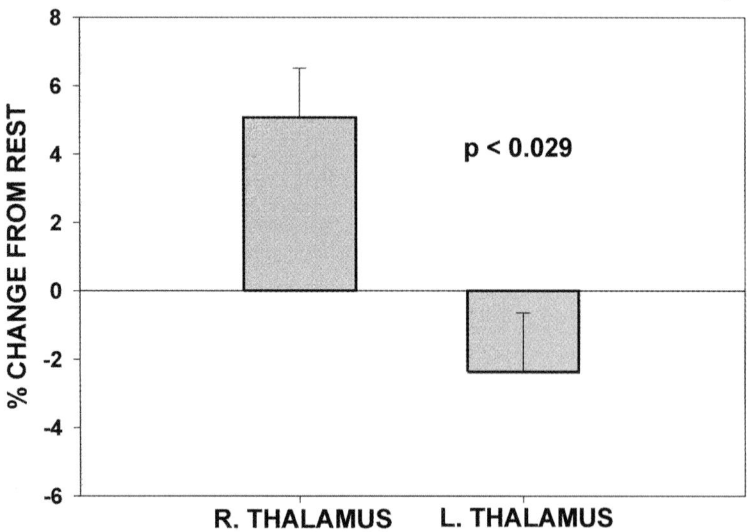

Fig. 1. Top: Anatomical MRI scan shows lacunar infarction adjacent to the right thalamus (arrow) in a patient with bilaterally elevated heat pain threshold (49°C) and central pain syndrome involving the left side of the body. Sequential PET regional cerebral blood flow (rCBF) images show hypoactivity of the right thalamus at rest with increasing hemodynamic activity at increasing intensities of contralateral (left arm) contact heat stimulation (49°, 52°, and 55°C; 5 seconds). Flame bar at right shows the difference (*Z* score) from normalized global cerebral blood flow. Bottom: Volume of interest analysis of right and left thalamic hemodynamic responses (percentage change from resting normalized rCBF) to contact heat stimulation of the contralateral arm at the highest stimulus intensity. The right thalamus, which was relatively hypoactive at rest, shows increased responsiveness compared to the left (t test; $P < 0.029$), which shows a tendency for reduced responsiveness.

two patients with hyperpathia when the abnormal, but not the normal, side was stimulated. Peyron and colleagues (1998) also reported increased contralateral thalamic responsiveness during cold allodynia in patients with lateral medullary infarction (Wallenberg syndrome). Sensory stimulation evokes considerable inhibitory activity in the mammalian thalamus (Salt 1989; Roberts et al. 1992). Inhibitory interneurons and synaptic profiles comprise a significant population of primate thalamic neurons (Ohara et al. 1989; Williamson et al. 1994), and these are highly susceptible to pathological changes following spinal cord injury (SCI) (Ralston et al. 1996). It seems likely that further analyses of clinical cases such as those presented here will reveal the complexity of physiological and anatomical changes that are triggered by injury to the central or peripheral nervous system (Pons et al. 1991; Kaas et al. 1997; Jones and Pons 1998).

SUPRASPINAL CONSEQUENCES OF EXCITOTOXIC SCI: ANIMAL IMAGING STUDIES

Spinal cord injury in humans and animals often results not only in variable motor deficits but also in the development of chronic central pain syndromes. It is also clear from the scholarly clinical and basic science reports presented in the chapters of this book that our understanding of the neural mechanisms of central pain in SCI is incomplete. These abnormal pain states frequently include spontaneous chronic pain as well as an increased responsiveness to previously innocuous (allodynia) and noxious (hyperalgesia) somatic stimuli. One area of research that has been largely ignored with respect to the varied consequences of spinal injury comprises the pathophysiological and neurochemical changes at sites remote to the site of injury, specifically cortical and subcortical supraspinal regions. Because spinal injury leads to partial or complete deafferentation of supraspinal structures, it is likely that, secondary to the disruption of spinal pathways, these supraspinal regions may undergo significant reorganization. It is therefore reasonable to conclude that SCI-induced changes in the activation pattern of supraspinal structures may be partly responsible for the development or maintenance of some aspects of a central pain state. However, few studies have looked at changes in supraspinal processing following spinal injury.

Animal studies employing metabolic or regional blood flow mapping techniques allow the simultaneous study of changes in neuronal activation induced by nociceptive input in large populations of neurons in different CNS structures of the same animal (Coghill and Morrow 2001). Some 2-deoxyglucose (2-DG) studies have shown a functional correlation of acute and chronic pain nociception with activation of a large array of spinal and supraspinal regions including the spinal cord, brainstem, and thalamic, cortical, and limbic regions (Coghill et al. 1991; Porro et al. 1991a,b; Price et al. 1991; Mao et al. 1992; Porro and Cavazzuti 1996; Neto et al. 1999; Schadrack et al. 1999). Recent studies in our laboratory have demonstrated that autoradiographic estimates of rCBF can be used to simultaneously identify acute and chronic pain-specific alterations in the activation of multiple forebrain structures (Morrow et al. 1998, 2000; Paulson et al. 2000). At present, autoradiographic 2-DG or rCBF imaging in animals allows considerably greater resolution of CNS structures than can be achieved with either PET or fMRI in humans, making imaging in animals an ideal platform for investigating the CNS mechanisms of SCI-induced central pain syndromes. Accordingly, we conducted several studies using the Yezierski model of excitotoxic SCI (Yezierski 1996; Yezierski et al. 1998) to determine the extent and nature of SCI-triggered supraspinal changes in rats, using rCBF as an indicator of neuronal activity. For this model, a spinal lesion is produced by a microinjection of quisqualic acid into the dorsal horn on one side of the spinal cord in rats. We computed a mean index of activation for each of 25 sampled regions of interest across all animals in an experimental group (for detailed methods see Morrow et al. 1998).

SCI-INDUCED CHANGES IN BASELINE (UNSTIMULATED) FOREBRAIN ACTIVATION

We found increases in activation in unstimulated Long Evans SCI rats that suggest that pathophysiological changes may have occurred not only at spinal levels but also in supraspinal structures. As compared to controls, Long Evans SCI rats exhibited bilateral increases in the baseline (unstimulated) activation of both cortical and subcortical structures traditionally associated with the processing of somatosensory information (Morrow et al. 2000), including the S1 and S2 cortex and the thalamic posterior group (PO), ventral lateral thalamus (VL), ventral posterior lateral thalamus (VPL), and ventral posterior medial thalamus (VPM) (see Fig. 2). A role in nociceptive processing for many of the thalamic, cortical, and adjacent brain regions activated in the present study is well documented (for review see Willis and Westlund 1997). Ness et al. (1998) also described increased activation in the thalamus and cortex using PET in SCI patients during the perception of chronic pain. Nociceptive activation of the S1 and S2 cortex also has been reported in animal and human studies of acute pain (Willis 1985; Price 1988; Talbot et al. 1991; Casey et al. 1994; Coghill et al. 1994).

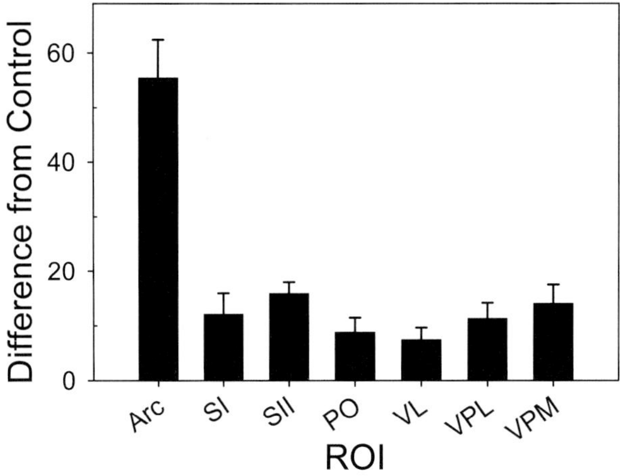

Fig. 2. Regions of interest showing significant baseline (unstimulated) increases in activation because of excitotoxic SCI in Long Evans rats ($P \leq 0.05$, ANOVA). Arc = arcuate nucleus; SI = primary somatosensory cortex; SII = secondary somatosensory cortex; PO = posterior group; VL = ventral lateral thalamus; VPL = ventral posterior lateral thalamus; VPM = ventral posterior medial thalamus.

INFLUENCE OF GENETIC STRAIN ON THE PATTERN OF FOREBRAIN ACTIVATION AFTER SCI

In another study, we found that SCI-induced changes in the basal (unstimulated) pattern of forebrain activation can vary significantly with the strain of rat used. Fig. 3 shows that in contrast to the Long Evans strain, excitotoxic SCI in Sprague-Dawley rats produced robust bilateral increases in rCBF primarily within limbic forebrain structures, although the S1 and S2 cortex also showed an increase in activation above control levels similar to Long Evans rats. Such strain differences in cerebral activation should not be unexpected and may account in part for reported variations in the development neuropathic pain behaviors when different strains of rats or mice are used. Strain-related differences in the onset of neuropathic pain behaviors have been reported after nerve injury (Panerai et al. 1987; Cohn and Seltzer 1991; Defrin et al. 1996; Mogil 1999) and SCI (Popovich et al. 1997; Gorman et al. 2001). In addition, the development of both allodynia and hyperalgesia in rats or mice with partial nerve injury are also strain-dependent (Mogil and Adhikari 1999; Mogil et al. 1999a,b,c; Yoon et al. 1999). Such behavioral data, coupled with our findings of strain-related variations in the SCI-induced pattern of forebrain activation, highlight the importance of genetic factors when using animal models of central pain either to investigate neural mechanisms or to evaluate potential interventions.

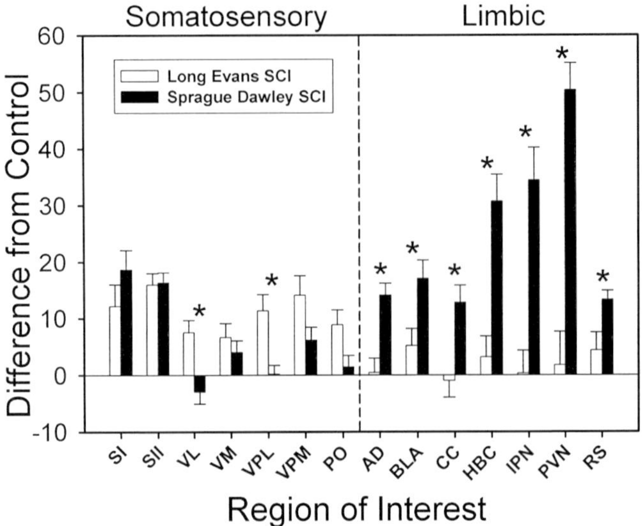

Fig. 3. Effect of genetic strain on SCI-induced differences from control in baseline (unstimulated) brain activation. Long Evans rats showed increases in activation primarily in somatosensory structures, whereas Sprague Dawley rats exhibited SCI-induced increases in activation primarily in limbic forebrain structures. Asterisks (*) denote a significant difference between Long Evans and Sprague Dawley rats ($P \leq 0.05$, ANOVA). SI = primary somatosensory cortex; SII = secondary somatosensory cortex; VL = ventral lateral thalamus; VM = ventral medial thalamus; VPL = ventral posterior lateral thalamus; VPM = ventral posterior medial thalamus; PO = posterior group; AD = anterior dorsal thalamic group; BLA = basolateral amygdala; CC = cingulate cortex; HBC = habenacular complex; IPN = interpeduncular nucleus; PVN = periventricular nucleus; RS = retrosplenial cortex.

STIMULUS-EVOKED FOREBRAIN ACTIVATION IN SCI RATS

Excitotoxic SCI is known to produce abnormal behavioral responses to thermal stimuli in the innocuous range (thermal allodynia) as well as the noxious range (thermal hyperalgesia) (Yezierski et al. 1998). As compared to preoperative baseline values and the responses of control subjects, SCI Sprague-Dawley rats exhibited enhanced behavioral responses to noxious 47°C stimuli (thermal hyperalgesia) applied to the hindfoot on the side of the spinal lesion (see Fig. 4) that were paralleled by increases in the stimulus-evoked activation

---

Fig. 4. Bar graph shows the hyperalgesic behavioral response to a noxious 47°C stimulus applied to the hindfoot on the same side as the spinal cord lesion. Color-enhanced brain images are single brain sections from one stimulated control and one stimulated SCI rat. Note the significantly increased activation to the same 47°C stimulus in thalamic and cortical structures of the SCI rat. ROD = relative optical density. ⟶

Control 47°C Stimulus

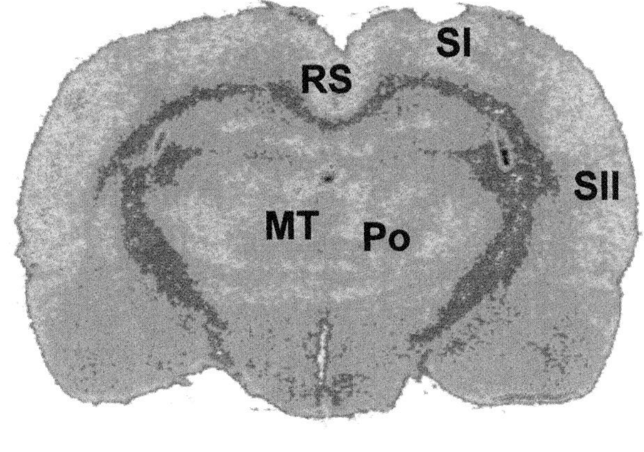

ROD
2.41
0.92
0.61
0.43
0.30
0.21
0.13
0.06
0.00

SCI 47°C Stimulus

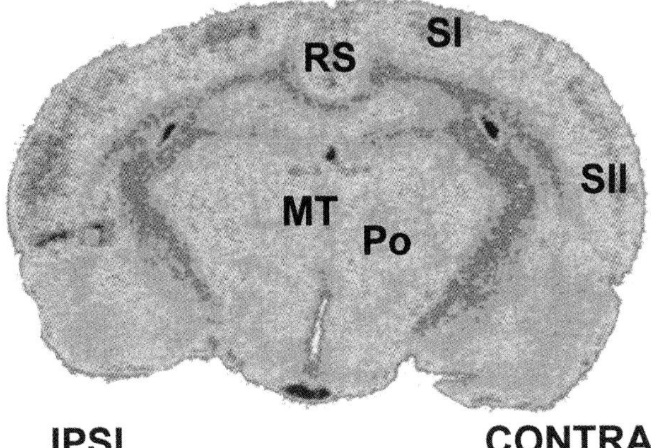

IPSI **CONTRA**

Withdrawal Latency (seconds)

5
4
3
2
1
0

Control
SCI

*

47°C Stimulus

in several forebrain somatosensory structures. Although Fig. 4 shows only single brain images of a coronal section from one stimulated control and one stimulated SCI rat, it clearly highlights the hyperactivation by noxious thermal stimuli in thalamic and cortical structures of the SCI rat as compared to the control. Such increases in the activation of cortical and thalamic structures has also been reported in patients with SCI pain (Ness et al. 1998). Electrophysiological investigations have described spontaneous and evoked hyperactivity in the VPL nucleus of the cat following an ipsilateral transection of the spinothalamic tract (Koyama et al. 1993). Lenz et al. (1994) reported similar findings in a study examining thalamic neuronal activity in patients with SCI. Faggin et al. (1997) also showed that deafferentation produces an immediate and simultaneous change in neuronal activity in rat thalamus and cortex. Furthermore, a recent case report using PET in a patient experiencing central pain due to a supraspinal lesion (Casey et al. 1999; see also human studies described earlier in this chapter) identified hyperactivation in the thalamus on the involved side during noxious thermal stimulation on a background of thalamic hypoactivation.

The changes in forebrain activation described here constitute remote responses to injury and suggest that widespread functional alterations occur within cortical and subcortical regions following injury to the spinal cord. Based on the data presented here and evidence from other studies, it is reasonable to speculate that following SCI, the onset and especially the maintenance of chronic pain-related behaviors is in part the result of alterations in the pattern of neuronal activation in these supraspinal structures. Contributing to this elevated state of activation would be the relay of discharges from spinal generators of abnormal activity as well as the effects produced secondary to deafferentation of supraspinal structures. To address this hypothesis it will be important to record neuronal activity from different brain regions areas identified as having elevated levels of rCBF in these animal imaging studies. Future studies will be necessary to gain a better understanding of the extent of "remote" supraspinal changes and specifically the functional reorganization in the somatotopic map secondary to spinal injury.

In conclusion, the results presented here show that brain imaging can be a powerful tool for investigating the neural mechanisms of central pain syndromes in human patients as well as animal models. Finally, the combined evidence from human and animal studies suggests that one common feature in the development of a central pain syndrome involves thalamic and possibly cortical hyperexcitability.

REFERENCES

Apkarian AV, Functional imaging of pain: new insights regarding the role of the cerebral cortex in human pain. *Semin Neurosci* 1995; 7:279–293.

Casey KL. Forebrain mechanisms of nociception and pain: analysis through imaging. *Proc Natl Acad Sci USA* 1999; 96:7668–7674.

Casey KL, Minoshima S. Can pain be imaged? In: Jensen TS, Turner JA, Wiesenfeld-Hallin Z (Eds). *Proceedings of the 8th World Congress on Pain,* Progress in Pain Research and Management, Vol. 8. Seattle: IASP Press, 1997, pp 855–866.

Casey KL, Minoshima S, Berger KL, et al. Positron emission tomographic analysis of cerebral structures activated specifically by repetitive noxious heat stimuli. *J Neurophysiol* 1994; 71:802–807.

Casey KL, Minoshima S, Morrow TJ, Koeppe RA. Comparison of human cerebral activation patterns during cutaneous warmth, heat pain, and deep cold pain. *J Neurophysiol* 1996; 76:571–581.

Casey KL, Cross DJ, Morrow TJ, Minoshima S. Thalamocortical disinhibition in a case of central pain: a PET study. *Abstracts: 9th World Congress on Pain.* Seattle: IASP Press, 1999, pp 435–436.

Casey KL, Morrow TJ, Lorenz J, Minoshima S. Temporal and spatial dynamics of human forebrain activity during heat pain: analysis by positron emission tomography. *J Neurophysiol* 2001; 85(2):951–959.

Cesaro P, Mann MW, Moretti JL, et al. Central pain and thalamic hyperactivity: a single photon emission computerized tomographic study. *Pain* 1991; 47:329–336.

Coghill RC, Morrow TJ. Functional imaging of animal models of pain: high-resolution insights into nociceptive processing. In: Casey KL, Bushnell MC (Eds). *Pain Imaging.* Seattle: IASP Press, 2001, pp 211–239.

Coghill RC, Price DD, Hayes RL, Mayer DJ. Spatial distribution of nociceptive processing in the rat spinal cord. *J Neurophysiol* 1991; 65:133–140.

Coghill RC, Talbot JD, Evans AC, et al. Distributed processing of pain and vibration by the human brain. *J Neurosci* 1994; 14:4095–4108.

Coghill RC, Sang CN, Maisog JH, Iadarola MJ. Pain intensity processing within the human brain: a bilateral, distributed mechanism. *J Neurophysiol* 1999; 82:1934–1943.

Cohn S, Seltzer Z. Inherited propensity for neuropathic pain is mediated by sensitivity to injury discharge. *Neuroreport* 1991; 2:647–650.

Cross DJ, Minoshima S, Ladabaum U, et al. Cerebral representations of somatic versus visceral pain as revealed by PET. *Neurosci Abstracts* 1999.

Defrin R, Zeitoun I, Urca G. Strain differences in autotomy levels in mice: relation to spinal excitability. *Brain Res* 1996; 711:241–244.

Derbyshire SWG. Meta-analysis of thirty-four independent samples studied using PET reveals a significantly attenuated central response to noxious stimulation in clinical pain patients. *Curr Rev Pain* 1999; 3:265–280.

Derbyshire SW, Jones AK, Gyulai F, et al. Pain processing during three levels of noxious stimulation produces differential patterns of central activity. *Pain* 1997; 73:431–445.

Faggin BM, Nguyen KT, Nicolelis MA. Immediate and simultaneous sensory reorganization at cortical and subcortical levels of the somatosensory system. *Proc Natl Acad Sci USA* 1997; 94:9428–9433.

Gorman AL, Yu C-G, Ruenes GR, Daniels L, Yezierski RP. Conditions affecting the onset, severity, and progression of a spontaneous pain-like behavior after excitotoxic spinal cord injury. *J Pain* 2001; 2:229–240.

Hsieh J-C, Belfrage M, Stone-Elander S, Hansson P, Ingvar M. Central representation of chronic ongoing neuropathic pain studied by positron emission tomography. *Pain* 1995; 63:225–336.

Iadarola MJ, Max MB, Berman KF, et al. Unilateral decrease in thalamic activity observed with positron emission tomography in patients with chronic neuropathic pain. *Pain* 1995; 63:55–64.

Jones EG, Pons TP. Thalamic and brainstem contributions to large-scale plasticity of primate somatosensory cortex. *Science* 1998; 282:1121–1125.

Kaas JH, Florence SL, Neeraj J. Reorganization of sensory systems of primates after injury. *Neuroscientist* 1997; 3:123–130.

Koyama S, Katayama Y, Maejima S, et al. Thalamic neuronal hyperactivity following transection of the spinothalamic tract in the cat: involvement of *N*-methyl-D-aspartate receptor. *Brain Res* 1993; 612:345–350.

Ladabaum U, Minoshima S, Owyang C. Pathobiology of visceral pain: molecular mechanisms and therapeutic implications v. central nervous system processing of somatic and visceral sensory signals. *Am J Physiol Gastrointest Liver Physiol* 2000; 279:1–6.

Lenz FA, Kwan HC, Martin R, et al. Characteristics of somatotopic organization and spontaneous neuronal activity in the region of the thalamic principal sensory nucleus in patients with spinal cord transection. *J Neurophysiol* 1994; 72:1570–1587.

Mao J, Price DD, Coghill RC, Mayer DJ, Hayes RL. Spatial patterns of spinal cord [^{14}C]-2-deoxyglucose metabolic activity in a rat model of painful peripheral mononeuropathy [published erratum appears in *Pain* 1992; 51(3):389]. *Pain* 1992; 50:89–100.

Mogil JS. The genetic mediation of individual differences in sensitivity to pain and its inhibition. *Proc Natl Acad Sci USA* 1999; 96:7744–7751.

Mogil JS, Adhikari SM. Hot and cold nociception are genetically correlated. *J Neurosci* 1999; 19:13–17.

Mogil JS, Wilson SG, Bon K, et al. Heritability of nociception I: responses of 11 inbred mouse strains on 12 measures of nociception. *Pain* 1999a; 80:67–82.

Mogil JS, Wilson SG, Bon K, et al. Heritability of nociception II. 'Types' of nociception revealed by genetic correlation analysis. *Pain* 1999b; 80:83–93.

Morrow TJ, Paulson PE, Danneman PJ, Casey KL. Regional changes in forebrain activation during the early and late phase of formalin nociception: analysis using cerebral blood flow in the rat. *Pain* 1998; 75:355–365.

Morrow TJ, Paulson PE, Brewer KL, Yezierski RP, Casey KL. Chronic, selective forebrain responses to excitotoxic dorsal horn injury. *Exp Neurol* 2000; 161:220–226.

Ness TJ, San Pedro EC, Richards JS, et al. A case of spinal cord injury-related pain with baseline rCBF brain SPECT imaging and beneficial response to gabapentin. *Pain* 1998; 78:139–143.

Neto FL, Schadrack J, Ableitner A, et al. Supraspinal metabolic activity changes in the rat during adjuvant monoarthritis. *Neuroscience* 1999; 94:607–621.

Ohara PT, Chazal G, Ralston III HJ. Ultrastructural analysis of GABA-immunoreactive elements in the monkey thalamic ventrobasal complex. *J Comp Neurol* 1989; 283:541–558.

Pagni CA, Canavero S. Functional thalamic depression in a case of reversible central pain due to a spinal intramedullary cyst. *J Neurosurg* 1995; 83:163–165.

Panerai AE, Sacerdote P, Brini A, Bianchi M, Mantegazza P. Autotomy and central nervous system neuropeptides after section of the sciatic nerve in rats of different strains. *Pharmacol Biochem Behav* 1987; 28:385–388.

Paulson PE, Morrow TJ, Casey KL. Bilateral behavioral and regional cerebral blood flow changes during painful peripheral mononeuropathy in the rat. *Pain* 2000; 84:233–245.

Paulson PE, Minoshima S, Morrow TJ, Casey KL. Gender differences in pain perception and patterns of cerebral activation during noxious heat stimulation in humans. *Pain* 1998; 76:223–229.

Peyron R, Garcia-Larrea L, Gregoire MC, et al. Allodynia after lateral-medullary (Wallenberg) infarct. A PET study. *Brain* 1998; 121:345–356.

Ploghaus A, Tracey I, Gati JS, et al. Dissociating pain from its anticipation in the human brain. *Science* 1999; 284:1979–1981.

Pons TP, Garraghty PE, Ommaya AK, et al. Massive cortical reorganization after sensory deafferentation in adult macaques. *Science* 1991; 252:1857–1860.

Popovich PG, Wei P, Stokes BT. Cellular inflammatory response after spinal cord injury in Sprague-Dawley and Lewis rats. *J Comp Neurol* 1997; 377:443–464.

Porro CA, Cavazzuti M. Functional imaging studies of the pain system in man and animals. *Prog Brain Res* 1996.110:47–62.

Porro CA, Cavazzuti M, Galetti A, Sassatelli L. Functional activity mapping of the rat brainstem during formalin-induced noxious stimulation. *Neuroscience* 1991a; 41:667–680.

Porro CA, Cavazzuti M, Galetti A, Sassatelli L, Barbieri GC. Functional activity mapping of the rat spinal cord during formalin-induced noxious stimulation. *Neuroscience* 1991b; 41:655–665.

Price DD. *Psychological and Neural Mechanisms of Pain.* New York: Raven Press, 1988, pp 1–241.

Price DD, Mao J, Coghill RC, et al. Regional changes in spinal cord glucose metabolism in a rat model of painful neuropathy. *Brain Res* 1991; 564:314–318.

Rainville P, Duncan GH, Price DD, Carrier M, Bushnell MC. Pain affect encoded in human anterior cingulate but not somatosensory cortex. *Science* 1997; 277:968–971.

Ralston HJ III, Ohara PT, Meng XW, Wells J, Ralston DD. Transneuronal changes of the inhibitory circuitry in the macaque somatosensory thalamus following lesions of the dorsal column nuclei. *J Comp Neurol* 1996; 371:325–335.

Roberts WA, Eaton SA, Salt TE. Widely distributed GABA-mediated afferent inhibition processes within the ventrobasal thalamus of rat and their possible relevance to pathological pain states and somatotopic plasticity. *Exp Brain Res* 1992; 89:363–372.

Rosen SD, Camici PG. The brain-heart axis in the perception of cardiac pain: the elusive link between ischaemia and pain. *Ann Med* 2000; 32:350–364.

Salt TE. Gamma-aminobutyric acid and afferent inhibition in the cat and rat ventrobasal thalamus. *Neuroscience* 1989; 28:17–26.

Schadrack J, Neto FL, Ableitner A, et al. Metabolic activity changes in the rat spinal cord during adjuvant monoarthritis. *Neuroscience* 1999; 94:595–605.

Svensson P, Minoshima S, Beydoun A, Morrow TJ, Casey KL. Cerebral processing of acute skin and muscle pain in humans. *J Neurophysiol* 1997; 78:450–460.

Talbot JD, Marrett S, Evans AC, et al. Multiple representations of pain in human cerebral cortex. *Science* 1991; 251:1355–1358.

Williamson AM, Ohara PT, Ralston DD, Milroy AM, Ralston HJ III. Analysis of gamma-aminobutyric acidergic synaptic contacts in the thalamic reticular nucleus of the monkey. *J Comp Neurol* 1994; 349:182–192.

Willis WD Jr. *The Pain System: The Neural Mechanisms of Nociceptive Transmission in the Mammalian Nervous System.* Basel: Karger, 1985, pp 1–346.

Willis WD, Westlund KN. Neuroanatomy of the pain system and of the pathways that modulate pain. *J Clin Neurophysiol* 1997; 14:2–31.

Yezierski RP. Pain following spinal cord injury: the clinical problem and experimental studies. *Pain* 1996; 68:185–194.

Yezierski RP, Liu S, Ruenes GL, Kajander KC, Brewer KL. Excitotoxic spinal cord injury: behavioral and morphological characteristics of a central pain model. *Pain* 1998; 75:141–155.

Yoon YW, Lee DH, Lee BH, Chung K, Chung JM. Different strains and substrains of rats show different levels of neuropathic pain behaviors. *Exp Brain Res* 1999; 129:167–171.

Correspondence to: Thomas J. Morrow, PhD, Neurology Research Laboratories, Veterans Affairs Hospital, Research 11R, 2215 Fuller Road, Ann Arbor, MI 48105, USA. Tel: 734-761-7956; Fax: 734-761-7693; email: ruscat@umich.edu.

Spinal Cord Injury Pain: Assessment, Mechanisms, Management. Progress in Pain Research and Management, Vol. 23, edited by Robert P. Yezierski and Kim J. Burchiel, IASP Press, Seattle, © 2002.

16

Cortical Pathophysiology of Neuropathic Pain: Human Brain Imaging Studies and Theories of Neuropathic Pain

A. Vania Apkarian

Department of Physiology and Neuroscience Institute, Department of Surgery, and Department of Anesthesia, Northwestern University Medical School, Chicago, Illinois, USA

Research over the last two decades has revolutionized our understanding of mechanisms underlying neuropathic pain conditions, especially for processes in the periphery and the spinal cord. Both in the periphery and in the spinal cord a neuropathic injury causes drastic reorganization of nociceptive coding. Many of these changes are directly relevant to spinal cord injury (SCI) pain conditions, as elaborated in many chapters in this book. This reorganization includes changes in the phenotype of large-fiber afferents, in the responsiveness of silent nociceptors, in the receptor and neurotransmitter expression of different afferents and of spinal cord cells, and in the response properties of spinal cord cells. Such changes will clearly affect spinocephalad information transmission and result in changes in cortical representation of pain. SCI pain, which often is due to a complete severance of the cord and is accompanied by chronic pain in body sites below the site of the injury, must be considered a major subcategory of phantom pain. This consideration implies that at least some forms of SCI pain must be primarily due to supraspinal networks, involving the cortex not merely as a final transmission site of spinal cord inputs, but rather as a source of the perception per se. This chapter deals with the issue of the relative importance of cortical circuitry as opposed to spinal cord reorganization and transmission of the reorganized spinal information in neuropathic chronic pain conditions. Work in my laboratory over multiple years has concentrated on identifying the cortical networks underlying chronic neuropathic pain conditions in humans. We have not studied SCI pain patients, and to our knowledge no studies have directly examined the human brain network engaged in SCI pain.

This chapter reviews progress in our laboratory in identifying cortical regions involved in chronic pain, emphasizing the results from ongoing work. I argue that ongoing steady pain is a sine qua non of chronic neuropathic conditions. As a result, the identification of cortical circuitry underlying such conditions provides direct insight into the mechanisms—e.g., reorganization of nociceptive pathways and of changes in cortical dynamics and cortical biochemistry—that may be critical for the ongoing pain. Moreover, information about brain regions engaged in ongoing pain should be similar across multiple neuropathic pain conditions. Thus, these results should also shed light on the brain circuitry in ongoing SCI pain. Our studies using functional magnetic resonance imaging (fMRI) and hydrogen spectroscopy (^{1}H-MRS) provide a consistent picture of the cortical elements critical for such conditions. Overall, we observe that the prefrontal cortex is involved in two distinct clinical chronic pain conditions. The details of the specific prefrontal regions engaged in each condition seem distinct, which has important consequences regarding the subjectivity of various clinical pain conditions. Biochemical analysis of chronic pain patients in comparison to age- and sex-matched normal subjects indicates that the prefrontal cortical neurons undergo use-dependent atrophy in a pattern that reflects the specifics of the dimensions of pain experienced by these patients. I will review current theories of neuropathic pain to determine their consistency with the experimental results and to outline a plausible mechanism of chronic pain, bearing in mind the limited number of clinical conditions that have been studied so far.

A main emphasis of research in our laboratory has been the search for noninvasive brain imaging techniques that can be used to study clinical pain conditions. I will outline two separate approaches, fMRI and ^{1}H-MRS, and describe their properties in measuring human brain activity and human brain biochemistry, especially from the viewpoint of understanding the cortical circuitry of clinical chronic pain conditions.

MEASURING FUNCTIONAL BRAIN ACTIVITY

Functional MRI is becoming the main method for measuring brain activity in humans. Functional MRI is a noninvasive method with which scientists can indirectly monitor brain activity in awake humans while the participants are subjected to some stimulus or are instructed to perform some task. Functional MRI detects small fluctuations in tissue magnetization properties secondary to neuronal activity. Because fMRI is noninvasive and, as far as we know, harmless, there is no limit to the number of fMRI tests that can be performed. Changes in neuronal activity are accompanied by changes in cerebral blood flow, blood volume, level of oxygenation, and tissue metabolic rate. Transient changes in these parameters alter the balance between paramagnetic deoxyhemoglobin and diamagnetic oxyhemoglobin in red cells. Changes in this balance result in transient local magnetization changes, which can be monitored directly by fMRI (Kwong et al. 1992). This method has been used to visualize brain activations in a large set of stimulus and task conditions, including thermal painful stimuli (e.g., Davis et al. 1995, 1998, 2000; Gelnar et al. 1998, 1999; Apkarian et al. 1999, 2000). In such studies the participant is subjected to a stimulus-control condition, repeated many times. By assuming that the stimulus and control situations are reproducible and represent different brain states, researchers can determine the brain regions where local magnetization differs between the two states and infer that these regions participate in the perceptual change accompanying stimulus-control sequences. This type of analysis is also used in positron emission tomography (PET), where radionucleotide-tagged metabolic markers are injected into participants. The differential distribution of these radioactive markers between the two states indicates the distinctive brain regions involved.

Several laboratories have determined the temporal properties of brain hemodynamics (Cohen et al. 1997; Bandettini and Cox 2000). These studies indicate that the brain hemodynamic response has a characteristic time course and generally can be viewed as a typical response to a transient input, which in linear systems theory is equivalent to the impulse response function. This characterization in turn has led to new experimental designs that present very brief stimuli and look for related hemodynamic responses in the MR images; this approach is called event-related fMRI design and analysis. A main advantage of event-related design is its ability to present short stimuli with randomly varying intervals between events, which reduces predictability and expectation by the volunteers. The main assumption in functional brain imaging is that subjects' responses to a given stimulus are reproducible and time-locked with the application of the stimulus, but in chronic pain this assumption usually does not hold true, which necessitates alternative designs. fMRI is a noninvasive tool that can readily identify cortical networks involved in certain tasks or stimuli. It delineates the brain network difference between the stimulus and control conditions examined. The longer-term organization of these networks may be examined by fMRI, although such designs are complicated and rarely used.

TEMPORAL PROFILE OF PAIN CONSCIOUSNESS

Unlike touch, vision, or audition, neural systems underlying pain perception are slow. As a result, pain perception can often be dissociated from the stimulus. There is a complex relationship between the intensity of pain experienced and its temporal properties. Hardy et al. (1968) showed that when a thermal painful stimulus is mild, the reported pain may be delayed by several seconds from the start of the stimulus and may be transient. These authors also showed individual variability in temporal changes in pain perception as well as differences in temporal properties of pain as a function of intensity. As the intensity of the thermal painful stimulus is increased, its perception becomes more constant and outlasts the stimulus. However, this temporal pattern seems to differ among individuals. Such temporal dissociations between stimulus and perception may become far more dramatic in pain abnormalities, as shown by Gracely et al. (1996). Neuropathic pain patients show a long delay between the start of a painful stimulus and their perceived pain, as well as a strong sensitization that far outlasts the second stimulus when the stimulus is repeated within a few seconds.

We have taken advantage of this temporal dissociation between a painful stimulus and the subjective perception of pain to analyze the brain circuitry of pain (Apkarian 1999). Within the parietal cortex, spanning from the anterior commissure to just behind the posterior commissure, a monotonic change occurs in the brain response to painful thermal stimulation such that the more anterior regions are better related to the stimulus itself while the more posterior portions of the region are better related to the perception of the pain. We extended the method to directly image brain regions involved in the ongoing spontaneous pain of clinical neuropathic pain conditions (Apkarian et al. 2001b).

The conceptual novelty of our fMRI studies is the notion that we can take advantage of the unique temporal properties of pain to identify cortical regions specifically involved in the *subjective, conscious perception of pain* and to be able to apply this to *directly* study cortical regions involved in clinical pain syndromes.

MEASURING THE SUBJECTIVE EXPERIENCE OF PAIN

The need to study the subjective experience of pain was eloquently stated years ago by Donald D. Price. In the first chapter of his book (1988), he states:

> The definition of pain as "an unpleasant sensory and emotional *experience* associated with actual or potential tissue damage..." (Merskey 1986) leaves us in a very interesting philosophical position with regard to the study of pain. *If pain is defined subjectively as an experience, then the scientific study of pain ultimately has to study and even measure that experience.* [italics are my emphasis]

This challenge is exactly what we have achieved. It should first be stated that all prior brain-imaging studies of pain have examined brain activity patterns between two states. By comparing a painful state to a nonpainful state, researchers have defined brain regions involved in pain perception in PET and fMRI studies. This approach does not distinguish between stimulus coding and pain perception in the brain.

In our earlier fMRI study of cortical regions activated by a thermal painful stimulus, we simply compared the brain areas significantly activated during the painful state as compared to the nonpainful warm control state (Gelnar et al. 1999). This cortical pattern was compared to that seen when subjects performed a vibrotactile or motor task. The study showed that multiple brain regions are activated in an experimental painful task, including the primary and secondary somatosensory cortices, the primary and supplementary motor cortices, the posterior parietal cortex, the insula, and the anterior cingulate cortex. This pattern of brain activity has been demonstrated by many brain imaging studies (for details see Apkarian et al. 1995; Bushnell et al. 1999; Treede et al. 1999, 2000). Because fMRI has a higher spatial resolution than PET, it enables researchers to further subdivide these activated regions with respect to specific Brodmann's areas and in relation to activations seen in the vibrotactile or motor tasks. These comparisons point to the conclusion that thermal painful stimulation activates brain regions uniquely responding to this stimulus, such as the secondary somatosensory cortex, the anterior cingulate cortex, and portions of the primary somatosensory and motor cortices, as well as regions that overlap with vibrotactile sensation and motor performance.

Subsequently, we analyzed the fMRI thermal painful stimulus results in relation to the time course of the stimulus and pain perception (Apkarian et al. 1999). We determined the time course of pain perception in another group of subjects who were required to continuously rate the intensity of subjectively perceived pain when they were presented with the same thermal painful stimulus as used in the fMRI study. These ratings showed that although the thermal painful stimulus was constant, the subjectively perceived pain varied. Painful heat was applied for 35 seconds (with 35-second controls) and was constant through the stimulus period. The subjective pain reports, however, continuously increased during each stimulus period, over 35 seconds. Moreover, the time variation was greater in the peak pain perceived. By taking advantage of this temporal dissociation between stimulus characteristics and pain perception, we analyzed brain activity with both time curves and identified cortical regions more closely related to either the stimulus or the perception (Apkarian et al. 1999). This analysis showed a gradual transition of information processing anteroposteriorly in the parietal cortex. Within this region, activity in the anterior areas more closely reflected thermal stimulus parameters, while activity more posteriorly was better related to the temporal properties of pain perception. Within the brain region analyzed, the posterior parietal cortex best reflects the time-varying conscious subjective report of pain. We tentatively conclude that this area may be critical in pain consciousness. The region is clinically significant because lesions of this part of the brain, especially in the right hemisphere, lead to hemi-neglect. Therefore, the normal conscious awareness of pain may be critically linked to the normal awareness of body image. Overall, these results indicate that we have developed an approach with which we can differentiate and relate cortical regions to the subjective conscious perception of pain, fulfilling Price's wish.

AN OBJECTIVE MEASURE OF PAIN

In an article published on the occasion of the 25th anniversary of the International Association for the Study of Pain, Allan Basbaum (1998), writing on "New techniques, targets and treatments for pain: what promise does the future hold?" stated that "a better objective measure of a patient's pain will have enormous value."

Seemingly paradoxically, our results indicate that the examination of brain activity by correlating subjective reports of pain perception to the fMRI signal provides an objective measure of the presence of pain. The relevant parameter, especially in patients suffering from pain, is not stimulus representation in the brain but rather the extent to which their consciousness is preoccupied by pain. The latter can only be known by first determining which brain regions are specifically involved in the subjective knowledge of pain and then examining the extent to which these areas are active when the patients indicate a high level of pain. Our methodology directly targets the latter, and as a result it has the potential of becoming an objective measure of pain.

An example may better illustrate why our approach is objective. We have been studying a patient with syringomyelia who psychophysically performs thermal discrimination at chance level. However, she thinks that she can feel warm and cold stimuli. During the fMRI study of cortical activity, she did rate the stimulus as warm some of the time (the stimulus is accompanied by a tactile cue). When her brain activity was examined in relation to the stimulus, contralateral somatosensory regions were activated. When the brain activity was examined in relation to the ratings, only motor regions were active ipsilateral to the stimulus and contralateral to the hand with which the ratings were performed. Thus, the perception-related activity simply shows rating of related finger movements. The subject is attempting to perform a task that she cannot do, and the perception-related activity indicates this fact. Therefore, although the method uses subjective ratings of perception, if these ratings do not match the subject's conscious state the resultant brain activity pattern will show the discrepancy.

SOMATOTOPY FOR ACUTE/EXPERIMENTAL PAIN

Several groups have used fMRI to examine cortical circuitry underlying experimental and acute pain conditions. These studies show close similarity to results reported by PET studies, where similar thermal painful stimuli were used to map cortical activations (e.g., Jones et al. 1991; Talbot et al. 1991; Casey et al. 1994; Coghill et al. 1994; Hsieh et al. 1996; Derbyshire et al. 1997). Multiple reviews have discussed these results and compared them between tasks and among laboratories (Apkarian 1995; Bushnell et al. 1999; Ingvar 1999; Treede et al. 1999, 2000). In a recent study we examined the cortical somatotopy of thermal pain (Darbar et al. 1999). We examined segregation of cortical activity to painful thermal stimuli when the stimulus was applied to either the hand or the foot, as compared to vibrotactile stimuli applied to the hand. We observed somatotopic activations within the primary somatosensory cortex. Within the superior operculum of the lateral sulcus we observed multiple topographic maps for thermal pain, some of which were bilaterally activated. More anteriorly, at the junction of the insula and the inferior frontal gyrus, we observed bilateral activity that clearly lacked somatotopy. A weak somatotopy was observed in the anterior cingulate cortex; this portion of the midline cortex is most consistently activated across pain tasks and laboratories and seems to be involved in the perception of pain unpleasantness (Rainville et al. 1997), yet its specific role in pain perception remains uncertain (see Davis et al. 2000). Below I will compare these thermal pain activations with the cortical networks we have identified in chronic pain patients.

APPLICATION OF fMRI TO CLINICAL CHRONIC PAIN STATES

COMPLEX REGIONAL PAIN SYNDROME

An important distinction between chronic and acute pain conditions is the general inability of researchers to control and manipulate chronic pain conditions. Thus it is more complicated to apply brain imaging methods to the delineation of cortical networks underlying such states. In standard fMRI methods the primary assumption is that the stimulus and control conditions are well defined and clearly separate. However, chronic pain interacts with any painful stimulus applied in chronic pain patients. An fMRI study of patients with complex regional pain syndrome type I (CRPS-I) was designed specifically to isolate the brain network involved in the ongoing chronic pain from that of a painful stimulus (Apkarian et al. 2001a). This study recruited patients with CRPS-I with clear evidence for sympathetically mediated pain (SMP) because sympathetic blocks can be used to decrease chronic SMP (Ribbers et al. 1997), and the effects of thermal painful stimuli can be tested before and after the block.

Temporary relief of SMP by peripheral sympathetic blockade also permits us to study related neural activity without perturbing sensory inputs. We used fMRI in examining thermal painful stimuli applied to the chronically painful body site, both before and after sympathetic blockade, to determine the cortical network of chronic pain. We began with the assumption that the dual states of chronic pain and pain due to thermal painful stimuli can be additively present in the brain, such that cortical activity represents both conditions together. Moreover, when the same thermal stimulus is applied after a sympathetic block that significantly reduces or abolishes the chronic spontaneous pain, brain activity now represents the thermal pain network alone. Therefore, the residual brain activity, after subtracting the brain activation before the block from that obtained after the block, reflects the brain network responsible for chronic pain perception. The result of this subtraction across the patients and multiple trials indicated that chronic CRPS-I with SMP was associated with a widely spread prefrontal hyperactivity, as well as activity in the anterior cingulate and decreased activity in the thalamus contralateral to the affected body side. The parietal and insular regions that were activated in control subjects for thermal stimuli and that were also activated prior to sympathetic block in the CRPS patients did not survive the subtraction.

Ineffective sympathetic blocks that did not diminish SMP did not change the cortical responses to the painful thermal stimulus, while effective placebo resulted in similar responses to those of effective blocks. Several groups of normal volunteers were used as a comparison to the activations in the CRPS patients. In one group of normal volunteers, thermal painful stimuli were applied before and after sympathetic blocks. In this group the sympathetic block decreased sensorimotor activity and had no effect on prefrontal activations. Thus, sympathetic blocks have disparate effects in CRPS and normal subjects, implying a reorganization in the relationship between the central nervous system and autonomic responses.

The pattern of brain activation in CRPS patients is relevant to that of SCI pain patients in multiple ways. First, some SCI pain patients exhibit CRPS-like symptoms. It is unclear whether this is limited to pain at the site of injury, or if it may also extend to pain at levels below the injury. In any case, CRPS-type brain activity is at least directly related to the brain activations one expects in the subset of SCI pain patients with clear CRPS symptoms. It remains unknown what portion of SCI pain patients belong to this subcategory. The second link between SCI pain and CRPS pain is more important because in both cases the main debilitating pain is the ongoing pain. In the study described above (Apkarian et al. 2001a), we attempted to isolate the brain circuitry underlying sympathetically mediated ongoing pain. The results imply that the brain region most commonly involved in ongoing pain across multiple patients and across a large number of scans is the prefrontal cortex. This finding does not imply that other brain regions are not involved in the spontaneous pain perception, but rather that this is the most consistent region on average. Variability among patients may be significant as to the specific cortical areas involved in the spontaneous pain, which one would expect given different patients' variability in pain behavior and pain affect. We hope that fMRI will allow us to delineate and identify this variability in the near future. Also, the frontal cortex is implicated in a large number of cognitive functions, and different portions of the prefrontal cortex are implicated in multiple diverse functions. The relationship between these cognitive functions and neuropathic pain activations are discussed below. In CRPS patients, prefrontal activity was concentrated in the most frontal pole and in the lateral portions of the prefrontal cortex.

The results obtained in the CRPS patients also carry important implications regarding nociceptive transmission pathways. The overall thalamic activity in the CRPS patients was similar between the thalamus contralateral to the painful body and the ipsilateral side when the comparison was made for thermal painful stimuli averaged over all stimulus and pre- and post-sympathetic block conditions. However, this comparison was very different in the subtraction of the pre- from post-sympathetic block conditions. In this case there was a large asymmetry, with the thalamus contralateral to the CRPS-affected hand showing a significant decrease in activity as compared to the ipsilateral thalamus. The first comparison simply shows that during thermal painful stimulation the overall thalamic activity is not different between its two sides. This result may simply reflect the small amount of change in a small portion of the thalamus during thermal stimulation, which is not detected in the average of the whole thalamus. The second comparison implies an overall decrease in the thalamus on the side where the spontaneous CRPS pain is experienced, in the condition where this is specifically isolated. Several groups have reported thalamic hypoactivity in chronic pain conditions (Di Piero 1991; Hsieh et al. 1995; Iadarola et al. 1995). This finding seems to be the most consistent result in brain imaging studies of chronic pain conditions. It has been interpreted by multiple diverse viewpoints, all of which attempt to preserve the notion that the pain condition must involve nociceptive transmission through the spinothalamic pathway. However, the simplest interpretation of thalamic hypoactivity is that the thalamus is disengaged from the chronic pain state. In turn, this view implies that the spinothalamic pathway is not critical and may in fact be actively inhibited in the spontaneous chronic pain state. Such inhibition is neither surprising nor contradictory to the behavioral manifestations of chronic pain conditions and may in fact be a mode of coping with the pain. Suppressed spinothalamic transmission may be a sign that the brain is actively attempting to block sensory information about the intensity, location, and modality of pain. In fact, a large body of clinical data shows that chronic pain is often accompanied by decreased sensory perception of both painful and nonpainful stimuli, especially at the site where the ongoing chronic pain is experienced (see, e.g., Casey 1991). This interpretation implies that the amount of suffering in chronic pain does not relate to the sensory information per se but rather to the negative affect as reflected in the frontal activations.

These results shed new insight on nociceptive transmission through spinocephalad pathways versus dynamic brain states for neuropathic pain perception. Given that the prefrontal cortex is the most consistently active brain region during spontaneous neuropathic pain and considering our conclusion that the spinothalamic pathway is inhibited in this condition, what are the options for interpreting these results regarding the coding and representation of chronic pain? The most simplistic interpretation would be that nociceptive information is transmitted to the prefrontal cortex through pathways outside the spinothalamic projections, i.e., pathways bypassing the thalamus and gaining access to the cortex directly. A number of pathways are candidates for these projections, which may be reinforced by the persistence of the pain. This interpretation is most consistent with the ideas proposed by Cassinari and Pagni (1969), although it also harks back to Cartesian "labeled line" notions of information coding, which we do not favor.

An alternative explanation takes into account the general role of the prefrontal cortex in cognitive control. As Miller and Cohen (2001) state, "the prefrontal cortex is important when 'top-down' processing is needed; that is, when behavior must be guided by internal states or intentions." Thus, the prefrontal cortex determines the relative salience that the brain attaches to external events relative to internal intentions. Therefore, the prefrontal hyperactivity during neuropathic pain may simply be the signature of this heightened salience that the prefrontal cortex attaches to pain, and particularly to the pain's affective or emotional salience. From this viewpoint the chronic pain state becomes a central sensitization state, where the sensitization is at the level of the cortex, and does not involve transmission from spinal sensitized pathways. Another interpretation would be that the change in salience is the establishment of a long-term memory trace that engages the whole consciousness of the organism. These lines of thought lead to specific hypotheses regarding cortical synchronization and changes in the dynamics of synchronization across cortical regions with the change from acute pain perception to chronic neuropathic pain perception. We are testing these ideas directly in animal models of acute and chronic pain conditions. Another aspect of these lines of thought is the link between chronic pain behavior and addictive behavior. Recent studies implicate the prefrontal cortex in addictive behavior in a manner very similar to our interpretation of its role in neuropathic pain behavior, namely as the site where salience to external inputs is modified (Volkow et al. 2000). Therefore, the mechanisms of neuropathic pain may share important characteristics with those of addiction, and therapy strategies for addiction may be useful in chronic pain as well.

CHRONIC BACK PAIN

It is not clear to what extent the assumption regarding linear additivity of chronic and acute pain conditions is tenable. Most likely the interaction between acute and chronic pain is nonlinear, and the subtractive analysis used above for identifying the ongoing pain of CRPS ignores the multiplicative term between the two states and only identifies the linear component. To improve on this approach we developed an alternative fMRI method that directly examines brain activity of chronic pain (Apkarian et al. 2001b). Subjects are equipped with a finger-spanning device to continuously rate and log their perceived pain during fMRI data collection. These ratings are convolved with a canonical hemodynamic response function to generate predictor waveforms with which related brain activity can be identified. The approach uses continuous logging of ongoing subjective pain reports and relates these ratings back to objective measures of brain activity. We studied patients with chronic low back pain. In one series of fMRI scans the patient simply lies in the scanner and indicates spontaneous fluctuations of the subjective pain. In another series of scans, the patient performs a straight-leg-raising procedure to exacerbate the back pain. In both conditions the patient continuously rates the pain, and in the second condition he or she is asked to ignore the leg movements. The results indicate the feasibility of differentiating between different pain states. We have argued that this approach can be generalized to identify brain circuitry underlying diverse clinical pain conditions (for details, see Apkarian et al. 2001b). The brain activity for spontaneous ratings of ongoing back pain in five patients was averaged across multiple repetitions of fMRI scans (Krauss et al. 1999). The preliminary results indicate activations primarily in the prefrontal cortex, similar to the chronic pain-related activity in CRPS, as well as in the insula.

COMPARING THE BRAIN PAIN NETWORK BETWEEN NORMAL VOLUNTEERS AND CHRONIC PAIN GROUPS

We recently described the extent of overlap in brain activations between the three groups of studies described above, evaluating the similarity of the cortical network of activity in normal subjects subjected to a thermal stimulus in comparison to the activity during spontaneous pain in CRPS patients, and to that in chronic back pain patients who are asked to continuously rate their ongoing pain (Apkarian et al. 2001c). This comparison questions the extent to which chronic and acute pain conditions depend on the same cortical circuitry, and as a result how much cortical reorganization underlies chronic pain conditions, as well as the extent to which diverse chronic pain conditions depend on the same cortical circuitry. Results indicated that the anterior cingulate cortex was the only region of overlap among the three groups. Thus, we concluded that in both chronic pain conditions cortical activity engages more prefrontal regions. Moreover, we argued that the details of the regions activated in the chronic pain conditions are unique to each condition.

These results imply that the subjective experiences of acute and chronic pain are significantly different because they engage different cortical circuitry. Moreover, although the two chronic pain conditions activate mainly prefrontal areas, they too differ from each other in their subjectivity. It is unlikely that this diversity is due to differences in the spinocephalad transmission lines. Rather, it must be attributed to the salience of the two chronic pain conditions. Once again, this argument implies that the cortical sensitization details give rise to a prefrontal cortex-driven network that in turn governs the subjectivity of the chronic pain.

MEASURING HUMAN BRAIN BIOCHEMISTRY

Nuclear magnetic resonance spectroscopy (MRS) is a method used in chemistry and physics laboratories to analyze molecular interactions and identify chemical compounds. Recently this approach was adapted for in vivo analysis of brain chemistry. The key to this method is to localize MR signals to a specific volume, an approach commonly used in anatomical MRI. In all biological tissues including the brain, water is the predominant chemical, so observation of weak signals from metabolites with concentrations thousands of times smaller than that of water requires methods for suppressing the water signal. Advances in MR technology in automating voxel positioning and suppressing the water signal have made MRS a relatively simple noninvasive approach for studying brain chemistry (see Salibi and Brown 1998). Proton spectra (^{1}H-MRS) enable the measurement of concentrations of various metabolites and excitatory and inhibitory neurotransmitters. ^{1}H-MRS has been used to examine the brain biochemistry of various neurological patient populations, such as patients suffering from stroke, various types of brain tumors, multiple sclerosis, Alzheimer's disease, and epilepsy.

^{1}H-MRS can be used to measure the chemical concentrations (i.e., peaks or intensities) of up to nine different compounds in the living brain: *N*-acetyl aspartate (NAA), choline (Cho), glutamate (Glu), glutamine (Gln), γ-aminobutyric acid (GABA), myo- and scyllo-inositol complex (Ins), glucose (Glc), lactate (Lac), and creatine (Cr). These measurements are performed as relative ratios among peaks (most commonly relative to Cr) or as absolute concentrations. Absolute concentration measurement requires an external or internal standard, which remains difficult to perform routinely, especially because the external standard method is sensitive to magnetic field inhomogeneities due to separation of the standard and the measured volume.

The ^{1}H-MRS spectra are usually characterized by three major peaks: NAA at 2.02 parts per million (ppm), Cr at 3.0 ppm, and Cho at 3.2 ppm. NAA is the dominant peak in normal adult brain spectra. The Cr spectrum is a combination of creatine and phosphocreatine (Michaelis et al. 1993). The proton Cho signal is a combination of Cho and Cho-containing compounds: choline plasmogen, glycerophosphorylcholine, phosphorylcholine, cytedine-diphosphate-choline, acetylcholine, and phosphatidylcholine (Michaelis et al. 1993).

Growing literature shows a depletion of brain NAA in neurodegenerative diseases (reviewed in Salibi and Brown 1998), suggesting that it is a neuronal marker (this chemical is present only in living, mature neurons and not in glia). Subsequent breakdown of NAA leads to aspartate, an excitatory amino acid neurotransmitter. Recent reports suggest that NAA is also required for brain lipid biosynthesis and that it is a marker for mitochondrial dysfunction (for further details, see Faull et al. 1999). Cr resonance is considered to be more stable than the NAA peak and is commonly used as a reference. However, this peak is abnormal with hypoxia, trauma, stroke, and tumor (Salibi and Brown 1998). The Cr level is involved in energy metabolism in the brain.

Brain chemistry varies regionally and with sex and age (Grachev and Apkarian 2000a), with an overall increase in regional chemical concentration (across all measured chemicals) from childhood to young adult (up to 25 years old) and then a decrease with further aging (Grachev and Apkarian 2000b). The age- and sex-dependent changes highlight an important difference between MRS and fMRI. MRS is usually measured in subjects while the subject simply lies in the scanner. We have tested whether MRS can detect task-dependent changes, but we failed to observe any consistent changes in MRS signal in the sensorimotor cortex during a finger apposition task or during a thermal painful task. It is thought that ^{1}H-MRS spectra remain unchanged under anesthesia. The only chemical measured by ^{1}H-MRS that would be expected to change with a cognitive task is glucose (this change may be detected if large data sets are collected). All other chemicals should be independent of the instantaneous changes in cognitive states. These observations imply that when ^{1}H-MRS spectra do show change they must reflect the long-term reorganization of brain circuitry.

BRAIN BIOCHEMISTRY REFLECTS SUBJECTIVE PROPERTIES OF CHRONIC PAIN

We used ^{1}H-MRS to study brain chemistry in chronic back pain patients compared to age- and sex-matched normal subjects. We made six separate single-voxel measurements in six different left-brain regions (Grachev et al. 2000). The hypothesis we tested was that, in chronic pain patients, brain areas that show hyperactivity in fMRI studies should also show abnormal brain chemistry. We tested three brain regions, the thalamus, cingulate cortex, and dorsolateral prefrontal cortex, where we quantified the concentrations of NAA, Cho, Glu, Gln, GABA, Ins, Glc, and Lac relative to the concentration of Cr, which is commonly used as an internal standard. All chronic back pain subjects received clinical evaluation and completed perceptual measures of pain and anxiety. The results show that chronic back pain alters human brain chemistry: NAA and Glc were reduced in the dorsolateral prefrontal cortex, whereas the cingulate and sensorimotor cortices and other brain regions showed no chemical concentration differences. Given that decreases in NAA are documented in various conditions involving neuronal cell damage and loss (Salibi and Brown 1998), our results provide evidence for a link between chronic pain and neuronal degeneration, specifically in the prefrontal cortex. These results also show the concordance between the fMRI studies and the MRS measures, both pointing to the prefrontal cortex as an important brain site for chronic pain.

The chronic back pain subjects completed perceptual measures of pain (the short form of the McGill Pain Questionnaire; Melzack 1987) and anxiety (the State-Trait Anxiety Inventory; Spielberger et al. 1983) minutes before brain imaging. These measures were correlated with brain regional chemical concentrations. There was a specific relationship between regional chemicals and perceptual measures of pain and anxiety. Chemicals in the prefrontal cortex of these patients showed the strongest relationship with the affective components of back pain. Therefore, this study indicates not only that brain chemistry is different in chronic pain patients but also that the abnormal changes reflect the specific perceptual parameters that define the details of the suffering that constitutes chronic back pain. This study also demonstrates that the relationship among various chemicals across the different brain regions was abnormal in the back pain patients as compared to normal subjects, indicating regional reorganization of brain biochemistry with chronic pain.

PREFRONTAL CORTEX AND CHRONIC PAIN

The above results highlight the importance of the engagement of the prefrontal cortex in chronic pain conditions. We observed prefrontal activation in chronic CRPS and back pain patients in functional imaging studies that concentrated on identifying the ongoing component of chronic pain. Also, the biochemical analysis of the chronic back pain patients shows the main shift in brain biochemistry to be localized to the prefrontal cortex. Thus, using disparate brain imaging methods and examining different clinical populations, we repeatedly observed the involvement of the prefrontal cortex in chronic pain. A cursory review of the literature indicates that most functional imaging studies of acute and experimental pain show substantial activity in the prefrontal cortex, although the significance of this activity has been usually ignored.

The prefrontal cortex is the neocortical region that is most elaborated in primates. It comprises a collection of interconnected neocortical areas that sends and receives projections from virtually all cortical sensory, motor, and subcortical structures (Miller and Cohen 2001). Tasks that uniquely require an intact prefrontal cortex, such as the Stroop task or the Wisconsin

Card Sorting Task, are described as tapping cognitive functions of either selective attention, behavioral inhibition, working memory, or rule-based or goal-directed behavior. Miller and Cohen (2001) argue that all these functions depend on representation of rules or goals in the form of prefrontal cortical activity patterns, which configure processing in other parts of the brain in accordance with current task demands. Different pathways in the prefrontal system, carrying different sources of information, compete for expression in behavior, and the winners are those with the strongest sources of support. Therefore, central reorganization in chronic pain simply becomes a manifestation of the change in representation rules specifically for nociceptive signals, where a long-term winner pattern enhances the affective significance of nociceptive processing. Consistent with these ideas, we have collected preliminary data in studies that evaluated chronic pain patients as to their ability in long-term planning—a task that is critically dependent on ventral orbital circuitry of the prefrontal cortex. The results indicate decreased ability of chronic pain patients in long-term planning, as compared to normal subjects (Kumar et al. 2000).

Different portions of the prefrontal cortex have been associated with distinct functional organizations. For example, orbital and medial areas are associated with behavioral inhibition, whereas ventrolateral and dorsal regions are associated with memory or attentional functions (Furster 1989). Moreover, both deficits and activation of the orbital prefrontal cortex have been mostly associated with tasks involving social, emotional, and appetitive stimuli (Swedo et al. 1989; Price 1999; O'Doherty et al. 2000), while more dorsal regions are reported to be activated in cognitive tasks. The differential extent of the involvement of these regions in distinct chronic pain conditions and in acute pain indicates that the salience of pain may vary subjectively along these pain conditions. These relationships imply that the extent to which different types of chronic pain impinge on attentional-cognitive tasks as compared to social-emotional tasks may be unique in different clinical conditions.

COMPARISON OF THE CURRENT MODEL WITH OTHER PROPOSED MECHANISMS

In this chapter we have presented the experimental data underlying the simple model we propose for chronic neuropathic pain conditions, including SCI pain. We propose that chronic neuropathic pain is associated with prefrontal activity and with prefrontal biochemical abnormalities. This is interpreted as a change in the "top-down" control of behavior where the salience of pain is increased at the cost of other cognitive and emotional behavioral abilities. This change most likely comes about by the establishment of new connectivity strengths, for example by changes in across brain synchronizations, where chronic pain may be viewed as a long-term memory that cannot be turned off, and thus it constantly interferes with attention to other tasks. Clearly this cortical network reorganization is driven, at least initially, by changes in the peripheral nervous system and spinal cord. However, the chronicity of the pain may simply reflect the extent of the change in "top-down" control of pain transmission circuitry. The details of the interaction between "top-down" and "bottom-up" control of pain perception remain to be studied.

In the only previous conference organized on the topic of central pain syndromes, Tasker et al. (1991) reviewed the historical literature as well as their clinical experience of the condition. They concluded that the most common property of central pain (i.e., neuropathic pain of central origin, which certainly includes SCI pain) is its steadiness. They estimated that 98.6% of their patients exhibit steady pain of various types: burning pain in 64.6%, aching in 38.6%, and dysesthesia in 31.6% (Tasker et al. 1991). Therefore, in this chapter we emphasize the brain imaging experiments that specifically aim to define the brain circuitry underlying the steady pain of chronic neuropathic conditions.

Since the first descriptions of central pain syndromes, many scientists have emphasized that the central underlying process involves the most direct nociceptive information pathway, the spinothalamic tract (see Chapters 13, 14). Lesions along this pathway either cause or, less frequently, relieve, pain conditions. Neurosurgeons have used deep brain stimulation along this pathway to relieve pain (see Chapter 13). Occasionally, stimulation within the lateral thalamus, at termination sites for the spinothalamic pathway, can replicate the pain. Our viewpoint is that differentiating between transmission pathways might be an altogether erroneous concept regarding chronic pain conditions. Instead, we emphasize changes in dynamic cortical network strength. Our model for chronic pain provides a new viewpoint regarding the success of deep brain stimulation procedures. Pain relief by such procedures may be a consequence of reestablishing inputs from this pathway to the cortex and thus counterbalancing the prefrontal network. In time this barrage of activity can reset the connectivity strengths of the cortical prefrontal "top-down" control to more normal levels.

ACKNOWLEDGMENTS

I would like to thank all the collaborators and students who made these studies possible. This research was funded by NIH/NINDS grant NS 35115 and by the Department of Neurosurgery at SUNY Health Science Center.
In memoriam to Dr. Johannes Brueggemann: During preparation of this manuscript Dr. Johannes Brueggemann unexpectedly passed away. He was a wonderful colleague, a very good friend, and a dedicated scientist. His influence and contribution to our work is exemplified by many of the first-rate papers that we published together. I will miss him enormously, especially regarding the lines of work that we had planned on pursuing together over the next decades.

REFERENCES

Apkarian AV. Functional imaging of pain: new insights regarding the role of the cerebral cortex in human pain perception. *Semin Neurosci* 1995; 7:279–293.

Apkarian AV, Darbar A, Krauss BR, Gelnar PA, Szeverenyi NM. Differentiating cortical areas related to pain perception from stimulus identification: temporal analysis of fMRI activity. *J Neurophysiol* 1999; 81:2956–2963.

Apkarian AV, Gelnar PA, Krauss BR, Szeverenyi NM. Cortical responses to thermal pain depend upon stimulus size: an fMRI study. *J Neurophysiol* 2000: 83(5):3113–3122.

Apkarian AV, Thomas PS, Krauss BR, Szeverenyi NM. Prefrontal cortical hyperactivity in sympathetically mediated chronic pain. *Neurosci Lett* 2001a; 311:193–197.

Apkarian AV, Krauss BR, Frederickson BE, Szeverenyi NM. Imaging the pain of low back pain: functional MRI in combination with monitoring subjective pain perception allows the study of clinical pain-states. *Neurosci Lett* 2001b; 299(1–2):57–60.

Apkarian AV, Grachev ID, Krauss BR, Szeverenyi NM. Imaging brain pathophysiology of chronic CRPS pain. In: Harden N, Baron R, Jänig W (Eds). *Complex Regional Pain Syndrome,* Progress in Pain Research and Management, Vol. 22. Seattle: IASP Press, 2001c, pp 209–225.

Bandettini PA, Cox RW. Event-related fMRI contrast when using constant interstimulus interval: theory and experiment. *Magn Reson Med* 2000; 43:540–548.

Basbaum AI. New techniques, targets and treatments for pain: what promise does the future hold? *Celebrating 25 Years.* Seattle: IASP, 1998, pp 16–18.

Bushnell MC, Duncan GH, Hofbauer RK, et al. Pain perception: is there a role for primary somatosensory cortex? *Proc Natl Acad Sci USA* 1999; 96:7705–7709.

Casey KL (Ed). *Pain and Central Nervous System Disease: The Central Pain Syndromes.* New York: Raven Press, 1991, pp 1–75.

Casey KL, Minoshima S, Berger KL, et al. Positron emission tomographic analysis of cerebral structures activated specifically by repetitive noxious heat stimuli. *J Neurophysiol* 1994; 71:802–807.

Cassinari V, Pagni CA. *Central Pain: A Neurosurgical Survey.* Cambridge, MA: Harvard University Press, 1969.

Coghill RC, Talbot JD, Evans AC, et al. Distributed processing of pain and vibration by the human brain. *J Neurosci* 1994; 14(7):4095–4108.

Cohen JD, Perlstein WM, Braver TS, et al. Temporal dynamics of brain activation during a working memory task. *Nature* 1997; 386:604–608.

Di Piero V, Jones AKP, Iannotti F, et al. Chronic pain: a PET study of the central effects of percutaneous high cervical cordotomy. *Pain* 1991; 46:9–12.

Darbar A, Szeverenyi NM, Apkarian AV. Somatotopy of thermal pain: dependence on dominance and body part stimulated. *Soc Neurosci Abstracts* 1999; 25.

Davis KD, Wood ML, Crawley AP, Mikulis DJ. fMRI of human somatosensory and cingulate cortex during painful electrical nerve stimulation. *Neuroreport* 1995; 7:321–325.

Davis KD, Kwan CL, Crawley AP, Mikulis DJ. Functional MRI study of thalamic and cortical activations evoked by cutaneous heat, cold, and tactile stimuli. *J Neurophysiol* 1998; 80:1533–1546.

Davis KD, Hutchison WD, Lozano AM, Tasker RR, Dostrovsky JO. Human anterior cingulate cortex neurons modulated by attention-demanding tasks. *J Neurophysiol* 2000; 83(6):3575–3577.

Derbyshire SWG, Jones AKP, Gyulai F, et al. Pain processing during three levels of noxious stimulation produces differential patterns of central activity. *Pain* 1997; 73:431–445.

Faull KF, Rafie R, Pascoe N, Marsh L, Pfefferbaum A. N-acetylaspartic acid (NAA) and N-acetylaspartylglutamic acid (NAAG) in human ventricular, subarachnoid, and lumbar cerebrospinal fluid. *Neurochem Res* 1999; 24:1249–1261.

Furster JM. *The Prefrontal Cortex*, Vol. 2. New York: Raven Press, 1989.

Gelnar PA, Krauss BR, Szeverenyi NM, Apkarian AV. Fingertip representation in the human somatosensory cortex: an fMRI study. *Neuroimage* 1998; 7:261–283.

Gelnar PA, Krauss BR, Sheehe PR, Szeverenyi NM, Apkarian AV. A comparative fMRI study of cortical representations for thermal painful, vibrotactile, and motor performance tasks. *Neuroimage* 1999; 10:460–482.

Gracely RH, Price DD, Roberts WJ, Bennett GJ. Quantitative sensory testing in patients with complex regional pain syndrome (CRPS) I and II. In: Jänig W, Stanton-Hicks M (Eds). *Reflex Sympathetic Dystrophy: A Reappraisal,* Progress in Pain Research and Management, Vol. 6. Seattle: IASP Press, 1996, pp 151–172.

Grachev ID, Apkarian AV. Chemical heterogeneity of the living human brain: a proton MR spectroscopy study on the effects of sex, age and brain region. *Neuroimage* 2000a; 11:554–563.

Grachev ID, Apkarian AV. Aging alters regional multichemical profile of the human brain: an *in vivo* ^{1}H MRS study of young versus middle-aged subjects. *J Neurochem* 2000b; 76:1–13.

Grachev ID, Fredrickson BE, Apkarian AV. Abnormal brain chemistry in chronic back pain: an *in vivo* proton magnetic resonance spectroscopy study. *Pain* 2000; 89(1):7–18.

Hardy JD, Stolwijk AJ, Hoffman D. Pain following step increase in skin temperature. In: Kenshalo DR (Ed). *The Skin Senses*. Springfield: Charles C. Thomas, 1968, pp 444–456.

Hsieh JC, Belfrage M, Stone-Elander S, Hansson P, Ingvar M. Central representation of chronic ongoing neuropathic pain studied by positron emission tomography. *Pain* 1995; 63:225–236.

Hsieh JC, Hannerz J, Ingvar M. Right-lateralised central processing for pain of nitroglycerin-induced cluster headache. *Pain* 1996; 67:59–68.

Iadarola MJ, Max MB, Berman KF, et al. Unilateral decrease in thalamic activity observed with positron emission tomography in patients with chronic neuropathic pain. *Pain* 1995; 63:55–64.

Ingvar M. Pain and functional imaging. *Philos Trans R Soc Lond B Biol Sci* 1999; 354(1387):1347–1358.

Jones AKP, Brown WD, Friston KJ, Qi LY, Frackowiak RSJ. Cortical and subcortical localization of response to pain in man using positron emission tomography. *Proc R Soc Lond* 1991; 244:39–44.

Krauss BR, Grachev I, Szeverenyi NM, Apkarian AV. Imaging the pain of back pain. *Soc Neurosci Abstracts* 1999; 25:59.11.

Kumar R, Grachev ID, Apkarian AV. Relationship between cognitive performance and brain chemistry in chronic back pain. *Soc Neurosci Abstracts* 2000; 26:160.9.

Kwong KK, Belliveau JW, Chesler DA. Dynamic magnetic resonance imaging of human brain activity during primary sensory stimulation. *Proc Natl Acad Sci USA* 1992; 89:5675–5679.

Melzack R. The short-form McGill Pain Questionnaire. *Pain* 1987; 30:191–197.

Merskey H (Ed). Classification of chronic pain: descriptions of chronic pain syndromes and definitions of pain terms. Prepared by the International Association for the Study of Pain Subcommittee on Taxonomy. *Pain* 1986; (Suppl 3):217–219.

Michaelis T, Merboldt KD, Bruhn H, Hanicke W, Frahm J. Absolute concentrations of metabolites in the adult human brain in vivo: quantification of localized proton MR spectra. *Radiology* 1993; 187:219–227.

Miller EK, Cohen JD. An integrative theory of prefrontal cortex function. *Annu Rev Neurosci* 2001; 24:167–202.

O'Doherty J, Rolls ET, Francis S, et al. Sensory-specific satiety-related olfactory activation of the human orbitofrontal cortex. *Neuroreport* 2000; 11:893–897.

Price DD. Physiological mechanisms of pain inhibition. In: *Psychological and Neural Mechanisms of Pain.* New York: Raven Press, 1988.

Price JL. Prefrontal cortical networks related to visceral function and mood. *Ann NY Acad Sci* 1999; 877:383–396.

Rainville P, Duncan GH, Price DD, Carrier B, Bushnell MC. Pain affect encoded in human anterior cingulated but not somatosensory cortex. *Science* 1997; 277:968–971.

Ribbers GM, Geurts AC, Rijken RA, Kerkkamp HE. Axillary brachial plexus blockade for the reflex sympathetic dystrophy syndrome. *Int J Rehabil Res* 1997; 20:371–380.

Salibi N, Brown MA. *Clinical MR Spectroscopy: First Principles.* New York: Wiley Liss, 1998.

Spielberger CD, Gorsuch RL, Lushene R, Vagg PR, Jacobs GA. *Manual for the State-Trait Anxiety Inventory.* Palo Alto, CA: Consulting Psychologists Press, 1983.

Swedo SE, Shapiro MB, Grady CL, et al. Cerebral glucose metabolism in childhood-onset OCD. *Arch Gen Psychiatry* 1989; 46:518–523.

Talbot JD, Marrett S, Evans AC, et al. Multiple representations of pain in human cerebral cortex. *Science* 1991; 251:1355–1358.

Tasker RR, de Calvalho G, Dostrovsky JO. The history of central pain syndromes, with observations concerning pathophysiology and treatment. In: Casey KL (Ed). *Pain and Central Nervous System Disease: The Central Pain Syndrome.* New York: Raven Press, 1991, pp 31–59.

Treede RD, Kenshalo DR, Gracely RH, Jones AK. The cortical representation of pain. *Pain* 1999; 79:105–111.

Treede R-D, Apkarian AV, Bromm B, Greenspan JD, Lenz FA. Cortical representation of pain: functional characterization of nociceptive areas near the lateral sulcus. *Pain* 2000; 87:113–119.

Volkow ND, Fowler JS. Addiction, a disease of compulsion and drive: involvement of the orbitofrontal cortex. *Cereb Cortex* 2000; 10(3):318–25.

Correspondence to: A. Vania Apkarian, PhD, Department of Physiology, Northwestern University Medical School, 303 E. Chicago Avenue, Ward M-211, Chicago, IL 60614, USA. Tel: 312-503-0404; Fax: 312-503-5101; email: a-apkarian@northwestern.edu.

Spinal Cord Injury Pain: Assessment, Mechanisms, Management. Progress in Pain Research and Management, Vol. 23, edited by Robert P. Yezierski and Kim J. Burchiel, IASP Press, Seattle, © 2002.

17

Proton Magnetic Resonance Spectroscopy following Spinal Cord Injury: Evaluation of Patients with Chronic Neuropathic Pain

Pradip M. Pattany,[a] Eva G. Widerström-Noga,[b] Brian C. Bowen,[a] Alberto Martinez-Arizala,[c] Bernardo R. Garcia,[a] Ernesto Cuevo,[b] Robert M. Quencer,[a] and Robert P. Yezierski[d]

[a]Department of Radiology, [b]The Miami Project to Cure Paralysis, and [c]Department of Neurology, University of Miami School of Medicine, Miami, Florida, USA; [d]Department of Orthodontics, College of Dentistry, University of Florida, Gainesville, Florida, USA

Recent studies reveal a high incidence of chronic pain following spinal cord injury (SCI), along with high pain intensity ratings (Störmer et al. 1997; Demirel 1998; Rintala et al. 1998; Siddall et al. 1999; Turner and Cardenas 1999; Finnerup et al. 2001; Turner et al. 2001; Widerström-Noga et al. 2001). Despite an increased understanding of the mechanisms responsible for the different types of pain observed after SCI (for recent reviews see Vierck et al. 2000; Siddall and Loeser 2001), no treatments are consistently effective for central neuropathic pain after SCI (pain located at or below the level of the lesion). Because chronic SCI pain is heterogeneous (Bowsher 1996; Eide 1998; Turner et al. 2001; Widerström-Noga et al. 2001), an extensive verbal pain evaluation and a neurological examination are needed to determine the specific type and severity of pain. One of the primary objectives in research on the central mechanisms of SCI pain has been the delineation of anatomical, neurochemical, and functional changes at or adjacent to the site of injury (Hao et al. 1992; Yezierski and Park 1993; Yezierski et al. 1993; Christensen et al. 1996). The many changes that occur after deafferentation of central neurons (Loeser and Ward 1967; Loeser et al. 1968; Roberts and Rees 1991) may play an important role in the development of SCI-induced pain. An important observation regarding the central mechanism of SCI pain appeared in a report describing an increase in spontaneous neuronal activity as well as burst discharges in the thalamic nuclei of a patient with chronic SCI pain (Lenz et al. 1987). Another study described significant increases in blood flow in specific thalamic nuclei during the sensation of pain, while during non-pain periods blood flow in these nuclei decreased (Ness et al. 1998).

While changes in blood flow can be used as a reflection of neuronal activity in different brain structures, another potential signature of pathophysiological changes in the brain is provided by the chemical changes that can be determined by magnetic resonance spectroscopy (MRS). MRS is a noninvasive means of measuring the in vivo concentration of metabolites in the human brain. To our knowledge no previous MRS study has assessed alteration in brain metabolites in SCI subjects with pain.

This chapter describes a study in which we used MRS to evaluate the region of the thalamus, a major sensory relay station that has been the focus of many pain studies. We tested the hypothesis that MRS can detect alterations in brain metabolites resulting from SCI-induced functional changes in thalamic nuclei.

MRS EVALUATION OF FUNCTIONAL CHANGES IN THE THALAMUS

SUBJECTS

Twenty-six male subjects participated in the study. Sixteen were paraplegic patients with SCI; seven of them (aged 46.2 ± 16.2 years, mean ± SD) had chronic pain, and nine (aged 34.8 ± 10.0 years) had no pain. Ten healthy males (aged 42.3 ± 10.5 years) served as controls. The time since injury was 7.6 ± 6.3 years for SCI subjects with chronic pain, and 11.3 ± 9.6 years for SCI subjects with no pain. Among the SCI subjects with chronic pain, one was injured at the C8 level and six were injured at the T9–L3 levels, and among subjects with no pain, four were injured at C4–C8 levels and five at T7–L3 levels. We obtained informed consent in accordance with the guidelines of the human subject committee of our institutional review board.

NEUROLOGICAL EXAMINATION AND PAIN EVALUATION

At the time of enrollment each patient received a complete neurological examination to determine sensory and motor levels of function and to derive an impairment score according to the guidelines of the American Spinal

Injury Association (ASIA). All but two patients had suffered traumatic SCI; one patient in the nonpain group had an ischemic SCI and one patient in the pain group had SCI secondary to a tumor. Most injuries in both groups were complete (ASIA level A), including 67% in the non-pain group and 74% in the pain group.

Pain was evaluated according to a previous study (Widerström-Noga et al. 2001). For the location of pain, subjects were asked to mark on a pain drawing those areas corresponding to the chronic pain they were presently experiencing. The pain drawing was divided into eight principal areas: (1) head, (2) neck and shoulders, (3) hands and arms, (4) frontal torso and genitals, (5) back, (6) buttocks, (7) thighs, and (8) legs and feet. The participants were asked to describe the location of pain and if possible, mark the pain perceived as most disturbing on a separate pain drawing.

To define the quality of their pain, subjects were asked to select words from a list that best described the pain they were presently experiencing. These sensory descriptors have been used in a previous study (Widerström-Noga et al. 2001).

Pain intensity was assessed using a numerical rating scale (NRS) ranging from no pain (0) to the most intense pain imaginable (10). Some of the analyses used "average pain intensity." This variable was obtained by averaging the most intense and least intense pain intensity. Pain intensity was evaluated immediately before, during, and immediately after the study.

MAGNETIC RESONANCE IMAGING AND SPECTROSCOPY

All subjects were scanned on a 1.5-Tesla whole-body MRI system that used quadrature body coil as a transmitter and quadrature head coil as a receiver, a combination that provides optimal signal to noise images and MRS data. Axial T1-weighted spin-echo images, T2-weighted fast spin-echo images, and fast fluid-attenuated inversion recovery (FLAIR) images were obtained with the same slice thickness (5 mm), gap (1.5 mm), field of view (FOV) (220 mm), and matrix (192 × 256). For the purpose of voxel placement, additional parasagittal and coronal T1-weighted, spin-echo pilot images with slice thickness of 5 mm, FOV of 220 mm, and a matrix of 128 × 256 were acquired in the region of the thalamus. Localized proton spectra were acquired from the left and right thalamus (Fig. 1) using an 8-mL voxel (Fig. 1). MRS data were acquired using a stimulated echo acquisition mode (STEAM) pulse sequence.

Spectral analysis was performed using the Linear Combination Model (LCModel) software (Provencher et al. 1993), a which employs a basis set of concentration-calibrated model spectra of individual metabolites to estimate

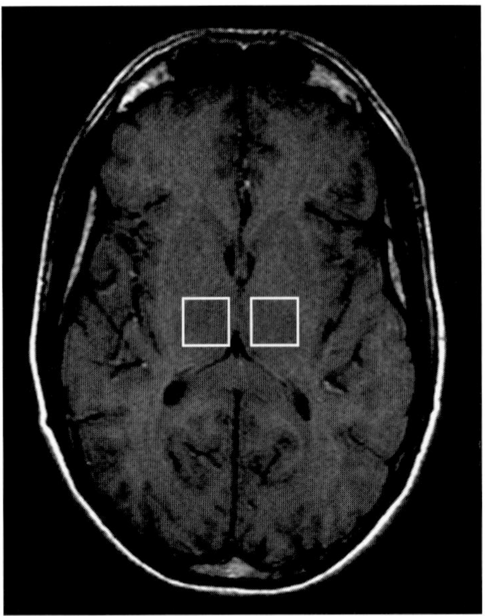

Fig. 1. The location of the 2 × 2 × 2 cm voxel in the region corresponding to the left and right thalamus. MRS data were acquired from each voxel separately for the three groups: SCI patients with pain, SCI patients without pain, and normal controls.

the absolute concentrations of similar brain metabolites from in vivo spectral data. This method exploits the full spectroscopic information of each metabolite rather than relying on isolated resonances (Fig. 2). The LCModel method yields concentrations for N-acetyl (NA), total creatine (Cr), choline compounds (Cho), glutamate (Glu), glutamine (Gln), Glu + Gln (Glx), and myo-inositol (Ins). To account for subject-to-subject variability in coil loading, the unsuppressed water signal for each subject was divided by the mean of the water signal for all subjects, and this ratio was multiplied by the concentration results for each subject. Each metabolite was correlated with measures of pain intensity (Pearson correlation matrix). Post hoc *t* tests were performed to test for differences between different groups, and *P* values of less than 0.05 were considered significant.

PAIN LOCATION, DESCRIPTORS, AND RATINGS

The location of pain marked on the pain drawings (Fig. 3) showed that 29% of the seven subjects with pain had pain in the neck and shoulder area, 43% in the upper extremities, 45% in the front and back, 43% in the buttocks, and 86% in the thigh and lower extremities (below the level of injury). The descriptors used the by the SCI subjects to describe the type of pain experienced showed that 57% had sharp pain sensations and 86% had burning, aching, and electric sensations.

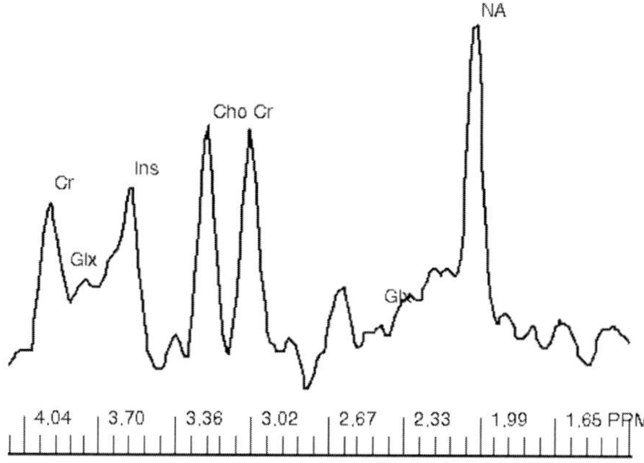

Fig. 2. Typical single-voxel stimulated echo acquisition mode (STEAM) spectrum from a normal male control. The assignment of peaks to various cerebral metabolites and the spectral analysis are described in the text.

The average of the least and most intense pain as rated on the NRS showed that 14% of the subjects had an average pain intensity of 5 or less and 86% had pain intensity greater than 5. The same questions were asked on the day of the MR study, and all seven subjects had pain intensity greater than 5.

MAGNETIC RESONANCE SPECTROSCOPY FINDINGS COMPARED

For all subjects, MRS data were acquired from the left and right thalamus, and statistical analysis showed no significant difference in metabolite concentrations between the two sides. As a result, we averaged the concentrations for each metabolite for each individual. For all 26 subjects we performed Pearson correlation analysis for each metabolite concentration to look for trends, and found that NA correlated negatively with average pain intensity (r = –0.678) and that Ins correlated positively (r = 0.520). We observed no correlation for the other metabolites (Cho, Cr, and Glx). The mean concentrations of NA and Ins and their standard deviations are shown in Table I for the three groups of subjects. We also computed the ratio of NA to Ins because these metabolites were showing opposite correlations as a function of pain intensity.

For NA the t test showed no significant difference between normal controls and SCI subjects without pain; however, there was a significant difference between SCI subjects with pain and those without pain (P = 0.006), and there was a trend toward significance between normal controls and SCI

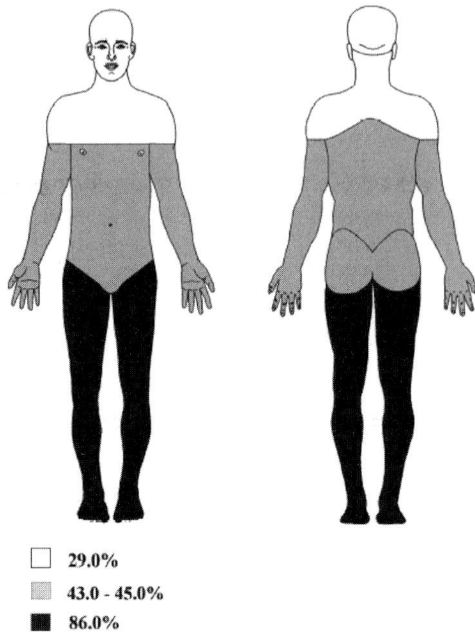

Fig. 3. Pain drawing used by subjects to indicate location of pain in eight body regions: head, neck and shoulders, upper extremity, frontal torso and genitals, back, buttocks, thighs, and legs and feet. The percentage of subjects who marked each region is indicated.

subjects with pain (P = 0.08). Similarly, for Ins there was no significant difference between normal controls and SCI subjects with or without pain. However, differences in Ins levels in SCI subjects with pain compared to those without pain approached significance (P = 0.06). The ratio of NA to Ins was significantly different in SCI subjects with pain compared to SCI subjects without pain (P = 0.004), and approached significance between normal controls and SCI subjects without pain (P = 0.06).

IMPORTANCE OF PAIN ASSESSMENT IN SCI PATIENTS

SCI has many consequences that can have a devastating impact on individuals dealing with the life-threatening complications of a traumatic injury to the central nervous system (Widerström-Noga et al. 1999, 2001). One of the consequences rated most difficult to deal with is the onset of chronic pain. In recent studies the prevalence of pain associated with SCI has been reported to range from 60% to 80% (Yezierski 1996; Störmer et al. 1997; Widerström-Noga et al. 1999, 2001a). More important, however, is the

Table I
Metabolite concentrations for patient and control groups (mean ± SD)

Groups	NA (mmol)	Ins (mmol)	NA/Ins Ratio
Control	6.305 ± 0.347	2.659 ± 0.542	2.474 ± 0.579
SCI without pain	6.566 ± 0.409	2.263 ± 0.313	2.957 ± 0.467****
SCI with pain	6.052 ± 0.206*	2.886 ± 0.699**	2.182 ± 0.418***

Note: Ins = myo-inositol; NA = N-acetyl.
*$P = 0.006$, compared to SCI without pain.
** $P = 0.06$, compared to SCI without pain.
*** $P = 0.004$, compared to SCI without pain.
**** $P = 0.06$, compared to normal controls.

influence of pain on quality of life. For example, pain interfered with daily activities including work, exercise, and social interactions in 83% of 800 subjects responding to a postal survey (Nepomuceuno et al. 1979). The significance of SCI pain is further underscored by the fact that nearly 40% of subjects in this study stated that they would trade any chance of physical recovery for relief of pain.

Of the different types of pain associated with SCI, the most challenging to patients and health professionals is neuropathic pain that appears within the first 6 months of injury. Not only is this type of pain present in parts of the body that lack normal sensation, but it has a spontaneous and persistent clinical profile. Descriptors used to describe this type of pain include burning, shooting, throbbing, and stabbing (Yezierski 1996). Although the condition of pain following SCI was first described more than a century ago, little is known about the pathophysiology underlying its onset and persistence. One of the primary objectives in understanding the central mechanism of SCI pain has focused on the delineation of anatomical, neurochemical, and functional changes at or adjacent to the site of injury (Hao et al. 1992; Yezierski and Park 1993; Yezierski et al. 1993; Christensen et al. 1996). While focusing on the spinal cord, however, investigators unfortunately have ignored what may be the most significant consequence of SCI—the impact of injury on certain regions of the brain, which become functionally and anatomically disconnected from the spinal cord. Considering the many changes that occur following deafferentation of central neurons (Loeser and Ward 1967; Loeser et al. 1968; Roberts and Rees 1991), it is possible that these alterations in the functional state, secondary to deafferentation, play an important role in the development of SCI-induced pain.

An important observation regarding the central mechanism of SCI pain appeared in a report describing the increase in spontaneous neuronal activity as well as burst discharges in thalamic nuclei of a patient with chronic SCI pain (Lenz et al. 1987). This study concluded that spinal injury resulted in the deafferentation of thalamic neurons and the emergence of abnormal seizure-like discharges. A second observation related to the role of thalamic structures in SCI pain was made using the technique of single photon emission computed tomography (SPECT) in a patient experiencing episodes of pain after SCI (Ness et al. 1998). During the sensation of pain, significant increases in blood flow occurred in thalamic nuclei, while during non-pain periods blood flow in these nuclei decreased. Given the fact that increased blood flow correlates with an increase in neuronal activity and/or abnormal discharges of central neurons (Iadecola 1993), the results of the SPECT study are consistent with the recording studies of Lenz and colleagues. Similarly, studies in rats have shown that SCI significantly increases blood flow in thalamic nuclei (Morrow et al. 2000).

Several MRS studies have shown decreased NA in patients with brain tumors, epilepsy, metabolic brain disorders, and neurological disorders such as Huntington's and Parkinson's disease and amyotrophic lateral sclerosis (ALS) (Bowen et al. 1995, 2000; Castillo et al. 1995). NA is thought to be localized in neurons and neuronal processes in the mature brain, and is decreased in several types of cerebral pathologies; such decreases are interpreted as reflecting neuronal dysfunction. In our study, patients with SCI pain had decreased NA compared both to controls and to SCI patients without pain. A possible explanation for decreased NA in those with SCI pain may be secondary changes of deafferentation that result in the dysfunction of inhibitory neurons. As a result NA levels would decrease, and pain would result from excitatory neurons without normal inhibitory controls. The location of pain and the descriptors provided showed that 86% of subjects had pain in the thigh and lower extremities, which is below the level of sensation based on the level of injury. Also, 86% of subjects had burning, aching, and electric sensations in the thigh and lower extremities, suggestive of neuropathic pain.

Inositol is thought to be a glial marker, acting as an organic osmolyte, with a major role in the volume and osmoregulation of astrocytes (Isaacks et al. 1994). Ins increases in ALS patients compared to normal controls (Bowen et al. 2000). Our results show that overall concentrations of Ins were lower in SCI subjects without pain compared to normal controls and SCI subjects with pain. The difference in Ins concentration between SCI subjects with pain and those without pain approached statistical significance, possibly due to the proliferation of glial cells (gliosis) in the thalamus.

Because concentrations of NA decrease and those of Ins increase with pain intensity, the ratio of NA/Ins shows promise as a clinically sensitive diagnostic tool for assessing pain in SCI patients. Also, it may be sensitive in assessing the efficacy of new therapeutic strategies for managing SCI pain.

Certain limitations hampered our study. First, the mean age of the SCI patients without pain was lower compared to the other two groups, a difference that may factor into our observed differences. But several studies (Huppi et al. 1991; Kreis et al. 1993; Kimura et al. 1995) have shown that metabolite changes only occur in the developing brain during the first 2 years of life. Another study (Pouwels et al. 1999) suggested that although major changes occur within the first year of life, slower changes occur thereafter, with full adult values not being reached until about 20 years of age. Based on the above-mentioned studies, we presume that the age differences would have no effect on the metabolite changes observed in our study. Second, the subjects enrolled in our study were all males, because Fillingim (2000) described gender differences in the perception of pain. In this study it was found that male subjects had a lower pain threshold than females. Third, for SCI subjects with chronic pain, the three most common drugs used were gabapentin, baclofen, and oxybutynin chloride. While their potential effect on the levels of MRS-detectable metabolites has not been fully investigated, we have reported previously (Bowen et al. 2000) that ALS patients treated with gabapentin had no difference in the metabolite levels, including NA and Ins, determined before and 2 weeks after gabapentin treatment. Experiments designed to assess the effects of each drug on metabolite concentrations would require large groups of subjects, which exceeds the scope of our investigation.

CONCLUSION

Our study shows that MRS can detect metabolic changes in the thalamus. Lower concentrations of NA suggest a higher degree of neuronal loss and dysfunction or dendritic pruning in SCI patients with pain when compared with SCI patients without pain and control subjects. Lower levels of Ins in SCI patients without pain when compared to SCI patients with pain and control subjects could be due to differences in glial reactions to injury. The observed differences in metabolites between SCI subjects with and without pain suggest that injury-induced functional changes may contribute to the central mechanism of chronic pain following SCI. The proposed method could be used to assess the effectiveness of potential neurochemical therapeutic targets developed for SCI patients with chronic neuropathic pain.

ACKNOWLEDGMENT

Supported in part by grants NS 40096 from the National Institutes of Health, National Institute of Neurological Disorders and Stroke, and Deans Pilot Project Award, University of Miami.

REFERENCES

Bowen BC, Block RE, Pattany PM, et al. Spectroscopy of the brain of 14 patients with Parkinson's Disease. *Am J Neuroradiol* 1995; 16:61–68.

Bowen BC, Pattany PM, Bradley WG, et al. MR imaging and localized proton spectroscopy of the precentral gyrus in amyotrophic lateral sclerosis. *Am J Neuroradiol* 2000; 21:647–658.

Bowsher D. Central pain: clinical and physiological characteristics. *J Neurol Neurosurg Psychiatry* 1996; 61:62–69.

Castillo M, Kwock L, Mukherji SK. Clinical applications of proton MR spectroscopy. *Am J Neuroradiol* 1995; 17:1–15.

Christensen MD, Everhart AW, Pickeman J, Hulsebosch CE. Mechanical and thermal allodynia in chronic central pain following spinal cord injury. *Pain* 1996; 68:97–107.

Demirel G, Yllmaz H, Gencosmanoglu B, Kesiktas N. Pain following spinal cord injury. *Spinal Cord* 1998; 36:25–28.

Eide PK. Pathophysiological mechanisms of central neuropathic pain after spinal cord injury. *Spinal Cord* 1998; 36:601–612.

Fillingim RB. Sex, gender and pain: women and men really are different. *Curr Rev Pain* 2000; 4:24–30.

Finnerup NB, Johannesen IL, Sindrup SH, Bach FW, Jensen TS. Pain and dysesthesia in patients with spinal cord injury: a postal survey. *Spinal Cord* 2001; 39:256–262.

Hao J-X, Xu X-J, Aldskogius H, Seiger Å, Wiesenfeld-Hallin Z. Chronic pain related syndrome in rats after ischemic spinal cord lesion: a possible animal model for pain in patients with spinal cord injury. *Pain* 1992; 43:279–290.

Huppi PS, Lazeyras F, Burri R, Bossi E, Herschkowitz N. Magnetic resonance in preterm and term newborns: 1h-spectroscopy in developing brain. *Pediatr Res* 1991; 30:574–578.

Iadecola C. Regulation of cerebral microcirculation during neural activity: is nitric oxide the missing link. *Trends Neurosci* 1993; 16:206–214.

Isaacks RE, Bender AS, Kim CY, Prieto NM, Norenberg MD. Osmotic regulation of myo-inositol uptake in primary astrocyte cultures. *Neurochem Res* 1994; 19(3):331–338.

Kimura FH, Fujii Y, Itoh S, et al. Metabolic alterations in the neonate and infant brain during development: evaluation with proton MR spectroscopy. *Radiology* 1995; 194:483–489.

Kreis R, Ernst T, Ross BD. Development of the human brain: in vivo quantification of metabolite and water content with proton magnetic resonance spectroscopy. *Magn Reson Med* 1993; 30:424–437.

Lenz FA, Tasker RR, Dostrovsky JO, et al. Abnormal single unit activity recorded in the somatosensory thalamus of a quadriplegic patient with central pain. *Pain* 1987; 31:225–236.

Loeser JD, Ward AA. Some effects of deafferentation on neurons of the cat spinal cord. *Arch Neurol* 1967; 17:629–636.

Loeser JD, Ward AA, White LE Jr. Chronic deafferentation of human spinal cord neurons. *J Neurosurg* 1968; 29:48–50.

Morrow TJ, Paulson PE, Brewer KL, Yezierski RP, Casey KL. Chronic, selective forebrain responses to excitotoxic dorsal horn injury. *Exp Neurol* 2000; 161:220–226.

Nepomuceuno C, Fine PR, Richards JS, et al. Pain in patients with spinal cord injury. *Arch Phys Med Rehabil* 1979; 60:605–609.

Ness TJ, San Pedro EC, Richards JS, et al. A case of spinal cord injury-pain with baseline rCBF brain SPECT imaging and beneficial response to gabapentin. *Pain* 1998; 78:139–143.

Pouwels PJ, Brockmann K, Kruse B, et al. Regional age dependence of human brain metabolites from infancy to adulthood as detected by quantitative localized proton MRS. *Pediatr Res* 1999; 46(4):474–485.

Provencher SW. Estimation of metabolites concentrations from localized in vivo proton NMR spectra. *Magn Reson Med* 1993; 30:672–679.

Rintala DH, Loubser PG, Castro J, Hart KA, Fuhrer MJ. Chronic pain in a community-based sample of men with spinal cord injury: prevalence, severity, and relationships with impairment, disability, handicap, and subjective well-being. *Arch Phys Med Rehabil* 1998; 79:604–614.

Roberts MHT, Rees H. Denervation supersensitivity in the central nervous system: possible relation to central pain syndromes. In: Casey KL (Ed). *Pain and Central Nervous System Disease.* New York: Raven Press, 1991, pp 219–321.

Siddall PJ, Loeser JD. Pain following spinal cord injury. *Spinal Cord* 2001; 39:63–73.

Siddall PJ, Taylor DA, McClelland JM, Rutkowski SB, Cousins MJ. Pain report and the relationship of pain to physical factors in the first 6 months following injury. *Pain* 1999; 81:187–197.

Störmer S, Gerner HJ, Gruninger W, et al. Chronic pain/dysaesthesiae in spinal cord injury patients: results of a multicentre study. *Spinal Cord* 1997; 35:446–455.

Turner JA, Cardenas DD. Chronic pain problems in individuals with spinal cord injuries. *Semin Clin Neuropsychiatry* 1999; 4:186–194.

Turner JA, Cardenas DD, Warms CA, McClellan CB. Chronic pain associated with spinal cord injuries: a community survey. *Arch Phys Med Rehabil* 2001; 82(4):501–509.

Vierck CJ, Siddall P, Yezierski RP. Pain following spinal cord injury: animal models and mechanistic studies. *Pain* 2000; 89:1–5.

Widerström-Noga EG, Cuervo E, Broton JG, et al. Perceived difficulty in dealing with consequences of spinal cord injury. *Arch Phys Med Rehabil* 1999; 80(5):580–586.

Widerström-Noga EG, Felipe-Cuervo E, Yezierski RP. Relationships among clinical characteristics of chronic pain following spinal cord injury. *Arch Phys Med Rehabil* 2001; 82:1191–1197.

Yezierski RP. Pain following spinal cord injury: the clinical problem and experimental studies. *Pain* 1996; 68:185–194.

Yezierski RP, Park SH. The mechanosensitivity of spinal sensory neurons following intraspinal injections of quisqualic acid in the rat. *Neurosci Lett* 1993; 157:115–119.

Yezierski RP, Santana M, Park DH, Madsen PW. Neuronal degeneration and spinal cavitation following intraspinal injections of quisqualic acid in the rat. *J Neurotrauma* 1993; 10:445–456.

Correspondence to: Pradip M. Pattany, PhD, Department of Radiology, MRI Center, University of Miami School of Medicine, 1115 NW 14th Street, Miami, FL 33136, USA. Tel: 305-243-3920; Fax: 305-243-4673; email: ppattany@med.miami.edu.

Spinal Cord Injury Pain: Assessment, Mechanisms, Management. Progress in Pain Research and Management, Vol. 23, edited by Robert P. Yezierski and Kim J. Burchiel, IASP Press, Seattle, © 2002.

18

Correlation of MRI Findings with Spinal Cord Injury Pain following Neural Tissue Grafting into Patients with Post-traumatic Syringomyelia

Edward D. Wirth III,[a,c] Charles J. Vierck, Jr.,[a,c] Paul J. Reier,[a,b,c] Richard G. Fessler,[a,b,c] and Douglas K. Anderson[a,b,c,d]

Departments of [a]Neuroscience and [b]Neurological Surgery, University of Florida College of Medicine, Gainesville, Florida; [c]McKnight Brain Institute, University of Florida, Gainesville, Florida; [d]Malcom Randall Veterans Affairs Medical Center, Gainesville, Florida, USA

Numerous studies in a variety of animal models have examined the capacity of fetal spinal cord (FSC) tissue grafts to facilitate structural and functional repair of the injured spinal cord (reviewed in Reier et al. 1994; Anderson et al. 1995). Early investigations in this field demonstrated that these FSC grafts survive, grow, differentiate, and integrate with the host spinal cord after placement into acute or chronic lesions (Reier et al. 1986; Houle and Reier 1988; Privat et al. 1988; Tessler et al. 1988; Anderson et al. 1991; Jakeman and Reier 1991; Reier et al. 1992; Itoh et al. 1996). Subsequent studies have shown that FSC transplants can assist recovery of locomotor function (Bernstein and Goldberg 1987; Stokes and Reier 1992; Bregman et al. 1993; Anderson et al. 1995; Howland et al. 1995, 1996; Ribotta et al. 1998) and modulate lumbar motor neuron excitability (Thompson et al. 1993).

Although more rigorous, quantitative studies in animal models are still needed to fully elucidate the mechanisms of graft-mediated functional recovery, we envisioned that a limited clinical study could guide the direction of basic science toward the more rapid development of an optimal clinical strategy. Accordingly, we initiated a pilot study to evaluate the feasibility and safety of intraspinal transplantation into human patients with spinal cord injuries (SCI). Grafting into SCI subjects with stable deficits would be ill-advised until we know more about the risk of causing further neurological impairment, so we only included subjects with progressive post-traumatic syringomyelia (PPTS). This syndrome is characterized by continual expansion of the lesion cavity and progressive neurological deterioration, and typically requires surgical intervention to stabilize the syrinx. Chronic pain is a prominent symptom and major debilitating component of PPTS, so the study design included detailed pain assessments of each subject at multiple pre- and postoperative time points. Outcome measures for pain included the numerical rating scale (NRS), visual analogue scale (VAS), McGill Pain Questionnaire, and pain drawings. The study design also included serial magnetic resonance imaging (MRI) examinations, which allowed for direct comparison of changes in syrinx morphology after transplantation with changes in pain outcome measures. To date, a total of eight patients with PPTS have received FSC transplants.

This chapter presents an overview of PPTS with a focus on the relationship between pain and anatomical findings as seen with MRI, followed by a discussion of the temporal course of the pain and MRI data after syrinx drainage and implantation of human FSC tissue. An overview of the study design and rationale was presented recently (Reier et al. 2000).

POST-TRAUMATIC SYRINGOMYELIA: PATHOPHYSIOLOGY, CLINICAL FEATURES, DIAGNOSTIC EVALUATION, AND CONVENTIONAL TREATMENT

Post-traumatic syringomyelia is a relatively infrequent, but potentially disastrous complication of SCI. This syndrome can cause intractable pain and loss of upper extremity function in paraplegic patients, and can be life-threatening if allowed to extend upward into the brainstem (Biyani and el Masry 1994; Piatt 1996). The reported incidence of progressive cystic degeneration after spinal cord trauma is 0.3–3.4% (Barnett et al. 1966; Umbach and Heilporn 1991; Biyani and el Masry 1994). However, the prevalence of asymptomatic cysts at the level of previous SCI may be over 50% (Backe et al. 1991; Nidecker et al. 1991). Why these cavities progressively enlarge and cause additional neurological damage in only a few patients is unknown.

This large disparity in the incidence of asymptomatic cysts and PPTS, combined with the typically long delay between injury and onset of new symptoms (Shannon et al. 1981; Vernon et al. 1982; Rossier et al. 1985), supports the theory of Williams and colleagues (1981) that syrinx formation is a two-stage process. The initial cavitation occurs at the time of injury as the result of a liquefying hematoma. Subsequent enlargement of the cavity most likely is due to the "slosh" and "suck" of cerebrospinal fluid (CSF) that is caused by acute rises in thoracic and abdominal pressure, such as a cough, which distend the epidural veins. This venous distension, in turn, compresses the dura and CSF pathways (Williams 1976). In the normal spinal canal, this compressive force dissipates freely up and down the subarachnoid space. However, the meningeal fibrosis that often results from injury may block this space, in which case the pressure wave is concentrated and is transmitted to the interior of the spinal cord (Piatt 1996). Fluids are noncompressible, so the intramedullary cavity expands cephalad along the path of least resistance ("slosh"), followed by a rebound in the caudal direction ("suck"), which accounts for syrinxes that extend both above and below the original injury site.

CLINICAL FEATURES OF PROGRESSIVE POST-TRAUMATIC SYRINGOMYELIA

The most common presenting complaint of PPTS is pain at or above the original injury level, localized to the chest wall or upper extremity, and frequently related to coughing or straining (Rossier et al. 1985; Piatt 1996). In some patients the pain may be worse in the sitting than in the lying position (Rossier et al. 1985). Pain generally presents as paresthesias (e.g., burning, tingling, or numbness) or dysesthesias that are not relieved by opioid analgesics. Paradoxically, pain and temperature sensation over lower dermatomes is usually *decreased* because the segmental pathways that subserve these sensations have been completely destroyed. Other common features are an ascending sensory level and increased motor weakness (Vernon et al. 1982; Rossier et al. 1985; Anton and Schweigel 1986; Biyani and el Masry 1994). Sensory deficits may be unilateral or bilateral (Vernon et al. 1982; Rossier et al. 1985). New onset of symptoms may occur from months to years after the original injury, with a mean latency of 4–9 years (Williams 1990; Piatt 1996).

Although the clinical signs and symptoms of PPTS are well documented, most studies involving therapeutic interventions have relied on subjective descriptions of changes in these characteristics as the primary outcome measures. The extreme variation in clinical presentation, severity, and response to treatment has thwarted attempts to quantitatively analyze and compare patient demographics and clinical outcome (Williams 1990; Oakes 1996). Despite these challenges, it is imperative that standardized pain assessments and scores of neurological function be used, whenever possible, to facilitate direct comparison of outcomes across studies and among different treatment paradigms.

DIAGNOSTIC EVALUATION

MRI is the modality of choice for detecting intraspinal cysts and for monitoring their response to surgical intervention (Kochan and Quencer 1991; Biyani and el Masry 1994). MR images accurately and easily show the location, size, and overall morphology of a post-traumatic syrinx (Kokmen et al. 1985; Lee et al. 1985; Barkovich et al. 1987; Samuelsson et al. 1987; Backe et al. 1991; Silberstein and Hennessy 1992; Oakes 1996). Additional advantages of MRI are its inherent capacity for multiplanar imaging and its noninvasive nature, which enables examinations to be performed on an outpatient basis. MRI also is valuable in selecting the site of myelotomy and shunt placement, and in assessing the outcome of treatment of PPTS (Biyani and el Masry 1994). Its drawbacks include artifacts from nonferromagnetic implants and difficulty distinguishing cysts from myelomalacia.

Sagittal T1-weighted images are accurate in measuring the cranial-caudal size of the cyst and are best for visualizing fibroglial septations (Kochan and Quencer 1991). Axial MRI helps to determine the laterality and eccentricity of a cyst and shows good correlation with clinical and pathological features (Milhorat et al. 1995). Cysts contain CSF and are seen on T1-weighted images as well-circumscribed areas of low signal intensity within the intermediate signal of the spinal cord. In contrast, T2-weighted imaging and gradient echo imaging yield very high signal intensity from CSF and are sensitive to turbulent flow within the cyst (Barkovich et al. 1987).

The correlation between morphological findings on MR images and neurological impairment in syringomyelia is unclear. Most studies have reported little or no direct association between cyst dimensions and clinical symptoms (Grant et al. 1987; Backe et al. 1991; Nidecker et al. 1991; Masur et al. 1992), although with eccentric cavities signs such as pain and sensory loss may be specifically related to the level and side of cavitation (Milhorat et al. 1995).

STANDARD SURGICAL TREATMENT

The first attempt at surgical treatment of syringomyelia was made over 100 years ago by Abbé and Coley (1892). Since that inaugural effort, most surgical therapies for syringomyelia have focused on removing the fluid from the syrinx, either via a permanent opening in the spinal cord wall (i.e., syringostomy) or through a tube (sometimes called a shunt or wick) whose distal end is affixed in a low-pressure space (i.e., subarachnoid, pleural, or peritoneal) (Shannon et al. 1981; Tator et al. 1982; Vernon et al. 1983; Barbaro et al. 1984; Van Calenbergh and Van den Bergh 1993; Biyani and el Masry 1994; Sgouros and Williams 1995; Wiart et al. 1995). Alternative approaches have aimed to disable the filling mechanism by transection or artificial meningocele rather than to drain the cavity (Williams 1990). Fetal neural grafts grow to fill a cavity and fuse with the host spinal cord, so this method should also disable the filling mechanism. Furthermore, evidence from animal studies suggests that suspensions of FSC actively infiltrate degenerating areas in the adjacent host cord.

All of the aforementioned conventional techniques have yielded good short-term results, with a decrease of clinical symptoms in 75–100% of patients during the first year (Phillips and Kindt 1981; Shannon et al. 1981; Peerless and Durward 1983; Vernon et al. 1983; Barbaro et al. 1984; Suzuki et al. 1985; Silberstein and Hennessy 1992; Hida et al. 1994). However, in those few reports with follow-up periods greater than 1 year, only about 50% of patients have sustained this improvement (Barbaro et al. 1984; Rossier et al. 1985; Anton and Schweigel 1986; La Haye and Batzdorf 1988; Aschoff and Kunze 1993; Sgouros and Williams 1995). Furthermore, conventional surgical treatment seldom leads to functional recovery (Anton and Schweigel 1986; Williams 1990). The poor long-term success with shunting is largely due to occlusion of the drain tubes, which often requires one or more subsequent operations (Suzuki et al. 1985; Sgouros and Williams 1995). Shunt tubes placed into the spinal canal may also cause bleeding, mechanical damage, and adhesions that can further traumatize the spinal cord (Steinmetz et al. 1993; Van Calenbergh and Van den Bergh 1993; Sgouros and Williams 1995; Wiart et al. 1995).

The effects of conventional PPTS surgery on SCI pain are also variable. For example, one seemingly paradoxical finding was that patients who had higher preoperative syrinx pressures had greater neurological improvement after shunting, but also had a higher incidence of postoperative dysesthetic pain (Milhorat et al. 1997). Another report on a single individual suggested that placement of an FSC graft in conjunction with a shunt may improve pain status (Falci et al. 1997).

CHANGES IN SCI PAIN AND SYRINX MORPHOLOGY AFTER NEURAL TISSUE GRAFTING INTO PATIENTS WITH PROGRESSIVE POST-TRAUMATIC SYRINGOMYELIA

STUDY DESIGN

Patients were considered for participation in the study if they presented with both clinical and radiological evidence of progressive syringomyelia, with the syrinx located primarily in the thoracic spinal cord (extension up to the C6 vertebral level was acceptable), and were free of serious medical complications that would increase the risk of surgery and/or immunosuppression.

Subjects were required to be at least 18 years old and to fulfill criteria for Grades A–C on the American Spinal Injury Association (ASIA) impairment scale or for Grade D with significant loss of function. Excluded were patients with MRI-incompatible implants, a history of intraspinal neoplasm or congenital spinal defect, or serious medical disease (e.g., AIDS, hepatitis) that would be complicated by immunosuppression. At the initial visit, patients were evaluated by the neurosurgeon (R.G. Fessler), who also discussed the study and obtained informed consent. Each patient then began the initial comprehensive assessment protocol: ASIA neurological exam, functional independence measure for disability, comprehensive pain assessment, psychosocial assessment, MRI scan, electrical studies of spinal conduction and reflexes, and quantitative testing for spasticity.

Patients returned 1 month after the initial visit for a second round of testing, so that an average baseline score could be computed for each outcome measure. Approximately 1 month after the second round of preoperative tests, patients were admitted for syrinx drainage and implantation of FSC tissue. Follow-up clinical, neurophysiological, and MRI evaluations were performed before discharge and at 1.5, 3, 6, 9, 12, and 18 months after discharge.

PATIENT HISTORIES

Six men and two women, ranging between 45 and 66 years of age, have been entered into this trial. The first seven subjects had sustained a spinal injury at thoracic levels 12–31 years prior to their first pretransplant clinical visit, whereas the eighth subject had sustained a low-cervical injury. The first diagnosed onset of PPTS in each subject ranged from 2 to 17 years after the initial SCI, which is consistent with published accounts of this syndrome.

Each subject was evaluated at least twice prior to surgery and at multiple postoperative intervals for up to 24 months. All subjects had dysesthesias associated with their syrinx preoperatively. The most common symptoms were burning (five of eight subjects), tingling or numbness (three of eight), spasms (three of eight), and stabbing (two of eight). These dysesthesias were found in dermatomes overlying the syrinx in all subjects, and extended distally in seven of eight subjects. In two cases, pain drawings included areas above the uppermost syrinx level.

TISSUE PROCUREMENT AND SURGICAL PROCEDURES

Human fetal spinal cord (FSC) tissue was procured after elective abortions in accordance with federal and state laws and ethical guidelines. Informed consent for donation of the fetal tissue was obtained only after informed consent was given for the abortion. Only donor tissue of 6–9 weeks' gestational age was used in this study. Each FSC was stored for 2–3 days at 8°C in sterile hibernation medium to allow screening for infectious organisms. Immediately prior to transplantation, the donor spinal cords were cut into smaller pieces, with consideration given to the intended graft site in each recipient. The donor tissue was minced into fragments of approximately 0.75 mm^3 for multilocular cysts, whereas larger pieces approximately 10 mm in length × 1 mm in diameter were used for larger cavities.

The anesthetic regimen and opening and closing procedures were performed in the usual fashion for conventional surgical treatment of syringomyelia.

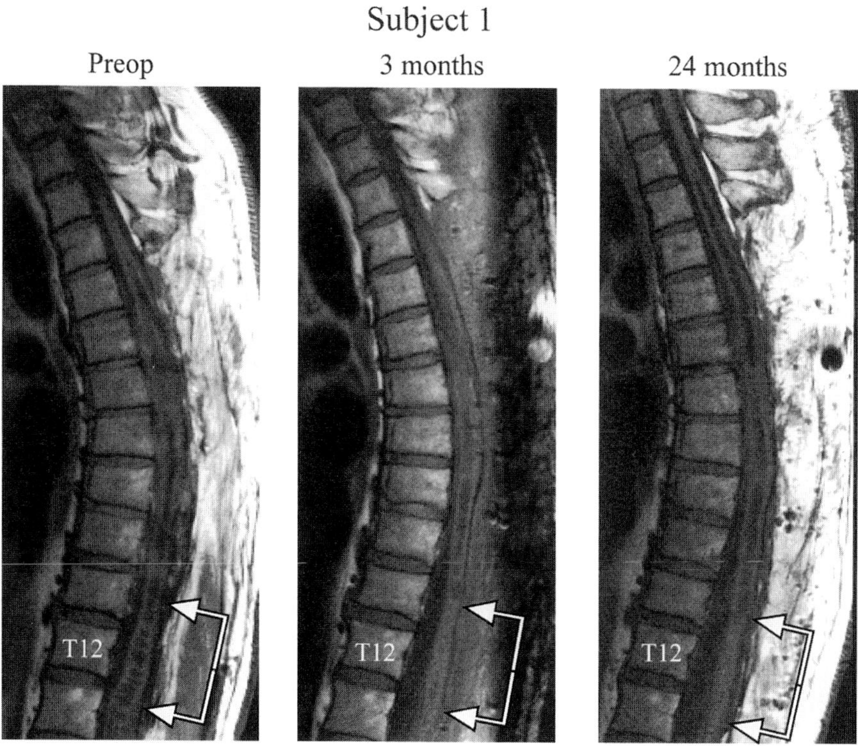

Fig. 1. T1-weighted sagittal MR images of Subject 1 acquired preoperatively and at 3 and 24 months after surgery. The syrinx is clearly visible as an elongated region of low signal extending from T4 to L1, and is multilocular over the T11–L1 levels. Most of the donor tissue was injected at three sites in the T11–L1 levels (double arrow), although a small amount of fetal spinal cord (FSC) tissue was also implanted at T7. Serial postoperative MR images show that adjacent syrinx regions that did not receive donor tissue refilled with CSF by 3 months and did not change subsequently. In contrast, syrinx closure was observed in areas where donor tissue was placed, although it is difficult to distinguish graft from host tissue.

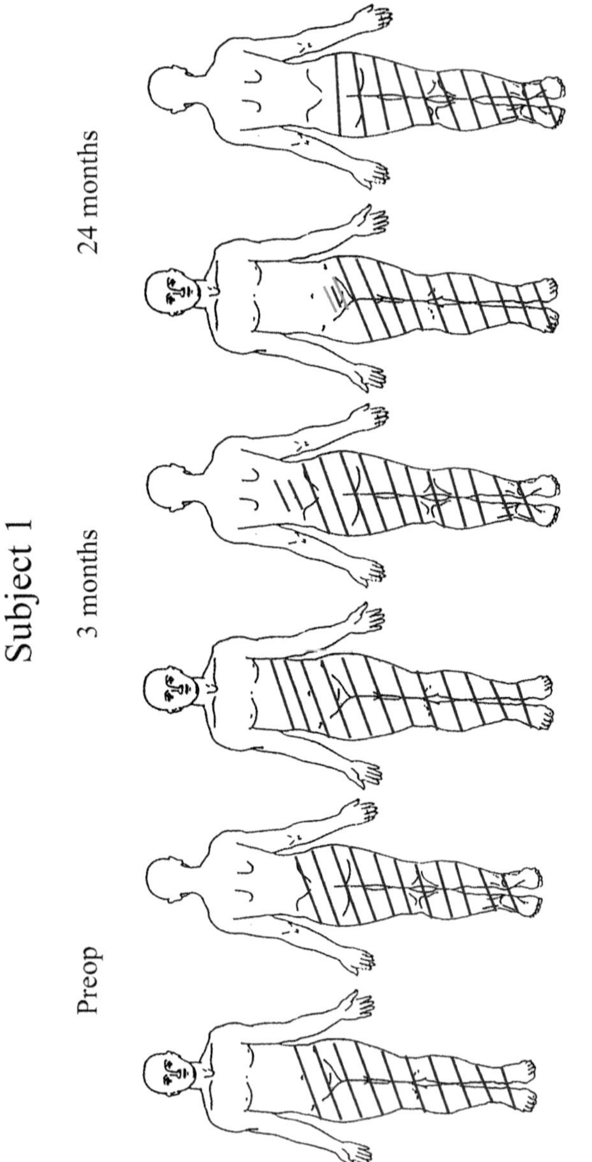

Fig. 2. Pain drawings by Subject 1 from preoperatively through 24 months postoperatively. The drawings show a stable pain distribution, except for the delayed onset of bladder spasms, as indicated on the 24-month drawing.

Fig. 3. Pain drawings by Subject 2 through 24 months postoperatively. A profound change in the pain's distribution and character are evident. This patient reported that the burning on his upper back and right arm was relieved almost immediately following surgery. However, he reported delayed onset of several new areas of pain in his mid- and lower torso. ⟶

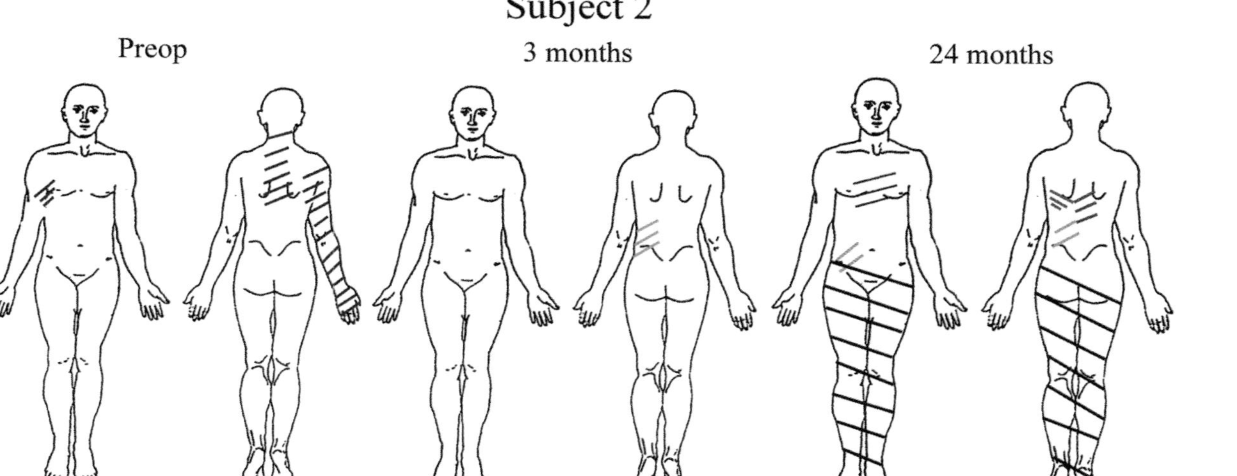

Pain 1: Burning sensation between shoulder blades and right arm

Pain 2: Left flank (kidney area) stabbing pain

Pain 3: T5-T8 area “bones grinding” in vertebrae

Pain 4: Spasms from bladder area to toes

Pain 5: T5-T8 Continuous stabbing pain

Pain 6: Burning in front of chest

Briefly, the patients were sedated and maintained under general anesthesia with endotracheal intubation and were placed in the prone position. Electrodes were placed for monitoring of somatosensory evoked potentials (SSEPs), and the spinal column was then exposed through a standard midline incision followed by a combination of blunt and sharp dissection. Careful sharp and blunt dissection was then continued until the dura was exposed and freed from tightly adherent overlying scar tissue. At this point, the dura was opened and the underlying adhesions were carefully dissected to free the spinal cord. Once dissection of the intradural adhesions was complete, the location and extent of the syrinx were confirmed by intraoperative ultrasound. Next, the fluid within the cysts was either aspirated through an 18-gauge needle attached to a 5-mL syringe, or allowed to efflux freely via a small myelotomy in the dorsal midline. After the syrinx was decompressed, the donor spinal cord tissue was then slowly injected using an 18-gauge cannula attached to a 500-μL syringe. After the donor tissue was implanted and the meninges sutured, graft placement was verified by intraoperative ultrasound. The deep muscle layers, subcutis, and skin were then closed in the usual sterile fashion.

All subjects tolerated the procedure well and received the usual acute postoperative care for syringomyelia surgery. They were then discharged for the usual acute postoperative rehabilitation, resumed their preoperative analgesic regimen, and returned home. All subjects were also immunosuppressed with cyclosporine (3 mg/kg b.i.d.), which was initiated 3–4 days prior to surgery and continued for 6 months postoperatively. Detailed case reports of the postoperative course for the first two subjects in this study were presented recently (Thompson et al. 2001; Wirth et al. 2001).

MAGNETIC RESONANCE IMAGING

MRI examinations were performed at the initial preoperative visit 8 weeks before surgery, and at 1.5, 3, 6, 9, 12, and 18 months postoperatively. The MRI protocol was designed to visualize the entire syrinx and to obtain restricted views with higher magnification of the transplant site. Each MRI examination began with sagittal and axial T1- and T2-weighted spin-echo images obtained before and after administration of gadolinium (Gd-DTPA). In addition, sagittal fluid attenuation by inversion recovery (FLAIR)-weighted images were obtained at some time points. All images were acquired with a slice thickness of 3–4 mm and a 256 × 256 matrix size. In-plane resolution varied depending upon the field of view required to visualize the entire syrinx. Total scan time per subject at each session was approximately 1.5 hours.

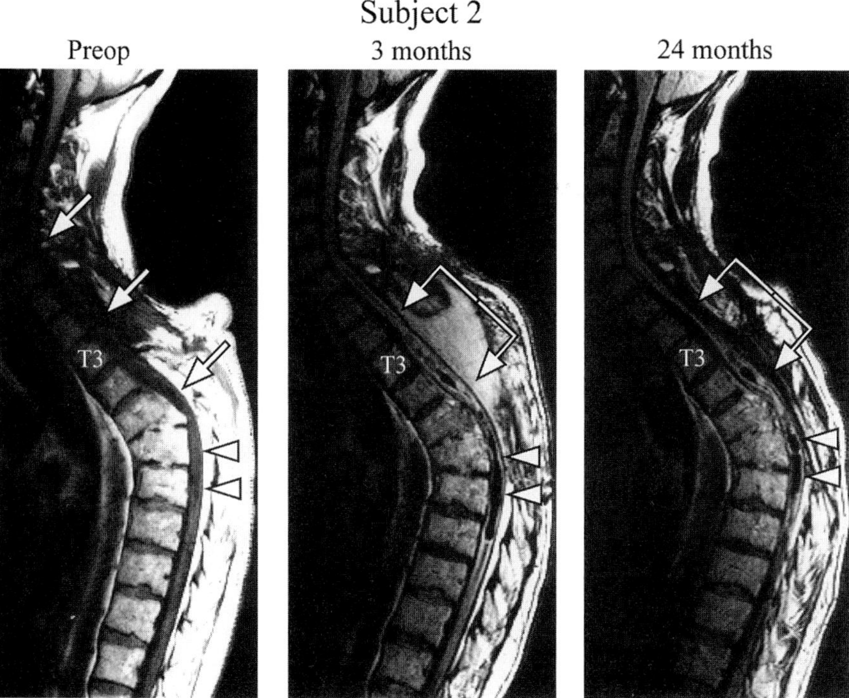

Fig. 4. T1- and FLAIR-weighted sagittal MR images of Subject 2 acquired preoperatively and at 3 and 24 months after surgery. FLAIR images (postoperative) provided sharper contrast between CSF in the syrinx and neural tissue than T1-weighted images (preoperative), which aided visualization of the graft site. On the preoperative MR image, an upper syrinx is visible from C6 to T5 (arrows), and a lower cyst is present from T6 to T8 (arrowheads). We confirmed intraoperatively that these two cysts were not in communication with each other. Most of the donor tissue was implanted at T2–T5 (double arrow), although a small amount of FSC tissue was injected at T7. Serial postoperative MR images show progressive closure of the syrinx at the T3 vertebral level, although it is difficult to clearly distinguish graft from host tissue. In contrast, the lower cyst exhibited progressive expansion after surgery.

POSTOPERATIVE PAIN AND MRI FINDINGS

After surgery, sustained collapse of the syrinx at the transplant site was noted on MR images in seven of eight subjects (Fig. 1). In order to determine whether the apparent cyst collapse on the sagittal MR images resulted from variations in slice position and/or partial volume averaging, consecutive transverse slices through the graft sites were also acquired at each evaluation interval. These axial images confirmed that the cysts were substantially obliterated at the graft sites, but relatively unaltered in nongrafted regions. Despite the clear evidence of cyst collapse at the graft sites, no

Subject 5

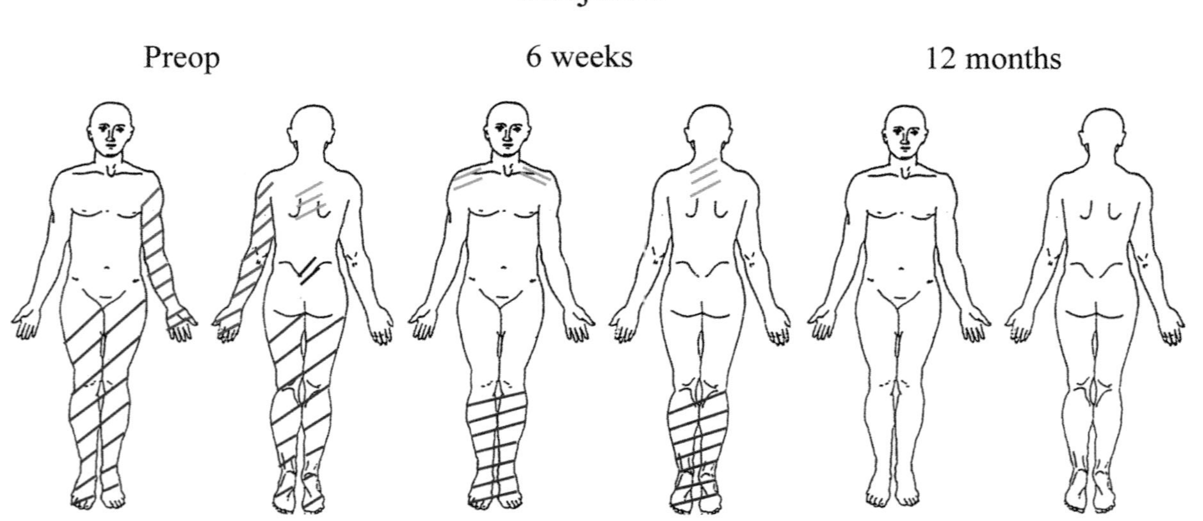

Pain 1: Bilateral legs—deep viselike gripping, sharp, stabbing that radiates to feet

Pain 2: Surgical site area—T1-T8 consistent knife stabbing

Pain 3: Arms—deep ache, hands—stabbing pain through fingers

Pain 4: L2-L3—Sharp to deep nagging ache (graft site)

specific boundaries between donor and host tissue were observed on T1- or T2-weighted images. Thus, it was not possible to determine whether any of the transplanted tissue had survived.

The pain intensity reports (NRS, VAS) from each subject often varied substantially from one postoperative interval to the next, whereas the distribution of dysesthesias on the pain drawings tended to be more stable (Fig. 2). Significant pain relief (i.e., complete disappearance of a dysesthesia) was only observed in two of the eight subjects. In Subject 2, the burning sensation in the dermatomes associated with the upper cyst (C6–T3) disappeared immediately after surgery and had not returned by the 24-month evaluation point (Fig. 3). MRI scans showed that this cyst was completely collapsed from C6 to T3 (Fig. 4). This cyst had received an FSC tissue graft without placement of a shunt.

Also notable in Subject 2 was the onset of stabbing pain in the T6–T9 dermatomes 3 months after surgery. This appeared to coincide with visible expansion of his lower cyst at T6–T9. The intensity of this pain and the size of this cyst both gradually increased through 18 months postoperatively. Approximately 27 months after the initial surgery, a second operation was performed to transplant FSC tissue into this lower cyst. Follow-up assessments through 1 year suggest a slight decrease in the stabbing pain, although pain intensity varied substantially. Transverse MRI scans of the corresponding spinal levels showed a decrease in the cyst diameter from ~10 mm to ~5 mm.

Subject 5 reported that the stabbing pain present throughout both of her legs before surgery was limited to below the knees at 6 weeks (Fig. 5). This pain had disappeared completely by 9 months, but returned to baseline levels at 18 months. MRI scans showed that her small (1 cm length) cyst was completely obliterated for the first 9 months postoperatively (Fig. 6). However, a slight (~5 mm diameter) reopening was noted at 12 months and persisted through 24 months.

Of the six subjects who experienced no significant change in their pain, five had substantial collapse of the cyst at the graft site but also had either (1) a persistent cyst above the graft site or (2) one or more shunt tubes at or above the graft site. In the remaining subject, no collapse of the cyst was noted on MRI scans.

← **Fig. 5.** Pain drawings by Subject 5 through 12 months postoperatively. A progressive and substantial decrease in pain was observed following surgery, with the subject reporting a complete absence of pain by 12 months.

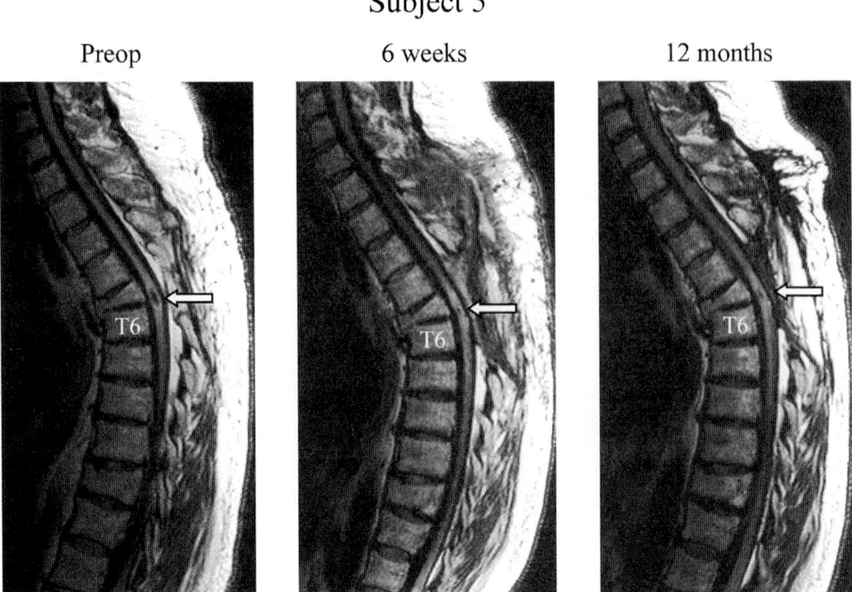

Fig. 6. T1-weighted sagittal MR images of Subject 5 acquired preoperatively, and at 6 weeks and 12 months after surgery. A small cyst, approximately 1 cm in length, was noted at the T5–T6 disk level (arrow). At 6 weeks postsurgery the cyst was completely filled, whereas a slight reaccumulation of CSF was seen at 12 months.

CONCLUSIONS

Although it is still too soon to draw any firm conclusions, these findings suggest that syringomyelia pain may be reduced substantially in some patients after syrinx drainage and FSC grafting. Despite clear MRI evidence of at least partial cyst obliteration in seven subjects, significant pain relief (i.e., complete disappearance of one or more pain symptoms) was noted only when *both* of the following conditions were met: (1) collapse of the most rostral portion of the cyst was achieved, and (2) no previous or new shunt tube was present in the cyst. Taken together, these findings further suggest that syringomyelia pain may result from or be exacerbated by irritation of the cord levels immediately rostral to the cyst. This irritation could alter segmental processing of afferent input in these rostral levels and may be due to either a mass effect secondary to increased cyst pressure and/or an inflammatory response resulting from tissue damage or the presence of a foreign body (i.e., the shunt tube). In support of this notion, sudden onset of pain immediately above the original injury level is the most common presenting complaint from patients who are subsequently diagnosed with syringomyelia, and often occurs in conjunction with a sudden increase in thoracic pressure (e.g., during a sneeze). Lastly, any beneficial effect on pain by cyst obliteration appears to be reversible insofar as a reopening of a collapsed cyst seems to cause return of the pain, as was observed in one subject in this study.

None of the patients in this study reported increased pain after surgery except for a delayed increase in one subject that appeared to be directly related to delayed expansion of a second cyst distant from the transplant site. Thus, it is encouraging that transplantation of FSC tissue in conjunction with syrinx drainage does not appear to exacerbate central dysesthetic pain.

ACKNOWLEDGMENTS

The authors are grateful to Michelle Forthofer, RN, for coordinating the study and to Thomas Freeman, MD, and Ray Moseley, PhD, who were instrumental in the study design. We would also like to thank Ellsworth J. Remson, MD, for his assistance with the ASIA exams, Don Price, PhD, and Michael Robinson, PhD, for their help in designing the pain assessment protocol, and Deborah Dalziel, Bryan Hains, and Venkatesh Nonabur, MD, for technical support. This work was supported by NIH clinical research center grant RR00082, University of Florida McKnight Brain Institute and College of Medicine, the Mark F. Overstreet and C.M. and K.E. Overstreet chairs in spinal cord regeneration, and the Foundation for Physical Therapy.

REFERENCES

Abbé R, Coley WB. Syringo-myelia, operation—exploration of cord—withdrawal of fluid—exhibition of patient. *J Nerv Ment Dis* 1892; 17:512–520.

Anderson DK, Howland DR, Reier PJ. Fetal neural grafts and repair of the injured spinal cord. *Brain Pathol* 1995; 5:451–457.

Anderson DK, Reier PJ, Wirth III ED, et al. Delayed grafting of fetal CNS tissue into chronic compression lesions of the adult cat spinal cord. *Restor Neurol Neurosci* 1991; 2:309–325.

Anton HA, Schweigel JF. Posttraumatic syringomyelia: the British Columbia experience. *Spine* 1986; 11:865–868.

Aschoff A, Kunze S. 100 years syrinx-surgery—a review. *Acta Neurochir Wien* 1993; 123:157–159.

Backe HA, Betz RR, Mesgarzadeh M, Beck T, Clancy M. Post-traumatic spinal cord cysts evaluated by magnetic resonance imaging. *Paraplegia* 1991; 29:607–612.

Barbaro NM, Wilson CB, Gutin PH, Edwards MS. Surgical treatment of syringomyelia: favorable results with syringoperitoneal shunting. *J Neurosurg* 1984; 61:531–538.

Barkovich AJ, Sherman JL, Citrin CM, Wippold FJ. MR of postoperative syringomyelia. *AJNR Am J Neuroradiol* 1987; 8:319–327.

Barnett HJ, Botterell EH, Jousse AT, Wynn Jones M. Progressive myelopathy as a sequel to traumatic paraplegia. *Brain* 1966; 89:159–174.

Bernstein JJ, Goldberg WJ. Fetal spinal cord homografts ameliorate the severity of lesion-induced hind limb behavioral deficits. *Exp Neurol* 1987; 98:633–644.
Biyani A, el Masry WS. Post-traumatic syringomyelia: a review of the literature. *Paraplegia* 1994; 32:723–731.
Bregman BS, Kunkel-Bagden E, Reier PJ, et al. Recovery of function after spinal cord injury: mechanisms underlying transplant-mediated recovery of function differ after spinal cord injury in newborn and adult rats. *Exp Neurol* 1993; 123:3–16.
Falci S, Holtz A, Akesson E, et al. Obliteration of a posttraumatic spinal cord cyst with solid human embryonic spinal cord grafts: first clinical attempt. *J Neurotrauma* 1997; 14:875–884.
Grant R, Hadley DM, MacPherson P, et al. Syringomyelia: cyst measurement by magnetic resonance imaging and comparison with symptoms, signs and disability. *J Neurol Neurosurg Psychiatry* 1987; 50:1008–1014.
Hida K, Iwasaki Y, Imamura H, Abe H. Posttraumatic syringomyelia: its characteristic magnetic resonance imaging findings and surgical management. *Neurosurgery* 1994; 35:886–891.
Houle JD, Reier PJ. Transplantation of fetal spinal cord tissue into the chronically injured adult rat spinal cord. *J Comp Neurol* 1988; 269:535–547.
Howland DR, Bregman BS, Tessler A, Goldberger ME. Transplants enhance locomotion in neonatal kittens whose spinal cords are transected: a behavioral and anatomical study. *Exp Neurol* 1995; 135:123–145.
Howland DR, Reier PJ, Anderson DK. Intraspinal transplantation of fetal tissue: therapeutic potential for spinal cord repair. In: Narayan RK, Wilberger JE, Povlishock JT (Eds). *Neurotrauma*. New York: McGraw-Hill, 1996, pp 1507–1520.
Itoh Y, Waldeck RF, Tessler A, Pinter MJ. Regenerated dorsal root fibers form functional synapses in embryonic spinal cord transplants. *J Neurophysiol* 1996; 76:1236–1245.
Jakeman LB, Reier PJ. Axonal projections between fetal spinal cord transplants and the adult rat spinal cord: a neuroanatomical tracing study of local interactions. *J Comp Neurol* 1991; 307:311–334.
Kochan JP, Quencer RM. Imaging of cystic and cavitary lesions of the spinal cord and canal—the value of MR and intraoperative sonography. *Radiol Clin North Am* 1991; 29:867–911.
Kokmen E, Marsh WR, Baker Jr HL. Magnetic resonance imaging in syringomyelia. *Neurosurgery* 1985; 17:267–270.
La Haye PA, Batzdorf U. Posttraumatic syringomyelia. *West J Med* 1988; 148:657–663.
Lee BC, Zimmerman RD, Manning JJ, Deck MD. MR imaging of syringomyelia and hydromyelia. *AJR Am J Roentgenol* 1985; 144:1149–1156.
Masur H, Oberwittler C, Fahrendorf G, et al. The relation between functional deficits, motor and sensory conduction times and MRI findings in syringomyelia. *Electroencephalogr Clin Neurophysiol* 1992; 85:321–330.
Milhorat TH, Johnson RW, Milhorat RH, Capocelli Jr AL, Pevsner PH. Clinicopathological correlations in syringomyelia using axial magnetic resonance imaging. *Neurosurgery* 1995; 37:206–213.
Milhorat TH, Capocelli ALJ, Kotzen RM, et al. Intramedullary pressure in syringomyelia: clinical and pathophysiological correlates of syrinx distension. *Neurosurgery* 1997; 41:1102–1110.
Nidecker A, Kocher M, Maeder M, et al. MR-imaging of chronic spinal cord injury: association with neurologic function. *Neurosurg Rev* 1991; 14:169–179.
Oakes WJ. Chiari malformations, hydromyelia, syringomyelia. In: Wilkins RH, Rengachary SS (Eds). *Neurosurgery*. New York: McGraw-Hill, 1996, pp 3593–3616.
Peerless SJ, Durward QJ. Management of syringomyelia: a pathophysiological approach. *Clin Neurosurg* 1983; 30:531–576.
Phillips TW, Kindt GW. Syringoperitoneal shunt for syringomyelia: a preliminary report. *Surg Neurol* 1981; 16:462–466.
Piatt JH Jr. Post-traumatic syringomyelia. In: Wilkins RH, Rengachary SS (Eds). *Neurosurgery*. New York: McGraw-Hill, 1996, pp 3063–3066.

Privat A, Mansour H, Geffard M. Transplantation of fetal serotonin neurons into the transected spinal cord of adult rats: morphological development and functional influence. *Prog Brain Res* 1988; 78:155–166.

Reier PJ, Bregman BS, Wujek JR. Intraspinal transplantation of embryonic spinal cord tissue in neonatal and adult rats. *J Comp Neurol* 1986; 247:275–296.

Reier PJ, Stokes BT, Thompson FJ, Anderson DK. Fetal cell grafts into resection and contusion/compression injuries of the rat and cat spinal cord. *Exp Neurol* 1992; 115:177–188.

Reier PJ, Anderson DK, Schrimsher GW, et al. Neural cell grafting: anatomical and functional repair of the spinal cord. In: Salzman SK, Faden AI (Eds). *The Neurobiology of Central Nervous System Trauma*. New York: Oxford University Press, 1994, pp 288–311.

Reier PJ, Thompson FJ, Fessler RG, Anderson DK, Wirth III ED. Spinal cord injury and fetal CNS tissue transplantation: an initial "bench-to-bedside" translational research experience. In: Ingoglia NA, Murray M (Eds). *Axonal Regeneration in the Central Nervous System*. New York: Marcel Dekker, 2000, pp 603–647.

Ribotta M, Orsal D, Feraboli-Lohnherr D, et al. Kinematic analysis of recovered locomotor movements of the hindlimbs in paraplegic rats transplanted with monoaminergic embryonic neurons. *Ann NY Acad Sci* 1998; 860:521–523.

Rossier AB, Foo D, Shillito J, Dyro FM. Posttraumatic cervical syringomyelia: incidence, clinical presentation, electrophysiological studies, syrinx protein and results of conservative and operative treatment. *Brain* 1985; 108:439–461.

Samuelsson L, Bergstrom K, Thuomas KA, Hemmingsson A, Wallensten R. MR imaging of syringohydromyelia and Chiari malformations in myelomeningocele patients with scoliosis. *AJNR Am J Neuroradiol* 1987; 8:539–546.

Sgouros S, Williams B. A critical appraisal of drainage in syringomyelia. *J Neurosurg* 1995; 82:1–10.

Shannon N, Symon L, Logue V, et al. Clinical features, investigation and treatment of post-traumatic syringomyelia. *J Neurol Neurosurg Psychiatry* 1981; 44:35–42.

Silberstein M, Hennessy O. Cystic cord lesions and neurological deterioration in spinal cord injury: operative considerations based on magnetic resonance imaging. *Paraplegia* 1992; 30:661–668.

Steinmetz A, Aschoff A, Kunze S. The iatrogenic tethering of the cord. *Acta Neurochir Wien* 1993; 123:219–220.

Stokes BT, Reier PJ. Fetal grafts alter chronic behavioral outcome after contusion damage to the adult rat spinal cord. *Exp Neurol* 1992; 116:1–12.

Suzuki M, Davis C, Symon L, Gentili F. Syringoperitoneal shunt for treatment of cord cavitation. *J Neurol Neurosurg Psychiatry* 1985; 48:620–627.

Tator CH, Meguro K, Rowed DW. Favorable results with syringosubarachnoid shunts for treatment of syringomyelia. *J Neurosurg* 1982; 56:517–523.

Tessler A, Himes BT, Houle J, Reier PJ. Regeneration of adult dorsal root axons into transplants of embryonic spinal cord. *J Comp Neurol* 1988; 270:537–548.

Thompson FJ, Reier PJ, Parmer R, Lucas CC. Inhibitory control of reflex excitability following contusion injury and neural tissue transplantation. *Adv Neurol* 1993; 59:175–184.

Thompson FJ, Parmer R, Ritter J, Reier PJ. Transplant-mediated improvement of lumbar reflex excitability and long tract conduction following chronic thoracic contusion spinal cord injury in the rat. *J Neurotrauma* 1996; 13:629.

Thompson FJ, Reier PJ, Uthman B, et al. Neurophysiological assessment of the feasibility and safety of neural tissue transplantation in patients with syringomyelia. *J Neurotrauma* 2001; 18:931–945.

Umbach I, Heilporn A. Review article: post-spinal cord injury syringomyelia. *Paraplegia* 1991; 29:219–221.

Van Calenbergh F, Van den Bergh R. Syringo-peritoneal shunting: results and problems in a consecutive series. *Acta Neurochir Wien* 1993; 123:203–205.

Vernon JD, Silver JR, Ohry A. Post-traumatic syringomyelia. *Paraplegia* 1982; 20:339–364.

Vernon JD, Silver JR, Symon L. Post-traumatic syringomyelia: the results of surgery. *Paraplegia* 1983; 21:37–46.

Wiart L, Dautheribes M, Pointillart V, et al. Mean term follow-up of a series of post-traumatic syringomyelia patients after syringo-peritoneal shunting. *Paraplegia* 1995; 33:241–245.

Williams B. Cerebrospinal fluid pressure changes in response to coughing. *Brain* 1976; 99:331–346.

Williams B. Post-traumatic syringomyelia, an update. *Paraplegia* 1990; 28:296–313.

Williams B, Terry AF, Jones F, McSweeney T. Syringomyelia as a sequel to traumatic paraplegia. *Paraplegia* 1981; 19:67–80.

Wirth ED, III, Reier PJ, Fessler RG, et al. Feasibility and safety of neural tissue transplantation in patients with syringomyelia. *J Neurotrauma* 2001; 18:911–929.

Correspondence to: Edward D. Wirth III, MD, PhD, Ruth-Presbyterian-St. Luke's Medical Center, Dept. of Neurosurgery, Room 1491 Jelke, 1635 West Congress Parkway, Chicago, IL 60612, USA. Tel: 312-942-4948; Fax: 312-563-3358; email: ed_wirth@rush.edu.

Part IV

Treatment

Spinal Cord Injury Pain: Assessment, Mechanisms, Management. Progress in Pain Research and Management, Vol. 23, edited by Robert P. Yezierski and Kim J. Burchiel, IASP Press, Seattle, © 2002.

19

Clinical Trials for Spinal Cord Injury Pain

Jennifer A. Haythornthwaite[a] and Stephen Wegener[b]

Departments of [a]Psychiatry and Behavioral Science and [b]Physical Medicine and Rehabilitation, Johns Hopkins University, Baltimore, Maryland, USA

Clinical trials are increasingly providing useful information for the treatment of chronic painful conditions. For some conditions, primarily neuropathic pain syndromes such as postherpetic neuralgia and diabetic neuralgia, extensive clinical trial data provide a basis for meta-analytic summaries of the treatment literature (Sindrup and Jensen 1999). However, for other conditions, including pain following spinal cord injury (SCI), limited clinical trial data provide only suggestions as to what therapeutic interventions might be initiated for a specific patient (see Chapter 20).

CLINICAL TRIAL METHODS

Randomized clinical trials have become the standard methodology for evaluating pharmacological and psychological interventions for managing chronic painful conditions. In addition to randomized assignment to treatment group, controlled trials include a placebo group or attentional control group in the case of pharmacological and psychological interventions, respectively. Standardized measures assess outcome, typically including serial pain ratings and ratings of pain relief, patient or physician ratings of global improvement, and patient ratings of function or quality of life. Appropriate study designs control bias and include sufficient sample size and statistical power so that meaningful conclusions can be drawn (Institute of Medicine 2001).

How can existing clinical trial data be used to make decisions about designing new trials with patients with SCI pain or about treating an individual patient? Two indices have been developed to help investigators and clinicians evaluate the impact of a treatment on pain and function—effect size (ES; Cohen 1988) and number needed to treat (NNT; Cook and Sackett 1995). Each provides an index of the effect of active treatment relative to a control and allows comparison of the results of one trial to those of another. The ES is typically calculated as a ratio of the difference between active treatment and control treatment relative to an index of variability, such as the standard deviation (SD; see Table I). If the SDs for the two groups are equivalent, then the SD for either group can be used. If there is a significant difference between the active and control groups in the SD of the outcome measure, an "average" of the two is calculated using the root mean square of the two values (Cohen 1988):

$$SD_{NEW} = \sqrt{}(SD_{ACTIVE}^2 + SD_{CONTROL}^2)/2$$

In formal analyses, such as meta-analyses, the ES is adjusted for sample size because small samples can lead to overestimates of the population ES. As an index with no measurement units, the ES allows comparison of study results across different outcome measures and even across different types of intervention. For example, the ES has been used to examine the relative efficacy of pharmacological, psychological, and physical medicine interventions for fibromyalgia (Rossy et al. 1999).

In addition to effect size, another index that is being used with increasing frequency in the pain literature to index and compare the impact of interventions is the number needed to treat (NNT; Cook and Sackett 1995). A clinical outcome—either harm or benefit—is defined, and the rate of that

Table I
Formula for estimating effect size and number needed to treat

Parameter	Formula	Sample Calculation
Effect Size		
Change due to new treatment	$D_{ACTIVE} = X_{PRE} - X_{POST}$	7.5 – 5.9 = 1.6
Change due to control treatment	$D_{CONTROL} = X_{PRE} - X_{POST}$	7.5 – 7.1 = 0.4
Effect size	$D_{ACTIVE} - D_{CONTROL}$/(pooled SDs)	(1.6 – 0.4)/2.4 = 0.50
Number Needed to Treat		
Proportion improved due to new treatment	$P_{ACTIVE} = N_{IMPROVED}/N_{TOTAL}$	40/60 = 0.67
Proportion improved due to control treatment	$P_{CONTROL} = N_{IMPROVED}/N_{TOTAL}$	10/60 = 0.17
NNT	$1/(P_{ACTIVE} - P_{CONTROL})$	1/(0.67 – 0.17) = 2.0

Notes: Effect size (Cohen 1988) can be calculated on any outcome measure for which a mean and standard deviation (SD) are available, and number needed to treat (NNT; Cook and Sackett 1995) is calculated using a dichotomous outcome, such as 50% pain relief. D = difference, X = mean, P = proportion, N = sample size.

outcome in the active treatment group is compared to the rate in the control group. In the pain literature, NNT is typically calculated as the number of patients who report at least 50% pain relief following an active treatment relative to the number who report at least 50% pain relief following a control treatment (see Table I; McQuay et al. 1995), although other clinical outcomes can be used. The NNT has rarely been used to examine functional outcomes of pain treatment. The ES index has the advantage of being easily applied to published data, which typically include means and SDs for treatment groups. However, means and SDs can be reliably converted into dichotomous scores reflecting 50% pain relief (Moore et al. 1996), which then can be used for calculating the NNT. Moore and his colleagues (1997a,b) provided formulas for converting mean total pain relief to the proportion with 50% or greater pain relief.

There are a number of ways investigators can use the effect size to design studies that provide meaningful information about pain treatments. The larger the ES, the smaller the sample size needed to detect a meaningful treatment effect (other things being equal, such as power or criterion for significance). One way of increasing the ES is to increase the potency of the active intervention, so that changes in pain ratings are large. If the sample active treatment included in Table I yielded an average reduction in pain ratings of 2.0 (instead of 1.2) and no increase in variability of measurement, the ES would increase from 0.50 to 0.83. Another way to increase the ES is to reduce variability in the outcome measure. This can often be accomplished by studying homogenous groups of patients, by studying a stable pain state, or by using highly reliable measures. Pain ratings show fairly high variability, so an index that summarizes pain over a number of observational periods or measures will typically have greater reliability of measurement than an index obtained from a single pain rating (Jensen and McFarland 1993). If the variability of measurement presented in Table I was reduced to 1.4 (from 2.4), the same treatment response—a reduction in pain ratings of 1.2—would yield an increase in ES from 0.50 to 1.43.

The application of clinical trial data to an individual patient at the doctor's office should be attempted with great caution and careful knowledge of the clinical trial literature. Effect size is much more difficult to use in this circumstance, but the NNT was designed for this purpose. However, the application of the NNT to an individual patient requires careful comparison of that individual's characteristics and presentation to the sample used in the referenced clinical trial. For example, the patient's clinical history and presentation must be comparable to the study sample, including inclusion and exclusion criteria. To the extent that the patient differs from the study sample, a correction factor must be added to the calculation of NNT (Cook and Sackett 1995).

INCREASING THE EFFICIENCY OF TRIALS: DESIGNS THAT ALLOW FOR SMALLER SAMPLES

Clinical trials addressing SCI pain frequently use small samples of patients. In studying rare conditions, it is important to increase the efficiency of clinical trials so that meaningful conclusions can be derived from small samples. Ways to increase the efficiency of a clinical trial include studying a single active treatment relative to a placebo or control group or using crossover trials for these comparisons whenever possible. In crossover trials, potential carryover effects of the active intervention must be minimal, and these designs cannot be used to test most psychological interventions. Use of highly sensitive outcome measures will also increase the efficiency of a clinical trial. In the pain literature, pain relief and global ratings of outcome generally appear to be more sensitive measures than serial pain ratings (Fischer et al. 1999). Several authors have argued for the use of dichotomous outcome standards (e.g., at least 50% pain relief; Moore et al. 1996) and standards that translate into clinical significance (e.g., the decision not to use a rescue medication; Farrar 2000; Farrar et al. 2000).

Other ways to increase the efficiency of a clinical trial, thereby providing adequate power to use smaller samples, include using selection methods that create homogeneous groups. Homogeneity in diagnosis, pain level, or treatment response can be used to select subjects for the clinical trial. The difficulty in identifying homogeneous groups of persons with SCI pain has been a significant barrier to pain research in this population (see Chapter 2). One selection method commonly used in the pain literature is the requirement that trial enrollees report at least a minimum level of pain, usually at least a 3 on a 10-point scale. Another method is to only include preselected responders for enrollment in the clinical trial, perhaps by conducting an open-label phase that is followed by a randomized phase with placebo control for only those individuals who show a positive response to the open-label phase (Schnitzer et al. 2000). There is also interest in using the results of infusion studies to select individuals who are likely to have a positive response to oral treatment (e.g., Attal et al. 2000). However, the results of infusion studies do not show good prediction of oral medication response. In the trial by Attal and colleagues (2000), 12 patients received a lidocaine infusion followed by a 4–12-week oral mexiletine trial. Only 2 of 8 (25%) patients who responded with pain relief to the lidocaine infusion went on to have a positive response to the mexiletine trial. Further, the "false-positive" rate of the lidocaine infusion (75%) was too high to provide any useful screening information. The "false-negative" rate of the lidocaine infusion was 33%; that is, of the three nonresponders to lidocaine infusion, one went on to have a positive response to oral mexiletine.

Finally, the efficiency of clinical trials can be increased by minimizing factors that contribute to placebo and nonspecific effects associated with conducting such trials (Turner et al. 1994). Patients are likely to seek treatment or enroll in a study at a time when their symptoms are at their worst. The natural effects of time may yield a "regression to the mean." When this occurs, repeated observations and the passage of time will typically result in the individual moving in a seemingly positive direction—away from the extreme distress down to a more typical level of symptoms. Trials that have a long baseline period may decrease the occurrence of regression to the mean. Further, the nonspecific effects of being in a clinical trial, including physician attention, expectations for treatment outcome, and characteristics of the setting, may affect how patients feel and what they report. These nonspecific effects are often what are meant by "placebo" effects (Turner et al. 1994). Also, trials that include a single-blind selection phase that allows for identification and exclusion of "placebo responders" will increase efficiency by reducing placebo response rates. Trials that minimize the nonspecific effects of treatment are also likely to reduce placebo response rates and increase the efficiency of the study.

DECREASING THE EFFICIENCY OF TRIALS: DESIGNS THAT REQUIRE LARGER SAMPLES

Recent statistical simulations (Moore et al. 1998) provide convincing evidence that random factors—unrelated to trial method, setting, or sampling—cause significant variability in both treatment effects (even for effective treatments) and placebo effects when samples are in the range of 30 patients per treatment group, which is typical of studies in the chronic pain literature. Moore and his colleagues (1998) advocate caution in applying the results of any single small-scale trial to everyday clinical practice and clarify why inconsistent results may be seen across studies of a single intervention. In essence, random factors have a much greater impact when samples are small. While pooling across studies involving small samples will improve outcome estimates, large-scale trials—involving as many as 500 patients in each treatment group–are needed to determine the clinical significance of a treatment when the treatment effect is in the range of most analgesics (Moore et al. 1998).

Great variability is seen in placebo response rates across analgesic trials (McQuay et al. 1996; Moore et al. 1998), despite the common misperception that the placebo effect is 30% (Turner et al. 1994). Use of control conditions is inconsistent in the psychological treatment outcome literature (Morley et al. 1999). Given these observations, more stringent standards are needed than typically have been applied in most analgesic studies. Active placebos should be used more frequently in pharmacology studies (Turner et al. 1994), and more carefully designed and executed control groups are necessary for tests of psychological interventions (Morley et al. 1999).

Some of the more interesting questions in clinical pain management will require clinical trials with large samples. Understanding whether one medication is more effective than another is an important issue facing most pain clinicians. Trials that compare different medications, such as whether opioids are more or less effective than antidepressants in treating neuropathic pain (Rowbotham 1999), face the enormous challenge of demonstrating a superior effect of one active treatment over another. Similar challenges are raised in comparing pharmacological and psychological treatments and in identifying the separate and combined effects of these interventions. Large samples are also needed to examine subgroup responses to treatment (Rowbotham et al. 1998), an issue that is very applicable to patients who experience SCI pain. For example, testing differential treatment responses of groups based on the International Association for the Study of Pain's new classification system for SCI pain (see Chapter 2) will require significantly larger samples of patients than are typically included in clinical trials of SCI pain.

Finally, the logistics of participation in a clinical trial most likely affects the efficiency of the trial. Some factors known to affect the placebo response, such as increased attention by the clinical staff, may decrease the efficiency of a single trial (by increasing the placebo response rate) and are likely to increase the sample size needed to demonstrate the benefits of an active treatment. In contrast to clinical practice, clinical trials increase the demands on participants in terms of time and effort, usually requiring multiple visits to the clinic and completion of multiple measures. Such trials select for persons willing and able to meet these demands, thus possibly biasing the study results. Dropouts can be high in clinical trials, necessitating analyses that include "intention to treat" models. For example, a recent trial of oxycodone in osteoarthritis (Roth et al. 2000) reported only 40–60% completion rates in the various treatment groups, although the requested participation was quite short—only 2 weeks. The challenges of completing clinical trials in other populations are compounded in the SCI population due to the limitations in mobility and transportation common to such individuals. Studies of SCI patients often require participation of the individual's support system, which increases the demands and complexity of executing the trial.

WAYS TO INCREASE THE QUALITY AND EFFICIENCY OF CLINICAL TRIALS IN SCI PAIN

These insights lead to several conclusions regarding the design of clinical trials of pain treatment for persons with SCI. First, multiple baseline observations made several weeks prior to beginning a new intervention will increase the reliability of the baseline pain assessment and reduce the likelihood of regression to the mean. There are significant feasibility and logistical challenges in implementing this recommendation. In studies that require drug washout during an observation period prior to the beginning of treatment, the availability of rescue medication at this time may affect baseline ratings, and the use of such medication may or may not serve as a reliable and valid outcome measure (Farrar et al. 2000). Second, active placebos must be used consistently across studies (Turner et al. 1994). Third, clinical trials must include multiple measures of outcome, including serial ratings of pain intensity and relief and physician and patient ratings of global outcome. The advent of palm-sized electronic monitoring systems (Jamison et al. 2001) provides a technology that will allow collection of repeated measurements of pain and function. Measurement of all outcome variables that require interaction with a person should ideally be completed by someone who is blind to the patient's treatment condition and independent of the clinical care team. In many circumstances, ongoing and evoked pain must be assessed. Fourth, data analyses must include the "intention to treat" methods so widely applied in the clinical trials literature. And finally, given the many challenges pain researchers face, multicenter trials are essential in establishing whether a pharmacological or psychological intervention is efficacious in treating SCI pain.

ACKNOWLEDGMENT

Preparation of this manuscript was supported in part by grants from the National Institutes of Health (P01 HD33990 and R01 AR47219).

REFERENCES

Attal N, Gaude V, Brasseur L, et al. Intravenous lidocaine in central pain: a double-blind, placebo-controlled, psychophysical study. *Neurology* 2000; 54:564–574.

Cohen J. *Statistical Power Analyses for the Behavioral Sciences*. Hillsdale, NJ: Lawrence Erlbaum, 1988.

Cook RJ, Sackett DL. The number needed to treat: a clinically useful measure of treatment effect. *BMJ* 1995; 310:452–454.

Farrar JT. What is clinically meaningful: outcome measures in pain clinical trials. *Clin J Pain* 2000; 16:S106–S112.

Farrar JT, Portenoy RK, Berlin JA, Kinman JL, Strom BL. Defining the clinically important difference in pain outcome measures. *Pain* 2000; 88:287–294.

Fischer D, Stewart AL, Bloch DA, et al. Capturing the patient's view of change as a clinical outcome measure. *JAMA* 1999; 282:1157–1162.

Institute of Medicine: Committee on Strategies for Small-Number-Participant Clinical Research Trials. *Small Clinical Trials: Issues and Challenges.* Washington, DC: National Academy Press, 2001.

Jamison RN, Raymond SA, Levine JG, et al. Electronic diaries for monitoring chronic pain: 1-year validation study. *Pain* 2001; 91:277–285.

Jensen MP, McFarland CA. Increasing the reliability and validity of pain intensity measurement in chronic pain patients. *Pain* 1993; 55:195–203.

McQuay H, Carroll D, Jadad AR, Wiffen P, Moore A. Anticonvulsant drugs for management of pain: a systematic review. *BMJ* 1995; 311:1047–1052.

McQuay HJ, Tramer M, Nye BA. A systematic review of antidepressants in neuropathic pain. *Pain* 1996; 68:217–227.

Moore A, McQuay H, Gavaghan D. Deriving dichotomous outcome measures from continuous data in randomised controlled trials of analgesics. *Pain* 1996; 66:229–237.

Moore A, Collins S, Carroll D, McQuay H. Paracetamol with and without codeine in acute pain: a quantitative systematic review. *Pain* 1997a; 70:193–201.

Moore A, McQuay H, Gavaghan D. Deriving dichotomous outcome measures from continuous data in randomised controlled trials of analgesics: verification from independent data. *Pain* 1997b; 69:127–130.

Moore RA, Gavaghan D, Tramer MR, Collins SL, McQuay HJ. Size is everything—large amounts of information are needed to overcome random effects in estimating direction and magnitude of treatment effects. *Pain* 1998; 78:209–216.

Morley S, Eccleston C, Williams A. Systematic review and meta-analysis of randomized controlled trials of cognitive behaviour therapy and behaviour therapy for chronic pain in adults, excluding headache. *Pain* 1999; 80:1–13.

Rossy LA, Buckelew SP, Dorr N. A meta-analysis of fibromyalgia treatment interventions. *Ann Behav Med* 1999; 21:180–191.

Roth SH, Fleischmann RM, Burch FX, et al. Around-the-clock, controlled-release oxycodone therapy for osteoarthritis-related pain: placebo-controlled trial and long-term evaluation. *Arch Intern Med* 2000; 160:853–860.

Rowbotham MC. The debate over opioids and neuropathic pain. In: Kalso E, McQuay HJ, Wiesenfeld-Hallin Z (Eds). *Opioid Sensitivity of Chronic Noncancer Pain,* Progress in Pain Research Management, Vol. 14. Seattle: IASP Press, 1999, pp 307–318.

Rowbotham MC, Petersen KL, Fields HL. Is postherpetic neuralgia more than one disorder? *Pain Forum* 1998; 7(a):231–237.

Schnitzer TJ, Gray WL, Paster RZ, Kamin M. Efficacy of tramadol in treatment of chronic low back pain. *J Rheumatol* 2000; 27:772–778.

Sindrup SH, Jensen TS. Efficacy of pharmacological treatments of neuropathic pain: an update and effect related to mechanism of drug action. *Pain* 1999; 83:389–400.

Turner JA, Deyo RA, Loeser JD, Von Korff M, Fordyce WE. The importance of placebo effects in pain treatment and research. *JAMA* 1994; 271:1609–1614.

Correspondence to: Jennifer A. Haythornthwaite, PhD, Department of Psychiatry and Behavioral Sciences, Johns Hopkins University, 218 Meyer, 600 N. Wolfe Street, Baltimore, MD 21287-7218, USA. Tel: 410-614-9850; Fax: 410-614-3366; email: jhaythor@jhmi.edu.

Spinal Cord Injury Pain: Assessment, Mechanisms, Management. Progress in Pain Research and Management, Vol. 23, edited by Robert P. Yezierski and Kim J. Burchiel, IASP Press, Seattle, © 2002.

20

Pharmacological Treatment of Spinal Cord Injury Pain

Nanna B. Finnerup,[a] Inger L. Johannesen,[b] Søren H. Sindrup,[c] Flemming W. Bach,[a] and Troels S. Jensen[a]

[a]*Department of Neurology and Danish Pain Research Center, Aarhus University Hospital, Aarhus, Denmark;* [b]*Department of Rheumatology, Viborg Hospital, Viborg, Denmark;* [c]*Department of Neurology, Odense University Hospital, Odense, Denmark*

Pain is a significant problem following spinal cord injury (SCI). While nociceptive pain is important, it can often be handled by changes in physical activities and posture and with physical therapy, simple analgesics, or anti-inflammatory medications. Treatment of neuropathic pain is usually more difficult, and no treatment algorithm has ever been established for neuropathic SCI pain (Finnerup et al. 2001a). This chapter will focus on pharmacological treatment of neuropathic SCI pain at or below the level of the lesion.

Drugs used in neuropathic pain rarely produce complete pain relief, and side effects often limit their use. A recent postal survey studied pain treatment satisfaction in SCI with an emphasis on shoulder pain and "dysesthetic" pain (Murphy and Reid 2001). Most patients reported dissatisfaction with the management of their pain, and in general they perceived treatment for "dysesthetic" pain to be less effective than that for shoulder pain. The respondents had tried only a few of the drugs available for neuropathic pain. In another postal survey in SCI patients, only 43% of 221 patients experiencing pain at or below the level of the lesion were taking analgesics (Finnerup et al. 2001b). The drugs used were simple analgesics, opioids, spasmolytics, and nonsteroidal anti-inflammatory drugs. Only 7% of patients were on antidepressants or anticonvulsants for pain relief. It is unknown whether antidepressants or anticonvulsants had previously been tried for neuropathic pain and had been unsuccessful or had unacceptable side effects, or whether patients or their physicians were hesitant to try these drugs. In both surveys pain had a substantial impact on patients' daily lives.

Below we will summarize the results from randomized, double-blind, placebo-controlled clinical trials on SCI pain. We did not survey unblinded and nonrandomized trials because these studies do not provide evidence for efficacy in SCI. Table I lists the studies on pharmacological treatments of SCI pain included in this chapter. Numbers needed to treat (NNTs) are used to provide clinically relevant measures of the analgesic efficacy of the drugs mentioned. NNT is defined as the number of patients that clinicians need to treat with a certain drug to provide one patient with a defined degree of pain relief (in this context, 50% pain relief) (Cook and Sackett 1995; McQuay et al. 1996). The 95% confidence interval (CI) of NNT is obtained as the reciprocal value of the 95% CI for the absolute risk difference. NNTs are estimated from dichotomized data, so an NNT with a range to infinity does not preclude significant relief of pain as measured with a more detailed pain or pain relief scale. Studies are generally based on small crossover trials with fewer than 20 patients, so the NNTs must be regarded as point estimates, and negative trials may have overlooked minor treatment effects.

ANTIDEPRESSANTS

Tricyclic antidepressants (TCAs) are increasingly popular in the management of chronic neuropathic pain, including pain after SCI, and controlled studies have clearly documented the benefit of antidepressants (ADs) in various peripheral and central neuropathic pain conditions (review in McQuay et al. 1996; Sindrup 1997; Sindrup and Jensen 1999). The principal mechanism by which TCAs relieves neuropathic pain is by blocking the reuptake of norepinephrine or serotonin (Sindrup 1997). However, TCAs have a wide range of other pharmacological actions with potential pain-relieving effects, including central *N*-methyl-D-aspartate (NMDA) receptor antagonist activity and sodium channel blockade. Side effects are mainly attributed to sedative and anticholinergic actions (e.g., dry mouth, constipation, and urinary retention). More selective ADs such as selective serotonin reuptake inhibitors (SSRIs) may have the advantage of fewer side effects, but they seem to be less effective than the less selective TCAs (McQuay et al. 1996; Sindrup 1997; Sindrup and Jensen 1999). No controlled study has examined the effect of TCAs on SCI pain. In the only controlled study of ADs for SCI pain, Davidoff and colleagues (1987) studied the effect of trazodone, an SSRI, on diffuse burning and tingling pain after traumatic SCI. Eighteen patients participated in a parallel double-blind study in which they received either trazodone at 150 mg/day or placebo for 6 weeks. Drug and

Table I
Randomized controlled trials of pharmacological treatment of pain in SCI patients

Study	Active Drug	Dose and Study Duration	No. SCI Patients (Total)	Design	Outcome	NNT (95% CI)
Davidoff et al. 1987	Trazodone hydrochloride	6 weeks, 150 mg/day	18	Parallel	Tra = pla	–
Loubser et al. 1991	Lidocaine s.a.	50–100 mg (titrated every 5 min in 25-mg aliquots)	21	Cross-over	Lid > pla	3.5 (1.8–37)
Attal et al. 2000	Lidocaine i.v.	5 mg/kg (over 30 min)	10 (16)	Cross-over	Lid > pla[a]	5[b] (1.6–∞)
Chiou-Tan et al. 1996	Mexiletine	2 × 4 weeks, 450 mg/day	11	Cross-over	Mex = pla	–
Drewes et al. 1994	Valproate	2 × 3 weeks, final dose 600–2400 mg/day	20	Cross-over	Val = pla	–
Finnerup et al., unpublished	Lamotrigine	2 × 9 weeks, final dose 200–400 mg/day	22	Cross-over	Ltg = pla [ltg > pla][c]	[12 (2–∞)][c]
Eide et al. 1995	Ketamine i.v. or alfentanil i.v.	Ketamine: bolus 60 µg/kg + 6 µg/kg/min (17–20 min); alfentanil: bolus 7 µg/kg + 0.6 µg/kg/min (17–20 min)	9	Cross-over	Ket > pla, alf > pla, ket = alf	NA
Siddall et al. 2000	Morphine i.t., and/or clonidine i.t.	Morphine: bolus 0.2–1.5 mg; clonidine: bolus 50–100 µg or 300–500 µg (over 6 hours); combination: half of each dose	15	Cross-over	Mor = pla, clo = pla, mor/ clo > pla	7.5[d] (2.1–∞)
Herman et al. 1992	Baclofen i.t.	Bolus 50 µg	7	Cross-over	Bac > pla	NA
Canavero et al. 1995[e]	Propofol i.v.	Bolus 0.2 mg/kg	8 (32)	Cross-over	Pro > pla[a]	NA

Abbreviations: i.t. = intrathecal; i.v. = intravenous; NA = not accessible from article; NNT = number needed to treat; pla = placebo; s.a. = subarachnoidal.
[a]Conclusion based on all patients in the study (SCI and stroke). [b]Based on SCI patients. [c]Patients with incomplete SCI (n = 12). [d]NNT for morphine in combination with clonidine. [e]Randomization procedure was not stated.

placebo groups showed no significant differences in pain measures according to the McGill Pain Questionnaire (MPQ), the Sternbach Pain Intensity Scale, and the Zung Pain and Distress Index. This result does not preclude the possible benefit of other ADs with a broader spectrum of action in the control of SCI pain. TCAs are still considered to be the drug of choice for many neuropathic pain conditions (Sindrup and Jensen 1999), and although ADs may be less effective in SCI pain than in other conditions such as poststroke pain (Boivie 1994), we need to conduct randomized controlled trials (RCTs) to estimate their effect on different types of SCI pain.

SODIUM CHANNEL BLOCKERS

Sodium channels play a key role in neuronal hyperexcitability and are thought to be one of the principal neurochemical mechanisms of neuropathic pain after SCI (Hao et al. 1992a; Yezierski 1996; Eide 1998; Vierck et al. 2000). Lidocaine, a nonspecific sodium channel blocker, may produce its analgesic effect by both a peripheral and a central action. Its peripheral action is indicated by its ability to reduce ectopic neuronal activity in damaged axons (Chabal et al. 1989; Devor et al. 1992) and by evidence that it can silence spontaneous discharges in dorsal root ganglion cells (Devor et al. 1992; Sotgiu et al. 1994). A central action of lidocaine and other local anesthetics is indicated by their ability to reduce a spinally mediated nociceptive withdrawal reflex in animals (Woolf and Wiesenfeld-Hallin 1985) and in humans (Bach et al. 1990), by their ability to suppress dorsal horn wide-dynamic-range neurons in the spinal cord (Hao et al. 1992b; Sotgiu et al. 1992), and by the ability of lidocaine injected in to the rostroventromedial medulla and the periaqueductal gray to attenuate allodynia in neuropathic rats (Pertovaara et al. 1996). Results from the study by Loubser and Donovan (1991) and from the recent study by Attal et al. (2000), discussed below, are compatible with a central action of lidocaine.

A crossover study monitored the effect of subarachnoidal lidocaine in 21 patients with at-level or below-level chronic pain secondary to traumatic SCI (Loubser and Donovan 1991). Lidocaine was significantly better than placebo at relieving pain ($P < 0.01$). Lidocaine relieved pain in 13 patients for 2 hours, whereas placebo was effective in only 4 patients, corresponding to an NNT for lidocaine of 3.5 (1.8–37). Where spinal anesthesia proximal to the SCI level was adequate, 9 of 11 patients had a positive response to lidocaine, compared to 4 of 10 patients who did not obtain anesthesia above the level of SCI because of spinal canal obstruction or a high level of lesion. These findings suggest a "neural pain generator" in the spinal cord. The authors considered that the negative response to subarachnoid lidocaine observed in two patients despite adequate spinal anesthesia cephalad to the lesion might suggest a more rostral pain mechanism or a psychogenic etiology in these cases.

In another crossover trial, Attal and colleagues (2000) studied the effect of intravenous (i.v.) lidocaine in 16 patients with chronic poststroke pain ($n = 6$) or SCI pain ($n = 10$). Spinal cord injuries included syringomyelia, post-traumatic myelomalacia, and cervical spondylosis with myelopathy. The 10 SCI patients had spontaneous ongoing at- or below-level neuropathic pain, and 5 of these patients also had evoked pain. Lidocaine (5 mg/kg) and saline were administered i.v. over a 30-minute period 3 weeks apart. Pain was assessed on a visual analogue scale (VAS). For all 16 patients, lidocaine significantly ($P < 0.05$) decreased spontaneous ongoing pain, brush-induced allodynia, and static mechanical hyperalgesia, but it was no better than placebo against thermal allodynia and hyperalgesia. Lidocaine also failed to elevate mechanical pain thresholds. The data for the SCI patients show an NNT of 5 (1.6–∞). The authors suggested that lidocaine has modality-specific analgesic effects, with specific antiallodynic/hyperalgesic properties, and that thermal and mechanical hyperalgesia in SCI and poststroke pain patients are mediated by different mechanisms. Lidocaine had no significant prolonged analgesic effect, which makes it inconvenient for prolonged treatment. After the trial, 12 patients received mexiletine orally titrated from 200 mg/day to the highest level possible without distressing side effects (400–800 mg/day). Most patients did not tolerate mexiletine, and only 25% obtained pain relief.

Chiou-Tan et al. (1996) studied the effect of mexiletine on SCI pain in a crossover trial. Eleven patients with at- or below-level chronic SCI pain completed the study, and nine of these had a complete injury. Mexiletine (450 mg/day) for 4 weeks had no significant effect on pain compared to placebo as assessed by VAS, MPQ, and Barthel function scores.

More selective blockers of sodium channels with fewer side effects that may be available in future may have a role in the treatment of central pain.

ANTIEPILEPTIC DRUGS

Antiepileptic drugs (AEDs) have been used in pain management since the 1960s. The exact mechanisms by which they exert their analgesic actions are unknown, but they probably involve multiple mechanisms that reduce excitation and enhance inhibition (for review, see Ross 2000). These mechanisms involve nonspecific blockade of voltage-dependent sodium channels, thus stabilizing neuronal membranes and reducing neuronal excitability. Other mechanisms involve blockade of calcium currents, blockade of NMDA receptors, and enhancement of γ-aminobutyric acid (GABA) (Ross 2000). Adverse events associated with the use of AEDs include dizziness, nausea, headache, fatigue, incoordination, and other CNS-related symptoms; in addition, bone marrow suppression and serious hypersensitivity reactions may be seen with carbamazepine and lamotrigine, respectively.

In the only controlled study on AEDs in SCI pain published so far, Drewes et al. (1994) studied the effect of doses of valproate of up to 2400 mg/day against placebo in a crossover trial with 3-week treatment periods. Valproate increases levels of GABA in the brain by inhibiting its degradation (Gram 1988). Outcome measures were the Pain Rating Index, Number of Words Chosen, and the Present Pain Index from the MPQ. Twenty patients completed the trial. Valproate was not significantly better than placebo in relieving pain, but there was a trend toward improvement in most of the MPQ subscores.

Gabapentin, an antiepileptic that binds to an $\alpha_2\delta$ subunit of voltage-gated Ca^{2+} channels, is effective in painful diabetic neuropathy (Backonja et al. 1998) and in postherpetic neuropathy (Rowbotham et al. 1998). Studies evaluating gabapentin and other second-generation antiepileptics such as topiramate and felbamate in SCI patients have not yet been published; however, see Chapter 23 for examples of the use of gabapentin in SCI pain, and Chapter 24 for an RCT of topiramate.

Lamotrigine is a novel antiepileptic drug that acts at voltage-sensitive sodium channels to stabilize neuronal membranes (Cheung et al. 1992; Lang et al. 1993; Deffois et al. 1996) and inhibit sodium influx- mediated pathological release of excitatory amino acid transmitters, principally glutamate (Leach et al. 1986; Teoh et al. 1995). RCTs have shown the efficacy of lamotrigine in peripheral neuropathic pain conditions (Zakrzewska et al. 1997; Luria et al. 2000; Simpson et al. 2000). In central neuropathic pain, only one controlled study has investigated lamotrigine (Vestergaard et al. 2001). This crossover trial with lamotrigine versus placebo in patients with central poststroke pain showed that 200 mg/day of this drug reduced pain significantly, with a mean reduction of 30%. We conducted a randomized, double-blind, placebo-controlled crossover trial to study the effect of lamotrigine in spinal cord injury pain (N.B. Finnerup et al., unpublished observations, 2001). Inclusion criteria were neuropathic pain or dysesthesia at or below the level of the lesion after traumatic SCI and pain intensity of at least 3 on a 0–10 point numeric rating scale. Thirty patients were included, and 22 completed the trial. A 1-week baseline period was followed by two treatment periods of 9 weeks' duration with lamotrigine or placebo, separated by a 2-week washout period. Drug dose was slowly increased to a maximum of 400 mg for the last 2 weeks. The primary efficacy variable was the change in the median value of the daily pain score (on a 0–10-point numeric rating scale) from baseline to the last week of each treatment period. Secondary efficacy variables included the effect of lamotrigine on different standardized sensory stimuli using quantitative somatosensory testing (QST). Overall, lamotrigine was not more effective than placebo at reducing pain. However, the study suggested that lamotrigine is effective in patients with incomplete SCI and evoked pain.

OPIOIDS, NMDA-RECEPTOR ANTAGONISTS, AND CLONIDINE

Previous articles have suggested that neuropathic pain is resistant to opioid treatment (e.g., Arner and Meyerson 1988), but several more recent studies have shown the efficacy of opioids in different neuropathic pain states (review in Sindrup and Jensen 1999). Central NMDA receptors activated by glutamate are involved in pain processing, neuronal plasticity, and central sensitization (Woolf and Thompson 1991; Dickenson et al. 1997; Sang 2000). These events are important in neuropathic pain, and NMDA-receptor antagonists have been used to treat different neuropathic pain states, although the clinical use of NMDA blockers has been limited by their side effects.

In a crossover trial, Eide and associates (1995) studied the effects of i.v. infusion of alfentanil (a μ-opioid receptor agonist), ketamine (an NMDA-receptor antagonist), or placebo on "dysesthesia" pain in nine patients with traumatic SCI. All patients had spontaneous and evoked pain. Alfentanil and ketamine significantly reduced the intensity of both continuous pain, as measured by a VAS, and evoked pain (allodynia and wind-up-like pain). Heat pain thresholds were unchanged. The differences between the two drugs were nonsignificant.

Siddall and colleagues (2000) studied the effect of intrathecal (i.t.) morphine and clonidine (an α_2-adrenergic agonist) on at- or below-level neuropathic pain after SCI. Morphine and clonidine in combination produced significantly greater pain relief than did saline placebo. The NNT for the combination of drugs was 7.5 (2.1–∞). Neither morphine nor clonidine alone produced significant pain relief. These results suggest that the two drugs have a synergistic action in reducing pain. Patients with at-level pain tended to have better pain relief than did those with pain below the SCI lesion level. The study further suggests that in patients with cerebrospinal fluid obstruction, i.t. drugs should be administered above the level of injury.

GABA-RECEPTOR AGONISTS

GABA is a widely distributed inhibitory neurotransmitter in the central nervous system that plays a key role in the control of pain-transmitting pathways (Stephenson 1995; Kontinen and Dickenson 2000). GABA activates the ligand-gated chloride ion $GABA_A$ receptor or the second-messenger-coupled $GABA_B$ receptor. Animal studies suggest that a decreased inhibitory influence of GABAergic neurotransmission contributes to neuropathic pain (Yezierski 1996), and both $GABA_A$ and $GABA_B$ agonists have been used in animal models of neuropathic pain.

The $GABA_B$-receptor agonist baclofen is widely used to suppress spasticity in SCI patients. Herman and colleagues (1992) conducted a crossover study to assess the effect of i.t. baclofen (50 μg) in seven patients with incomplete SCI who had "dysesthetic" pain (n = 6) and spasm-related pain (n = 6) from multiple sclerosis, spinal epidural abscess, and transverse myelitis. Baclofen significantly decreased "dysesthetic" pain and spasm-related pain, but did not influence pinch-induced or musculoskeletal (low back) pain. The effect on "dysesthetic" pain occurred before (and disappeared before) suppression of spasm-related pain.

Propofol, a $GABA_A$-receptor agonist, was studied in a crossover trial in 32 patients with nonmalignant pain, including 8 patients with SCI pain (Canavero et al. 1995). The report does not state whether the study was randomized. Propofol was injected as a single intravenous bolus of 0.2 mg/kg. All eight SCI patients had better pain relief with propofol than with placebo (P values were not reported). Five SCI patients had allodynia that was abolished by propofol injection, but unaltered by placebo.

DISCUSSION AND CONCLUSION

To summarize, i.v. or subarachnoidal lidocaine, i.v. ketamine, alfentanil, or propofol, and i.t. baclofen or morphine in combination with clonidine are effective in SCI pain. However, no oral treatment has so far proven to be effective, except for the suggestion that lamotrigine is effective in patients with incomplete SCI and evoked pain.

SCI pain represents heterogeneous pain conditions, and research has suffered from the lack of established clinical criteria for classifying them. Even in an individual patient it may be difficult to separate several types of pains produced by different mechanisms.

It has recently been suggested that classification of neuropathic pain based on underlying pain mechanisms rather than on etiology or anatomical location may improve pharmacological treatment (Woolf and Mannion 1999;

Jensen et al. 2001) because the treatment could be directed against a specific pain mechanism. While this concept is attractive from a theoretical point of view, it still needs to be validated in clinical neuropathic pain trials, and a diagnosis of mechanisms will be of value only if a specific therapy can target the particular mechanisms involved in each case. Combining our current understanding of the pathophysiological mechanisms behind different pain types with our knowledge of drug actions may help us to understand and treat neuropathic pain.

Because of the different pain mechanisms that seem to be involved in SCI pain, a combination of drugs with different profiles may improve treatment efficacy. Patients failing to respond to oral medication should be considered for i.t. treatment. Pharmacological treatment will probably provide only partial pain relief, so it seems rational to combine drug therapy with nonpharmacological approaches such as physical therapy and cognitive-behavioral therapy. There is obviously a need for additional large randomized, controlled trials comparing both pharmacological and nonpharmacological treatments, with a focus on their effect on different pain phenomena. Because of the relatively limited number of SCI patients at most centers, multicenter trials should be encouraged.

ACKNOWLEDGMENTS

Work behind this contribution is supported in part by grants from Ludvig og Sara Elsass' Foundation, the Institute of Experimental Clinical Research at Aarhus University, the Danish Medical Research Council (No. 9700764, No. 9700565) the Danish Society of Polio and Accident Victims (PTU), and GlaxoSmithKline Denmark.

REFERENCES

Arner S, Meyerson BA. Lack of analgesic effect of opioids on neuropathic and idiopathic forms of pain. *Pain* 1988; 33:11–23.

Attal N, Gaude V, Brasseur L, et al. Intravenous lidocaine in central pain: a double-blind, placebo-controlled, psychophysical study. *Neurology* 2000; 54:564–574.

Bach FW, Jensen TS, Kastrup J, Stigsby B, Dejgard A. The effect of intravenous lidocaine on nociceptive processing in diabetic neuropathy. *Pain* 1990; 40:29–34.

Backonja M, Beydoun A, Edwards KR, et al. Gabapentin for the symptomatic treatment of painful neuropathy in patients with diabetes mellitus: a randomized controlled trial. *JAMA* 1998; 280:1831–1836.

Boivie J. Central pain. In: Wall PD, Melzack R (Eds). *Textbook of Pain*. Edinburg: Churchill Livingstone, 1994, pp 871–902.

Canavero S, Bonicalzi V, Pagni CA, et al. Propofol analgesia in central pain: preliminary clinical observations. *J Neurol* 1995; 242:561–567.

Chabal C, Russell LC, Burchiel KJ. The effect of intravenous lidocaine, tocainide, and mexiletine on spontaneously active fibers originating in rat sciatic neuromas. *Pain* 1989; 38:333–338.

Cheung H, Kamp D, Harris E. An in vitro investigation of the action of lamotrigine on neuronal voltage-activated sodium channels. *Epilepsy Res* 1992; 13:107–112.

Chiou-Tan FY, Tuel SM, Johnson JC, et al. Effect of mexiletine on spinal cord injury dysesthetic pain. *Am J Phys Med Rehabil* 1996; 75:84–87.

Cook RJ, Sackett DL. The number needed to treat: a clinically useful measure of treatment effect. *BMJ* 1995; 310:452–454.

Davidoff G, Guarracini M, Roth E, Sliwa J, Yarkony G. Trazodone hydrochloride in the treatment of dysesthetic pain in traumatic myelopathy: a randomized, double-blind, placebo-controlled study. *Pain* 1987; 29:151–161.

Deffois A, Fage D, Carter C. Inhibition of synaptosomal veratridine-induced sodium influx by antidepressants and neuroleptics used in chronic pain. *Neurosci Lett* 1996; 220:117–120.

Devor M, Wall PD, Catalan N. Systemic lidocaine silences ectopic neuroma and DRG discharge without blocking nerve conduction. *Pain* 1992; 48:261–268.

Dickenson AH, Chapman V, Green GM. The pharmacology of excitatory and inhibitory amino acid-mediated events in the transmission and modulation of pain in the spinal cord. *Gen Pharmacol* 1997; 28:633–638.

Drewes AM, Andreasen A, Poulsen LH. Valproate for treatment of chronic central pain after spinal cord injury: a double-blind cross-over study. *Paraplegia* 1994; 32:565–569.

Eide PK. Pathophysiological mechanisms of central neuropathic pain after spinal cord injury. *Spinal Cord* 1998; 36:601–612.

Eide PK, Stubhaug A, Stenehjem AE. Central dysesthesia pain after traumatic spinal cord injury is dependent on N-methyl-D-aspartate receptor activation. *Neurosurgery* 1995; 37:1080–1087.

Finnerup NB, Yezierski RP, Sang CN, Burchiel KJ, Jensen TS. Treatment of spinal cord injury pain. *Pain: Clin Updates* 2001a; IX(2).

Finnerup NB, Johannesen IL, Sindrup EH, Bach FW, Jensen TS. Pain and dysesthesia in patients with spinal cord injury: a postal survey. *Spinal Cord* 2001b; 39:256–262.

Gram L. Experimental studies and controlled clinical testing of valproate and vigabatrin. *Acta Neurol Scand* 1988; 78:241–270.

Hao JX, Xu XJ, Yu YX, Seiger A, Wiesenfeld-Hallin Z. Transient spinal cord ischemia induces temporary hypersensitivity of dorsal horn wide dynamic range neurons to myelinated, but not unmyelinated, fiber input. *J Neurophysiol* 1992a; 68:384–391.

Hao JX, Yu YX, Seiger A, Wiesenfeld-Hallin Z. Systemic tocainide relieves mechanical hypersensitivity and normalizes the responses of hyperexcitable dorsal horn wide-dynamic-range neurons after transient spinal cord ischemia in rats. *Exp Brain Res* 1992b; 91:229–235.

Herman RM, D'Luzansky SC, Ippolito R. Intrathecal baclofen suppresses central pain in patients with spinal lesions: a pilot study. *Clin J Pain* 1992; 8:338–345.

Jensen TS, Gottrup H, Bach FW, Sindrup S. Clinical assessment of neuropathic pain. *Eur J Pharmacol* 2001; 429:1–11.

Kontinen VK, Dickenson AH. Effects of midazolam in the spinal nerve ligation model of neuropathic pain in rats. *Pain* 2000; 85:425–431.

Lang DG, Wang CM, Cooper BR. Lamotrigine, phenytoin and carbamazepine interactions on the sodium current present in N4TG1 mouse neuroblastoma cells. *J Pharmacol Exp Ther* 1993; 266:829–835.

Leach MJ, Marden CM, Miller AA. Pharmacological studies on lamotrigine, a novel potential antiepileptic drug: II. Neurochemical studies on the mechanism of action. *Epilepsia* 1986; 27:490–497.

Loubser PG, Donovan WH. Diagnostic spinal anaesthesia in chronic spinal cord injury pain. *Paraplegia* 1991; 29:25–36.

Luria Y, Brecker C, Daoud D, Ishay A, Eisenberg E. Lamotrigine in the treatment of painful diabetic neuropathy: a randomized controlled trial. *Proceedings of the 9th World Congress on Pain,* Progress in Pain Research and Management, Vol. 16. Seattle: IASP Press, 2000, pp 857–862.

McQuay HJ, Tramer M, Nye BA, et al. A systematic review of antidepressants in neuropathic pain. *Pain* 1996; 68:217–227.

Murphy D, Reid DB. Pain treatment satisfaction in spinal cord injury. *Spinal Cord* 2001; 39:44–46.

Pertovaara A, Wei H, Hamalainen MM. Lidocaine in the rostroventromedial medulla and the periaqueductal gray attenuates allodynia in neuropathic rats. *Neurosci Lett* 1996; 218:127–130.

Ross EL. The evolving role of antiepileptic drugs in treating neuropathic pain. *Neurology* 2000; 55:S41–S46

Rowbotham M, Harden N, Stacey B, Bernstein P, Magnus-Miller L. Gabapentin for the treatment of postherpetic neuralgia: a randomized controlled trial. *JAMA* 1998; 280:1837–1842.

Sang CN. NMDA-receptor antagonists in neuropathic pain: experimental methods to clinical trials. *J Pain Symptom Manage* 2000; 19:S21–S25

Siddall PJ, Molloy AR, Walker S, Rutkowski SB. The efficacy of intrathecal morphine and clonidine in the treatment of pain after spinal cord injury. *Anesth Analg* 2000; 91:1–6.

Simpson DM, Olney R, McArthur JC, et al. A placebo-controlled trial of lamotrigine for painful HIV-associated neuropathy. *Neurology* 2000; 54:2115–2119.

Sindrup SH. Antidepressants as analgesics. In: Yaksh TL, Lynch C, Zapol WM, et al. (Eds). *Anesthesia: Biological Foundations*. Philadelphia: Lippincott-Raven, 1997, pp 987–997.

Sindrup SH, Jensen TS. Efficacy of pharmacological treatments of neuropathic pain: an update and effect related to mechanism of drug action. *Pain* 1999; 83:389–400.

Sotgiu ML, Lacerenza M, Marchettini P. Effect of systemic lidocaine on dorsal horn neuron hyperactivity following chronic peripheral nerve injury in rats. *Somatosens Mot Res* 1992; 9:227–233.

Sotgiu ML, Biella G, Castagna A, Lacerenza M, Marchettini P. Different time-courses of i.v. lidocaine effect on ganglionic and spinal units in neuropathic rats. *Neuroreport* 1994; 5:873–876.

Stephenson FA. The GABA-A receptors. *Biochem J* 1995; 310:1–9.

Teoh H, Fowler LJ, Bowery NG. Effect of lamotrigine on the electrically-evoked release of endogenous amino acids from slices of dorsal horn of the rat spinal cord. *Neuropharmacology* 1995; 34:1273–1278.

Vestergaard K, Andersen G, Gottrup H, Kristensen BT, Jensen TS. Lamotrigine for central poststroke pain: a randomized controlled trial. *Neurology* 2001; 56:184–190.

Vierck CJ, Siddall P, Yezierski RP. Pain following spinal cord injury: animal studies and mechanistic studies. *Pain* 2000; 89:1–5.

Woolf CJ, Mannion RJ. Neuropathic pain: aetiology, symptoms, mechanisms, and management. *Lancet* 1999; 353:1959–1964.

Woolf CJ, Thompson SW. The induction and maintenance of central sensitization is dependent on N-methyl-D-aspartic acid receptor activation: implications for the treatment of post-injury pain hypersensitivity states. *Pain* 1991; 44:293–299.

Woolf CJ, Wiesenfeld-Hallin Z. The systemic administration of local anaesthetics produces a selective depression of C-afferent fibre evoked activity in the spinal cord. *Pain* 1985; 23:361–374.

Yezierski RP. Pain following spinal cord injury: the clinical problem and experimental studies. *Pain* 1996; 68:185–194.

Zakrzewska JM, Chaudhry Z, Nurmikko TJ, Patton DW, Mullens EL. Lamotrigine (Lamictal) in refractory trigeminal neuralgia: results from a double-blind placebo controlled crossover trial. *Pain* 1997; 73:223–230.

Correspondence to: Nanna B. Finnerup, MD, Danish Pain Research Center, Building 1A, Noerrebrogade 44, Aarhus University Hospital, DK-8000 Aarhus C, Denmark. Fax: 45-89-49-32-69; email: finnerup@akhphd.au.dk.

Spinal Cord Injury Pain: Assessment, Mechanisms, Management. Progress in Pain Research and Management, Vol. 23, edited by Robert P. Yezierski and Kim J. Burchiel, IASP Press, Seattle, © 2002.

21

Spinal Drug Administration in the Treatment of Spinal Cord Injury Pain

Philip J. Siddall

Pain Management and Research Centre, University of Sydney, Royal North Shore Hospital, Sydney, Australia

The use of spinal agents to treat pain following spinal cord injury (SCI) has a long history. A putative region of abnormal activity in the cord proximal to the spinal cord lesion, termed an "irritated focus" or "neural pain generator" (Loubser and Clearman 1993), may be responsible for generating abnormal neuronal impulses and pain (Loeser et al. 1968). Pollock and his colleagues (1951) reported that intrathecal (i.t.) administration of lidocaine at the level of injury resulted in good relief of SCI pain. However, lidocaine only provided short-term relief and was not proposed as a long-term solution. Nevertheless, there has been continued interest in the concept of a spinal generator of pain and in the use of spinal agents to control pain. Although there may be also be a supraspinal component to the pain, i.t. administration presents a method of delivering agents in relatively high doses at a spinal and possibly supraspinal level. Therefore, it may specifically target mechanisms at both of these levels that are involved in generating pain.

Studies using animal models of SCI pain have identified several changes that may be relevant to the administration of spinal agents in patients. Pain may stem from the loss of normally active GABAergic or glycinergic inhibitory mechanisms (Zimmerman 1991; Sivilotti and Woolf 1994). An ischemic model of neuropathic SCI pain showed that an acute period of hypersensitivity for 1–5 days following injury is associated with reduced γ-aminobutyric acid (GABA) immunoreactivity (Zhang et al. 1994). Also, spinal cord transection diminishes $GABA_B$-receptor binding in the spinal cord close to the site of damage (Kroin et al. 1993). Allodynia-like behavior in the ischemic model also is attenuated by systemic administration of the $GABA_B$-receptor agonist baclofen (Hao et al. 1992). Although baclofen's effect disappears after approximately a week, the study suggests that, at least initially, allodynia following SCI may be susceptible to administration of $GABA_B$ agonists.

Calcitonin gene-related peptide (CGRP), which is confined normally to laminae I and II of the dorsal horn, can be found in laminae III and IV after spinal cord hemisection (Christensen and Hulsebosch 1997). This finding suggests ingrowth of small-diameter primary afferent fibers into nuclear regions where they do not normally occur. This sprouting of small-diameter CGRP-immunoreactive neurons into laminae III and IV of the dorsal horn may provide a mechanism for the development of chronic pain. Administration of the selective CGRP antagonist CGRP 8-37 relieves mechanical and thermal allodynia following SCI (Bennett et al. 2000). Levels of nerve growth factor (NGF) also modulate the intensity of primary afferent sprouting. I.t. administration of an antibody to NGF prevents the sprouting of small-diameter afferents and lessens the increase in blood pressure induced by colonic distension after SCI (Krenz et al. 1999). This finding suggests a potential strategy for preventing spinal cord changes that occur after injury and could be related to the genesis of pain.

Adrenal chromaffin cells produce an array of neuroprotective and potentially analgesic agents, including the *N*-methyl D-aspartate (NMDA) antagonist histogranin as well as neurotrophic and growth factors (fibroblast growth factor 2 [FGF-2] and transforming growing factor α [TGF-α). These agents have significant effects on pain-related behaviors following SCI; for example, transplantation of adrenal chromaffin cells significantly decreases autotomy, overgrooming, and pain-related behavioral responses (Brewer and Yezierski 1998; Yu et al. 1998).

In summary, several mechanisms appear to be related to the development of neuropathic pain following SCI, including changes in opioid, α-adrenergic, GABA, glycine, NMDA, purinergic, and nitric oxide systems. These mechanisms suggest a number of potential therapeutic approaches, including pharmacological strategies targeting spinal mediators of cell signaling (e.g., glutamate) and cellular survival that determine the functional state of neurons.

SPINAL AGENTS FOR SCI PAIN

Before looking at the evidence for the effectiveness of spinal agents it may be worthwhile to ask a more general question: why consider spinal administration at all? In a group of patients who have experienced a spinal injury, why attempt to administer drugs by the spinal route when many more drugs are available for systemic administration? First, although many drugs are available for systemic administration, few, if any, provide consistent and adequate relief of pain. In fact, most of the drugs for the treatment of SCI pain that have been subjected to randomized controlled trials (RCTs) proved to be no better than placebo, and so we need alternative strategies. Second, as with treatment of other conditions, many of the drugs that are used for neuropathic SCI pain have generalized side effects that can be reduced by spinal administration. The third reason is that drugs have different efficacy depending on their route of administration. Wiesenfeld-Hallin's group has shown that drugs that are ineffective by the systemic route often are effective when given spinally (Hao et al. 1996; Yu et al. 1997). The reason for this difference is still not completely understood, but such studies indicate that complete dependence on the systemic route of administration may limit the availability of effective drugs.

LOCAL ANESTHETICS

Several case reports describe relief of SCI pain by spinal local anesthetic blockade (Pollock et al. 1951; Davis 1954; Loubser and Clearman 1993). In the first report (Pollock et al. 1951), spinal anesthesia above the level of injury eliminated pain. However, four patients with a "spinal fluid block" and spontaneous, diffuse, burning pain below the level of injury were unaffected by spinal anesthesia despite abolition of spasms and reflex activity below the level of injury. In the second report (Davis 1954), "spinal anesthesia" above the level of injury completely relieved spontaneous, diffuse, burning, below-level neuropathic pain. In the third report (Loubser and Clearman 1993), the patient had dysesthetic and cramping pain in both upper and lower limbs following a C6 incomplete injury. I.t. lidocaine (50 mg) produced a sensory block to light touch to the T8 level, with disappearance of both spasticity and pain.

In one RCT (Loubser and Donovan 1991), 21 patients with spontaneous burning pain and intermittent sharp pain received i.t. lidocaine, which provided a sensory level of anesthesia above the level of injury in those with lumbar and thoracic injuries and to T4 in those with cervical injuries. Lidocaine significantly reduced pain intensity when compared with placebo. Interestingly, analgesia lasted for a mean of 2 hours, which exceeds the expected duration of action for interruption of nociceptive messages. In two cases the response was negative despite sensory anesthesia rostral to the level of SCI; in these cases, a more rostral site may have been responsible for generating pain. Similarly, two patients with incomplete anterior cord syndromes failed to respond, although sensory block was in effect rostral to their level of injury.

This ability of spinal local anesthetic to attenuate neuropathic pain following SCI supports the concept of a "neural pain generator" located spinally at the distal end of the proximal segment. This suggestion is supported by Loubser and Donovan's finding that in five patients with evidence of spinal canal obstruction, a sensory block could not be achieved above the level of SCI. Four out of these five patients had no change in their pain level, and one obtained 20% relief of pain, in contrast with the remainder of the group, where 12 out of 16 patients obtained a mean of 65% relief of pain.

In summary, i.t. lidocaine significantly reduces pain in a proportion of SCI patients, but in most cases relief appears to depend on the drug being able to access the spinal cord above the level of injury. However, in some cases, relief is not obtained despite sensory block above the level of injury. Although good relief can often be obtained, the effect is only temporary, and there is no evidence that even multiple local anesthetic blocks result in long-term relief of pain. Therefore, although useful as a diagnostic tool, this approach appears to have limited usefulness in the long-term treatment of SCI pain.

OPIOIDS

A nonrandomized single-blind crossover study found that epidural morphine (5 mg) had a pain-relieving effect in 5 of 14 patients with neuropathic SCI pain (Glynn et al. 1986). In an uncontrolled study by Fenollosa and associates (1993), 8 of 12 patients obtained >50% relief of their pain and went on to have an i.t. infusion system implanted. Six patients were alive after 3 years of follow-up, and their final i.t. morphine doses were in the range of 1.6–6.0 mg/day.

In a double-blind study investigating the efficacy of i.t. morphine, clonidine, and a mixture of the two drugs, i.t. morphine (at a median dose of 0.75 mg) reduced pain scores to 80 ± 9% of baseline (mean ± SEM) (Siddall et al. 2000). However, only 4 of 15 patients had 50% or greater relief of their pain with i.t. morphine compared with 5 out of 15 with saline. In this small sample, those with incomplete injuries had a greater incidence of positive responses (3 out of 5 with incomplete injuries compared with 1 out of 10 with complete injuries).

In summary, spinal morphine, either by the epidural or i.t. route, at a dose of 0.5–1.0 mg/day, is initially effective against neuropathic SCI pain in some patients and may also reduce spasms. However, apart from the initially more promising results in those with incomplete injuries, little information indicates which particular subgroups are more likely to respond better.

CLONIDINE

Both epidural and i.t. administration of clonidine can relieve neuropathic SCI pain. In the single-blind study by Glynn et al. (1986), 10 of 15 patients obtained pain relief with epidural clonidine (150 μg), compared with 5 of 14 patients who obtained relief with epidural morphine.

A case series of 10 subjects found that three of six patients receiving epidural clonidine injections (150 μg) had 50% or greater relief of their pain (Glynn et al. 1992). All three patients with spasm had excellent relief with epidural clonidine, and one patient who received i.t. clonidine also obtained excellent relief. Those with higher concentrations in the cerebrospinal fluid (CSF) had better relief, which suggests a substantial spinal cord action of clonidine with a probable contribution from supraspinal sites.

As part of the RCT mentioned above (Siddall et al. 2000), all 15 patients with neuropathic SCI pain received i.t. clonidine (median dose 50 μg). Although clonidine administration relieved pain to 83 ± 10% of baseline (mean ± SEM), this result was not significantly different from the results for saline placebo. Three subjects had a positive response, defined as at least 50% relief, on clonidine compared to 5 of 15 patients receiving placebo (Siddall et al. 2000). Eight of the patients received clonidine by i.t. infusion (300–500 μg/6 hours), but there was no difference in effectiveness when the two methods of administration were compared.

In summary, clonidine administered either epidurally or intrathecally is efficacious in some patients, but responses were not better than placebo in our controlled study. It is not possible to state whether clonidine is more effective for some types of injury or pain. The reason for better success in the single-blind study may be the lack of a control. However, lack of efficacy may be due to low CSF concentrations beyond the level of injury and to the failure of the drug to reach supraspinal sites of action in patients with CSF block (Siddall et al. 2000).

BACLOFEN

Reasonably strong evidence from RCTs shows that i.t. administration of the GABA-receptor agonist baclofen is effective in managing spasticity associated with SCI (Penn and Kroin 1987; Taricco et al. 2000). The benefit of i.t. baclofen in the treatment of SCI pain, however, is less clear. Pain associated with muscle spasms should be relieved with control of the spasms, an expectation that is supported by several studies. An RCT by Penn et al. (1987) included 20 subjects with spasticity due to either multiple sclerosis or SCI. The reduction in muscle tone, rigidity, and spasm frequency was significant, and this improvement was maintained during the follow-up period of a mean of 19 months (range 10–33 months). One controlled trial has assessed the effect of acute i.t. baclofen on chronic spasm-related pain among patients with a mixture of pathologies causing spasticity, including traumatic SCI (Herman et al. 1992). I.t. baclofen (50 μg bolus) significantly suppressed reflex responses to cutaneous and muscle stimulation and abolished spasm-related pain. However, the drug had no effect on musculoskeletal pain in four of these patients.

In an uncontrolled study by Loubser and Akman (1996), 12 patients with spasticity and pain (6 with neuropathic pain, 3 with musculoskeletal pain, and 3 with both pain components) secondary to SCI were assessed prior to i.t. baclofen pump implantation and again 6 and 12 months postoperatively. At both 6- and 12-month intervals, all five patients with musculoskeletal pain related to muscle spasm had an improvement in their symptoms in conjunction with control of their spasticity. One patient with musculoskeletal low back pain unrelated to spasm had no change in the level of pain.

While i.t. baclofen appears to be efficacious in patients with SCI and muscle spasm pain, its efficacy in treating neuropathic SCI pain is disputed. Herman et al. (1992) found that acute i.t. baclofen (50 μg) significantly suppressed spontaneous dysesthetic pain in seven patients, including one with traumatic SCI who was not part of the double-blind component of the study. A case series study by Taira et al. (1995) investigated the effect of an i.t. bolus injection of baclofen in 14 patients, 6 of whom had neuropathic pain due to SCI. Nine reported "substantial" pain relief starting 1–2 hours after the injection and persisting for 10–24 hours. Allodynia and hyperalgesia, if present, were relieved as well.

Despite these reports of good results in patients with neuropathic pain, other results are less promising. In the study by Loubser and Akman (1996), seven of nine patients with neuropathic pain demonstrated no significant change in pain severity, while the two remaining patients had an increase in the level of their pain. The authors suggest that the efficacy seen in other studies is due to the higher doses achieved by bolus injections and that continuous infusion results in comparably lower CSF doses. Both studies describing positive results were also assessed over a short time frame (up to 24 hours). Therefore, it is possible that although i.t. baclofen produces short-term relief, it is not sustained due to long-term receptor changes or other factors that reduce or abolish efficacy.

In summary, good evidence shows that i.t. baclofen is efficacious in managing muscle spasm and spasm-related pain following SCI, and that this benefit is preserved with long-term administration. However, although some evidence indicates that i.t. baclofen may relieve neuropathic pain in the short term, there is no evidence that it is effective in the long term, and it may even make the pain worse. However, the evidence for this possible complication remains fairly limited, and further investigation would be valuable.

COMBINATIONS

Lidocaine, morphine, clonidine, and baclofen have been used as described above as single agents in the management of SCI pain. However, numerous studies suggest that some of these drugs may have a synergistic action (Mendez et al. 1990; Gordon et al. 1992; Plummer et al. 1992, 1995; Goudas et al. 1998). Some studies have suggested that tolerance to a combination of morphine and clonidine develops more slowly than when morphine is given alone (Yaksh and Reddy 1981; Plummer et al. 1995). Combinations of these drugs thus could provide greater efficacy with lower doses and a lower incidence of side effects.

One case report suggested that i.t. administration of clonidine in combination with morphine is effective in treating neuropathic SCI pain (Siddall et al. 1994). Another case report describes good results from a combination of i.t. baclofen and clonidine against painful anal spasms in a patient with anterior cord syndrome (Middleton et al. 1996). The controlled trial described above that examined the efficacy of i.t. morphine and clonidine also tested a combination of the two agents. While no significant pain relief was obtained with either morphine or clonidine alone, a mixture of half the effective dose of both agents provided significant pain relief of 63 ± 10% of baseline (mean ± SEM) (Siddall et al. 2000). Seven of the 15 patients in this study obtained at least 50% relief of pain. Many of those who received drugs below the level of their injury had very high lumbar but negligible cervical levels of the drug in the CSF, and there was a significant relationship between pain relief and levels of morphine in the cervical CSF. Morphine and clonidine thus appear to have a synergistic effect.

CONSIDERATIONS IN THE USE OF SPINAL AGENTS

SIDE EFFECTS

I.t. administration of drugs may result in significant side effects either in the short or long term. Studies focusing on SCI pain have documented numerous side effects; respiratory depression, hypotension, sedation, pruritus, nausea, and vomiting may occur shortly after spinal administration of opioids (Glynn et al. 1986; Fenollosa et al. 1993; Siddall et al. 2000). Spinal administration of clonidine may also be associated with hypotension and sedation (Glynn et al. 1986; Siddall et al. 2000). Unfortunately, coadministration of reduced doses of clonidine with morphine did not significantly reduce side effects (Siddall et al. 2000). Few side effects have been reported following spinal administration of baclofen in the management of SCI pain. The study by Penn and Kroin (1987) reported no problems with drowsiness or confusion. The main concern appears to be the possibility of the development or worsening of neuropathic pain (Loubser and Akman 1996).

CHRONIC INTRATHECAL ADMINISTRATION OF DRUGS

The reports reviewed above provide little information regarding the long-term use of i.t. drugs in the management of SCI pain. I.t. administration of lidocaine is only used as a short-term diagnostic strategy (Loubser and Donovan 1991; Loubser and Clearman 1993), and we lack information about the long-term use of this or other local anesthetics for this type of pain. Most of the other studies described above (Glynn et al. 1986, 1992; Herman et al. 1992; Siddall et al. 2000) only evaluate short-term efficacy. More information is available regarding the long-term use of morphine. Fenollosa et al. (1993) performed follow-up evaluation at 12, 18, 24, and 36 months after i.t. pump implantation. The authors noted that 8 of 12 patients were improved at 36 months, but they did not specify the degree of improvement. Although long-term use of i.t. baclofen (up to 33 months) continued to control muscle spasms, there is no direct evidence of its usefulness in controlling chronic pain. However, presumably control of spasm would be associated with relief of musculoskeletal pain secondary to muscle spasm.

TOLERANCE

One of the reported problems with long-term use of drugs with either systemic or spinal administration is the development of tolerance (Magora 1980). As mentioned above, information is scarce regarding long-term i.t. drug use and therefore we do not know the degree to which tolerance may develop, or its time course. Fenollosa et al. (1993) provide some long-term (3-year) data on dose increases. Some tolerance was evident with the daily i.t. morphine dose, which increased from a mean of 0.6 mg/day to 4.0 mg/day over 3 years. Although little information is available that specifically relates to pain following SCI, coadministration of other drugs such as clonidine may help to reduce the development of tolerance (Coombs et al. 1985).

BOLUS VERSUS INFUSION ADMINISTRATION

Information is also scarce regarding differences in efficacy related to the mode of administration. Diagnostic tests using lidocaine have used single (Pollock et al. 1951; Davis 1954; Loubser and Clearman 1993) or multiple (Loubser and Donovan 1991) bolus administration to achieve their effect. As is the case with diagnostic procedures, these studies have focused on short-term effects and have not examined the short- or long-term effects of infusion of local anesthetic. In contrast, case reports and studies that have examined the efficacy of morphine, clonidine, and baclofen have used differing modes of administration, including bolus (Glynn et al. 1986), infusion (Siddall et al. 1994; Loubser and Akman 1996; Middleton et al. 1996), or both (Herman et al. 1992; Fenollosa et al. 1993; Siddall et al. 2000). The logistical problems and risk of infection make repeated bolus injections unsuitable for long-term management of pain or spasm. A study in which clonidine was administered by both bolus and short-term infusion revealed no difference in efficacy related to the mode of administration (Siddall et al. 2000).

FACTORS RELATED TO SCI

Differences in the type or completeness of SCI have not yet been identified as determining factors in relation to the effectiveness of spinal administration of drugs. In one study, all those with incomplete injuries had a positive response (>50% relief) to i.t. drug administration, while less than a third of those with complete injuries had a positive response (Siddall et al. 2000). In regard to pathology, evidence is even more limited. Most studies have relatively low numbers, with a mix of pathologies. Therefore, it is not possible to determine whether response is linked to the pathology responsible for SCI, such as ischemia, syrinx, tumor, or trauma.

CEREBROSPINAL FLUID OBSTRUCTION

SCI results in considerable scarring and tethering of the cord, which may obstruct CSF flow. Administration of agents below the level of injury may result in very high levels of drug below that level but small and often undetectable quantities of drug above it (Siddall et al. 2000). The resulting pain relief is poor, suggesting that drugs need to access the spinal region immediately above the injury level or possibly supraspinal sites to have an adequate clinical effect. Therefore consideration should be given to administration above the level of injury.

FUTURE DIRECTIONS

The treatment of neuropathic SCI pain is limited to a large extent by the availability of suitable drugs. Animal studies suggest several approaches that are worth exploring. The changes in nitric oxide, GABA, glycine, and NMDA receptors in the traumatized spinal cord and responsiveness to some drugs acting on these pathways suggest that drugs that act on these receptors or that modulate the availability of endogenous transmitters may be useful. Many agents appear to have a synergistic action, and coadministration of currently available or new drugs is thus an option that may prove useful. The findings with administration of NGF suggest that agents that modify the effect of neurotrophins and prevent aberrant sprouting may be useful in preventing chronic pain syndromes (Krenz et al. 1999). However, how modification of neurotrophic actions would also interfere with "good" sprouting and attempts at regeneration is not clear. The results with implantation of adrenal tissue also raise the possibility of a novel approach to supplying endogenous neurotransmitters that decrease nociceptive transmission and modify neuropathic pain states (Brewer and Yezierski 1998; Yu et al. 1998). It will be interesting to see whether further work in this area results in approaches that are feasible in the clinical situation.

ACKNOWLEDGMENT

This work is supported by the National Health and Medical Research Council of Australia.

REFERENCES

Bennett AD, Chastain KM, Hulsebosch CE. Alleviation of mechanical and thermal allodynia by $CGRP_{8-37}$ in a rodent model of chronic central pain. *Pain* 2000; 86:163–175.

Brewer KL, Yezierski RP. Effects of adrenal medullary transplants on pain-related behaviors following excitotoxic spinal cord injury. *Brain Res* 1998; 798:83–92.

Christensen MD, Hulsebosch CE. Spinal cord injury and anti-NGF treatment results in changes in CGRP density and distribution in the dorsal horn of the rat. *Exp Neurol* 1997; 147:463–475.

Coombs DW, Saunders RL, Lachance D, et al. Intrathecal morphine tolerance: use of intrathecal clonidine, DADLE, and intraventricular morphine. *Anesthesiology* 1985; 62:358–363.

Davis L. Treatment of spinal cord injuries. *AMA Arch Surg* 1954; 69:488–495.

Fenollosa P, Pallares J, Cervera J, et al. Chronic pain in the spinal cord injured: statistical approach and pharmacological treatment. *Paraplegia* 1993; 31:722–729.

Glynn CJ, Jamous MA, Teddy PJ, Moore RA, Lloyd JW. Role of spinal noradrenergic system in transmission of pain in patients with spinal cord injury. *Lancet* 1986; ii:1249–1250.

Glynn CJ, Jamous MA, Teddy PJ. Cerebrospinal fluid kinetics of epidural clonidine in man. *Pain* 1992; 49:361–367.

Gordon NC, Heller PH, Levine JD. Enhancement of pentazocine analgesia by clonidine. *Pain* 1992; 48:167–169.

Goudas LC, Carr DB, Filos KS, Laurijssens BE, Kream RM. The spinal clonidine-opioid analgesic interaction: from laboratory animals to the postoperative ward. A review of preclinical and clinical evidence. *Analgesia* 1998; 3:1–2.

Hao JX, Xu XJ, Yu YX, Seiger A, Wiesenfeld-Hallin Z. Baclofen reverses the hypersensitivity of dorsal horn wide dynamic range neurons to mechanical stimulation after transient spinal cord ischaemia; implications for a tonic GABAergic inhibitory control of myelinated fiber input. *J Neurophysiol* 1992; 68:392–396.

Hao JX, Yu W, Xu XJ, Wiesenfeld-Hallin Z. Effects of intrathecal vs. systemic clonidine in treating chronic allodynia-like response in spinally injured rats. *Brain Res* 1996; 736:28–34.

Herman RM, D'Luzansky SC, Ippolito R. Intrathecal baclofen suppresses central pain in patients with spinal lesions: a pilot study. *Clin J Pain* 1992; 8:338–345.

Krenz NR, Meakin SO, Krassioukov AV, Weaver LC. Neutralizing intraspinal nerve growth factor blocks autonomic dysreflexia caused by spinal cord injury. *J Neurosci* 1999; 19:7405–7414.

Kroin JS, Bianchi GD, Penn RD. Spinal cord transection produces a long-term increase in $GABA_B$ binding in the rat substantia gelatinosa. *Synapse* 1993; 14:263–267.

Loeser JD, Ward AA, White LE. Chronic deafferentation of human spinal cord neurons. *J Neurosurg* 1968; 29:48–50.

Loubser PG, Akman NM. Effects of intrathecal baclofen on chronic spinal cord injury pain. *J Pain Symptom Manage* 1996; 12:241–247.

Loubser PG, Clearman RR. Evaluation of central spinal cord injury pain with diagnostic spinal anesthesia. *Anesthesiology* 1993; 79:376–378.

Loubser PG, Donovan WH. Diagnostic spinal anaesthesia in chronic spinal cord injury pain. *Paraplegia* 1991; 29:25–36.

Magora F. Observations of extradural morphine analgesia in various pain conditions. *Brit J Anaesth* 1980; 52:247–257.

Mendez R, Eisenach JC, Kashtan K. Epidural clonidine analgesia after cesarean section. *Anesthesiology* 1990; 73:848–852.

Middleton JW, Siddall PJ, Walker S, Molloy AR, Rutkowski SB. Intrathecal clonidine and baclofen in the management of spasticity and neuropathic pain following spinal cord injury: a case study. *Arch Phys Med Rehabil* 1996; 77:824–826.

Penn RD, Kroin JS. Long-term intrathecal baclofen infusion for treatment of spasticity. *J Neurosurg* 1987; 66:181–185.

Plummer JL, Cmielewski PL, Gourlay GK, Owen H, Cousins MJ. Antinociceptive and motor effects of intrathecal morphine combined with intrathecal clonidine, noradrenaline, carbachol or midazolam in rats. *Pain* 1992; 49:145–152.

Plummer JL, Cmielewski PL, Tallents S, et al. Development of tolerance to antinociceptive effects of an intrathecal morphine/clonidine combination in rats. *Naunyn Schmiedebergs Arch Pharmacol* 1995; 351:618–623.

Pollock LJ, Brown M, Boshes B, et al. Pain below the level of injury of the spinal cord. *Arch Neurol Psychiatry* 1951; 65:319–322.

Siddall PJ, Gray M, Rutkowski S, Cousins MJ. Intrathecal morphine and clonidine in the management of spinal cord injury pain: a case report. *Pain* 1994; 59:147–148.

Siddall PJ, Molloy AR, Walker S, et al. Efficacy of intrathecal morphine and clonidine in the treatment of neuropathic pain following spinal cord injury. *Anesth Analg* 2000; 91:1493–1498.

Sivilotti LG, Woolf CJ. The contribution of $GABA_A$ and glycine receptors to central sensitization: disinhibition and touch-evoked allodynia in the spinal cord. *J Neurophysiol* 1994; 72:169–179.

Taira T, Kawamura H, Tanikawa T, et al. A new approach to control central deafferentation pain: spinal intrathecal baclofen. *Stereotact Funct Neurosurg* 1995; 65:101–105.

Taricco M, Adone R, Pagliacci C, Telaro E. Pharmacological interventions for spasticity following spinal cord injury. *Cochrane Database of Systematic Reviews* 2000; 2:CD001131.

Yaksh TL, Reddy SVR. Studies in the primate on the analgetic effects associated with intrathecal actions of opiates, alpha-adrenergic agonists and baclofen. *Anesthesiology* 1981; 54:451–467.

Yu W, Hao JX, Xu XJ, Wiesenfeld-Hallin Z. Comparison of the anti-allodynic and antinociceptive effects of systemic, intrathecal and intracerebroventricular morphine in a rat model of central neuropathic pain. *Eur J Pain* 1997; 1:17–29.

Yu W, Hao JX, Xu XJ, et al. Long-term alleviation of allodynia-like behaviors by intrathecal implantation of bovine chromaffin cells in rats with spinal cord injury. *Pain* 1998; 74:115–122.

Zhang AL, Hao JX, Seiger A, et al. Decreased GABA immunoreactivity in spinal cord dorsal horn neurons after transient spinal cord ischaemia in the rat. *Brain Res* 1994; 656:187–190.

Zimmerman M. Central nervous mechanisms modulating pain-related information: do they become deficient after lesions of the peripheral or central nervous system? In: Casey KL (Ed). *Pain and Central Nervous System Disease: The Central Pain Syndromes*. New York: Raven Press, 1991, pp 183–199.

Correspondence to: Philip Siddall, MBBS, PhD, Pain Management and Research Centre, Royal North Shore Hospital, St. Leonards, NSW 2065, Australia. Fax: 61 2 9926 6548; email: phils@med.usyd.edu.au.

Spinal Cord Injury Pain: Assessment, Mechanisms, Management. Progress in Pain Research and Management, Vol. 23, edited by Robert P. Yezierski and Kim J. Burchiel, IASP Press, Seattle, © 2002.

22

Glutamate Receptor Antagonists in Central Neuropathic Pain following Spinal Cord Injury

Christine N. Sang

Clinical Trials Program, MGH Pain Center, and Department of Anesthesia and Critical Care, Massachusetts General Hospital; and Department of Anaesthesia, Harvard Medical School, Boston, Massachusetts, USA

The identification of potential new mechanisms of central and peripheral neuropathic pain and the development of novel selective compounds that target these specific mechanisms should now allow for a rational clinical approach. Even in heterogeneous chronic pain syndromes following spinal cord injury (SCI), we can now begin to target central and peripheral mechanisms that include peripheral transduction, changes in membrane excitability, disinhibition, and central sensitization. Central changes that involve excitation have been proposed to take place at several levels of the central nervous system in neuropathic pain following SCI. These include: (1) spinal neuron sensitization (Melzack and Loeser 1978), (2) supraspinal mechanisms (Koyama et al. 1993; Lenz et al. 1994; Jeanmonod et al. 1996), (3) plastic changes in molecular and/or neuroanatomic pathways (Bullitt 1991; McNeill et al. 1991), and (4) unmasking of latent pathways (Willis 1991).

Several recently developed animal models of central SCI pain have similar but slightly different features (Levitt and Levitt 1981; Hao et al. 1991; Yezierski et al. 1993; Christensen et al. 1996). Despite differences in specific lesion type, all rats developed spontaneous and evoked pain behaviors, including allodynia (Yezierski 1996), similar to the human experience in which different etiologies of spinal cord lesions (i.e., traumatic versus ischemic versus inflammatory) commonly result in similar symptoms.

Pharmacological assays in behavioral animal models of neuropathic pain show that *N*-methyl-D-aspartate (NMDA) receptor antagonists act specifically as antihyperalgesic agents. Animal data suggest that this class of compounds target what we know as central sensitization (Woolf and Thompson 1991), such that previously innocuous inputs now start to activate pain transmission and responses to noxious stimuli are augmented. NMDA receptor antagonists may selectively block symptoms that result from central sensitization rather than pain that is due to ongoing C-nociceptor drive, a feature that would be of therapeutic value in the treatment of specific central neuropathic pain symptoms. A wide body of data now demonstrates the sensitivity of various sensory methods in animals with allodynia and hyperalgesia to the NMDA-receptor antagonists. In patients, central sensitization may be also be manifested as the development of a wide area of dynamic allodynia with associated temporal and spatial summation, and we would predict that either the intensity or spread of allodynia in SCI patients may be sensitive to NMDA-receptor antagonists.

Pharmacological assays in animal models of SCI show a role for NMDA-mediated central sensitization (Xu et al. 1992, 1993; Bennett 1994; Bennett et al. 2000), as has the large body of data in animal models of peripheral neuropathic pain. In the ischemic SCI rat, mechanical allodynia was dose-dependently relieved by three systemic NMDA-receptor antagonists: MK-801, dextromethorphan, and CG 19755 (Hao et al. 1991; Hao and Xu 1996). Dextromethorphan was the only one of the three that did not compromise motor function.

Clinical studies have demonstrated that spinal and systemic administration of NMDA-receptor antagonists in patients with neuropathic pain reduces spontaneous pain and hyperalgesia following single-dose administration in experimental pain (Maurset et al. 1989; Price et al. 1994; Park et al. 1995; Andersen et al. 1996; Arendt-Nielsen et al. 1996; Ilkjaer et al. 1996, 1997; Warncke et al. 1997), postoperative pain (Maurset et al. 1989; Tverskoy et al. 1994; Stubhaug et al. 1997), and chronic neuropathic pain (Kristensen et al. 1992; Backonja et al. 1994; Eide et al. 1994, 1995; Felsby and Juelsgaard 1995; Max et al. 1995; Nikolajsen et al. 1996; Nelson et al. 1997). The ceiling analgesic effect seen with NMDA-receptor antagonists in clinical studies partly be due to dose-limiting side effects such as sedation, dysphoria, catatonia, and visual distortions. On the whole, clinical trials have consistently demonstrated efficacy and support a role for NMDA receptors in neuropathic pain, as described in this chapter. These findings would open the possibility for new treatments for SCI pain in humans.

NMDA-RECEPTOR ANTAGONISTS

KETAMINE AND CPP

Ketamine. In subanesthetic doses, the systemic oral, intramuscular, intravenous, or subcutaneous administration of ketamine has been shown in case reports and case series to relieve glossopharyngeal neuralgia (Eide and Stubhaug 1997), postherpetic neuralgia (Hoffmann et al. 1994; Eide et al. 1995; Klepstad and Borchgrevink 1997), postamputation stump and phantom limb pain (Stannard and Porter 1993; Nikolajsen et al. 1997), cancer pain (Mercadante et al. 1995), and mixed neuropathic pain syndromes (Persson et al. 1995; Oye et al. 1996). Several placebo-controlled trials have confirmed these reports in postherpetic neuralgia (Eide et al. 1994), acute postoperative hyperalgesia (Stubhaug et al. 1997), phantom pain (Nikolajsen et al. 1996), acute and chronic orofacial pain (Mathisen et al. 1995), chronic post-traumatic pain (Max et al. 1995), chronic ischemic pain (Persson et al. 1995), and mixed neuropathic pain syndromes (Backonja et al. 1994; Felsby et al. 1996). Eide et al. (1995) showed an effect of ketamine on spontaneous and evoked pain following SCI.

Orally administered ketamine may have a more favorable side effect profile than ketamine administered by other routes. Oral administration of this drug is associated with higher serum concentrations of norketamine, the major metabolite of ketamine and a noncompetitive NMDA-receptor antagonist (Grant et al. 1981; Clements et al. 1982; Ebert et al. 1997). Ketamine undergoes first-pass biotransformation by the liver with a plasma norketamine/ketamine area under the curve (AUC) ratio of 6.4, indicating extensive clearance of oral ketamine to norketamine (Shimoyama et al. 1999). The ability to achieve relatively high levels of norketamine in the brain (the norketamine/ketamine AUC ratio in the brain can reach as high as 2.9; Shimoyama et al. 1999), the demonstration that spinal norketamine is equipotent to ketamine in the phase 2 formalin test (Shimoyama et al. 1999), and the shorter duration of psychomotor effects of norketamine compared with ketamine (Leung and Baillie 1986) suggest that oral ketamine may provide a better therapeutic ratio for analgesia than the same drug administered by other routes. Case reports and case series have demonstrated the successful use of oral ketamine in experimental ischemic arm pain (Grant et al. 1981), postherpetic neuralgia (Hoffmann et al. 1994), neuropathic pain (Broadley et al. 1996; Enarson et al. 1999; Fisher and Hagen 1999), and postamputation stump pain (Nikolajsen et al. 1997). However, adverse effects limited the ability to evaluate analgesic effect in 21 patients receiving chronic oral ketamine therapy, causing most subjects to withdraw prematurely (Haines and Gaines 1999).

CPP. The competitive NMDA-receptor antagonist 3-(2-carboxypiperazin-4-yl)propyl-1-phosphonic acid (CPP) is a piperazine derivative (Lehmann et al. 1987). In one patient, Kristensen et al. (1992) demonstrated that intrathecal administration of CPP reduced the widespread area of pain evoked by low-threshold mechanical and thermal stimuli outside the territory of the injured nerve to a distribution consistent with the injured nerve territory. The authors suggested that CPP modulates pathological pain due to peripheral and central sensitization at the spinal level, and proposed that chronic protracted allodynia may involve mechanisms different from acute allodynia in experimental animal models. CPP is strongly hydrophilic (Hays et al. 1990), so that intrathecal administration at the lower lumbar level would be expected to result in rostral spread of CPP, which could have accounted for the psychotomimetic side effects that developed 4 hours following the last dose.

LOW-AFFINITY CHANNEL-BLOCKING NMDA-RECEPTOR ANTAGONISTS

The neurobehavioral toxicity of the dissociative anesthetics such as phencyclidine, ketamine, and dizocilpine has been attributed to their use-dependent blockade of the NMDA channel (Rogawski 1993). The "uncompetitive" NMDA antagonists with affinity at the phencyclidine site depend on the receptor channel to be gated in the open state. The newer phenylcyclohexylamines (primary amine analogues of phencyclidine) produce fewer neuropsychological deficits, attributed to the low micromolar affinity for the NMDA receptor. In the context of epilepsy, Rogawski (1993) has proposed that these low-affinity channel-blocking antagonists may, by exhibiting faster rates of block and unblock, contribute to their more favorable toxicity profile. These antagonists would be expected to reach equilibrium more rapidly to achieve the same degree of block as the higher affinity antagonists.

The low-affinity NMDA-receptor antagonists include dextromethorphan and dextrorphan, remacemide, amantadine, memantine and other adamantane analogues (Choi et al. 1987; Wong et al. 1988; Tortella et al. 1989). Dextrorphan has higher affinity than dextromethorphan (dextrorphan, 0.17 μM versus dextromethorphan, 1.5 μM) (Coughenour and Barr 2001), followed by memantine (0.54 μM) (Kornhuber et al. 1991) and remacemide (68 μM) (Palmer et al. 1992; Subramaniam et al. 1996).

Dextromethorphan. The *d* isomer of levorphanol, the antitussive dextromethorphan, and its O-demethylated metabolite dextrorphan both antagonize voltage-dependent calcium channels and NMDA-receptor-operated channels (Carpenter et al. 1988). The antitussive effect of dextromethorphan is not reversed by naloxone (Cavanaugh et al. 1976), and therefore must not be mediated by a μ-opioid-receptor mechanism. Dextromethorphan is primarily metabolized by the cytochrome P450 2D6 isoenzyme, and genetic polymorphism largely accounts for the wide variability in dose requirements (Capon et al. 1996). About 6% of Caucasians are slow metabolizers at this locus and may require longer dosing intervals to avoid severe sedation or dissociative reactions, and the situation is similar for patients taking 2D6 enzyme inhibitors such as quinidine, paroxetine, fluoxetine, or slowly eliminated metabolites such as norfluoxetine (Zhang et al. 1992; Preskorn 1997; Virani et al. 1997). Dextromethorphan increases serotonin levels at central synapses, and concomitant administration of antidepressants that block serotonin reuptake or monoamine oxidase inhibitors may cause a life-threatening serotonin syndrome (Bodner et al. 1995).

The effect of dextromethorphan or dextrorphan on mechanical allodynia in animals varies among neuropathic pain models (Tal and Bennett 1993, 1994; Chaplan et al. 1997), and data in humans have been equally conflicting. Nelson et al. (1997) and Sang et al. (1997) showed a significant analgesic effect of dextromethorphan at significantly higher doses in diabetic neuropathy, but were unable to detect a treatment effect in postherpetic neuralgia. In a case series, Suzuki et al. (1996) noted a similar response rate (36%) to that shown by Nelson (38%) in patients with postherpetic neuralgia. Studies evaluating dextromethorphan in SCI patients are reaching completion (Sang et al. 2002).

Steinberg and Bell (1991) showed that doses of 1440 mg/day are needed to achieve adequate brain tissue concentrations of dextromethorphan for neuroprotection. Although associated with psychotomimetic side effects at high doses, dextromethorphan is not associated with the potential for fatal overdose or organ toxicity (Bern and Peck 1992). Thus, inadequate dosing may have accounted for, in part, the inability of McQuay et al. (1994) to demonstrate a significant analgesic effect of 81 mg/day in patients with neuropathic pain.

Amantadine and memantine. The antiviral agent amantadine and the antiparkinsonian agent memantine are both 1-amino-3,5-dimethyl-adamantane derivatives. The adamantane analogues are lower affinity, uncompetitive NMDA-receptor antagonists (Bormann 1989; Chen at al. 1992; Blanpied et al. 1997). Amantadine and memantine reduce hyperalgesia in animal models (Carlton and Hargett 1995; Eisenberg et al. 1995; Chaplan et al. 1997), and cause fewer adverse effects than ketamine (Kornhuber et al. 1994).

Unfortunately, the efficacy of the adamantane analogues has not been consistently confirmed in clinical studies. Eisenberg and Pud (1998) noted that single-dose intravenous administration of amantadine completely resolved spontaneous pain, mechanical allodynia, and hyperalgesia in three patients with neuropathic pain following nerve injury or surgery. Pud et al. (1998) demonstrated that the same treatment was analgesic and antihyperalgesic in patients with cancer pain. However, neither Taira (1998), using the oral formulation in patients with neuropathic pain, nor Medrik-Goldberg et al. (1999), using the intravenous formulation in patients with sciatica, could demonstrate a similar effect.

Memantine has been evaluated for the treatment of diabetic neuropathy and postherpetic neuralgia in two clinical trials (Sang et al. 1997; Neurobiological Technologies, Inc. 1998; Pellegrino et al. 2000). Sang et al. (1997) were unable to detect a treatment effect in either diagnostic subgroup, when compared to the active placebo, lorazepam. Pellegrino et al. (2000) claim in an abstract that memantine relieved pain more than placebo in patients with diabetic neuropathy. Eisenberg et al. (1998) were also unable to detect a significant effect in patients with postherpetic neuralgia.

Remacemide. The anticonvulsant remacemide, 2-amino-*N*-(1-methyl-1,2-diphenyl)acetamide hydrochloride, and its pharmacologically active, more potent desglycine metabolite, ARL12495AA, are also low-affinity NMDA-channel antagonists (Palmer et al. 1992; Grant et al. 1996; Subramaniam et al. 1996). Remacemide not only has low-affinity uncompetitive blocking activity of the PCP site of the NMDA receptor, but also blocks fast sodium channels (Palmer and Hutchinson 1997). Clinical data support a role of remacemide for the treatment of refractory epilepsy (Scheyer et al. 1992; Chadwick et al. 2000; Richens et al. 2000). Phase II analgesic studies are currently underway.

OTHER AGENTS

Magnesium. Magnesium sulfate has been used clinically by obstetricians as a tocolytic and treatment for pre-eclampsia and eclampsia. Magnesium ions prevent extracellular calcium ions from entering the cell by exerting a physiological block of the ion channel coupled to the NMDA receptor. Felsby and Juelsgaard (1995) were unable to demonstrate a statistically significant reduction of pain and allodynia in patients with peripheral neuropathic pain at doses used in trials of myocardial infarction.

Riluzole. The exact mechanisms of riluzole has not been well elucidated (Doble et al. 1992), although research has shown that this agent prevents L-glutamate- and kainate-induced seizures. Researchers have suggested that riluzole noncompetitively inhibits the NMDA and kainate receptors (Debono et al. 1993), as well as inactivated sodium channels (Benoit and Escande 1991). Riluzole prolongs both the progression and survival of amyotrophic lateral sclerosis (Louvel 1997). It is currently in phase II trials in neuropathic pain.

EFFICACY AND TOXICITY

The clinically available channel-blocking NMDA-receptor antagonists have consistently been associated with phencyclidine-like cognitive effects (i.e., feelings of intoxication or delirium, dissociative effects, and/or vivid dreams). Moreover, both ketamine and dextromethorphan dose-dependently impair attention and memory (Ghoneim et al. 1985; Albers et al. 1992; Krystal et al. 1994; Hollander et al. 1994; Malhotra et al. 1996; Steinberg et al. 1996). Such adverse effects may have compromised the double-blinded nature of trials evaluating NMDA-receptor antagonists (Moscucci et al. 1987). Sang et al. (1997) incorporated an active placebo, lorazepam, into a trial evaluating the analgesic efficacy of dextromethorphan and memantine in an attempt to control for the influence of cognitive side effects on therapeutic response.

The potential for histopathological findings of neuronal injury has clouded the safety profile of the NMDA-receptor antagonists. Post-mortem histopathological changes of subpial spinal cord vacuolization has been noted following intrathecal ketamine (Karpinski et al. 1997). However, no other human autopsy studies note central nervous system changes such as neuronal vacuolization, as has been demonstrated in rat cortical neurons (Olney et al. 1989, 1991).

An approach to widening the therapeutic ratio of NMDA-receptor blockade includes the targeting of specific NMDA-receptor subunit combinations. Specifically, the development of the NR2B subtype antagonists may provide superior analgesia with the potential for a wider therapeutic ratio than that provided by nonspecific channel blockers such as dextromethorphan in patients with neuropathic pain (Taniguchi et al. 1997; Boyce et al. 1999). Immunocytochemical studies have demonstrated a distribution of the NR2B subunit in laminae I and II of the spinal cord dorsal horn, and the NR2B-subunit-selective antagonist CP101,606 is antihyperalgesic in neuropathic rats without impairing rotarod performance (Boyce et al. 1999). In addition, NMDA antagonists whose structure limits them to the periphery, where NMDA receptors are abundant (Davidson and Carlton 1998), may lack the sedative and psychotomimetic effects of currently available drugs.

The narrow therapeutic ratio associated with the use of the clinically available NMDA-receptor antagonists may be overcome by the use of drug combinations, by the development of newer low-affinity NMDA-channel antagonists and more selective systemic NMDA-receptor antagonists (which modulate binding sites within the NMDA complex, or have affinity at specific NMDA-receptor subtypes), and by the selective administration of available agents. The heterogeneity of the pain state following SCI may make treatment for each individual difficult, and may require an analgesic regimen that interacts at several selective sites with the potential for acting synergistically in terms of efficacy but not toxicity.

REFERENCES

Albers GW, Saenz RE, Moses JA. Tolerability of oral dextromethorphan in patients with a history of brain ischemia. *Clin Neuropharmacol* 1992; 15(6):509–514.

Andersen S, Dickenson AH, Kohn M, et al. The opioid ketobemidone has a NMDA blocking effect. *Pain* 1996; 67:369–374.

Arendt-Nielsen L, Nielsen J, Peterson-Felix S, et al. Effect of racemic mixture and the (S+)-isomer of ketamine on temporal and spatial summation of pain. *Br J Anaesth* 1996; 77:625–631.

Backonja M, Arndt G, Gombar KA, Check B, Zimmermann M. Response of chronic neuropathic pain syndromes to ketamine: a preliminary study. *Pain* 1994; 56:51–57.

Bennett AD, Everhart AW, Hulsebosch CE. Intrathecal administration of an NMDA or a non-NMDA receptor antagonist reduces mechanical but not thermal allodynia in a rodent model of chronic central pain after spinal cord injury. *Brain Res* 2000; 859(1):72–82.

Bennett GJ. Neuropathic pain. In: Wall PD. Melzack R (Eds). *Textbook of Pain*. Edinburgh: Churchill Livingstone, 1994, pp 201–224.

Benoit E, Escande D. Riluzole specifically blocks inactivated Na channels in myelinated nerve fibre. *Pflugers Arch* 1991; 419(6):603–609.

Bern J, Peck R. Dextromethorphan: an overview of safety issues. *Drug Safety* 1992; 7:190–199.

Blanpied TA, Boeckman FA, Aizeman E, Johnson JW. Trapping channel block of NMDA-activated responses by amantadine and memantine. *J Neurophysiol* 1997; 77:309–323.

Bodner RA, Lynch T, Lewis L, Kahn D. Serotonin syndrome. *Neurology* 1995; 45:219–223.

Bormann J. Memantine is a potent blocker of *N*-methyl-D-aspartate (NMDA) receptor channels. *Eur J Pharmacol* 1989; 166:591–592.

Boyce S, Wyatt A, Webb JK, et al. Selective NMDA NR2B antagonists induce antinociception without motor dysfunction: correlation with restricted localisation of NR2B subunit in dorsal horn. *Neuropharmacology* 1999; 38(5):611–623.

Broadley KE, Kurowska A, Tookman A. Ketamine injection used orally. *Palliat Med* 1996; 10(3):247–250.

Bullitt E. Abnormal anatomy of deafferentation: regeneration and sprouting within the central nervous system, in deafferentation pain syndromes: Pathophysiology and treatment. In: Nashold, Ovelmen-Levitt (Eds). New York: Raven Press, 1991.

Capon DA, Bochner F, Kerry N, et al. The influence of CYP2D6 polymorphism and quinidine on the disposition and antitussive effect of dextromethorphan in humans. *Clin Pharmacol Ther* 1996; 60:295–307.

Carlton SM, Hargett GL. Treatment with the NMDA antagonist memantine attenuates nociceptive responses to mechanical stimulation in neuropathic rats. *Neurosci Lett* 1995; 198:115–118.

Carpenter CL, Mark SS, Watson DL, Greenberg DA. Dextromethorphan and dextrorphan as calcium channel antagonists. *Brain Res* 1988; 439:371–375.

Cavanaugh RL, Gylys JA, Bierwagen ME. Antitussive properties of butorphanol. *Arch Int Pharmacodyn Ther* 1976; 220:258–268.

Chadwick D, Smith D, Crawford P, Harrison B. Remacemide hydrochloride: a placebo-controlled, one month, double-blind assessment of its safety, tolerability and pharmacokinetics as adjunctive therapy in patients with epilepsy. *Seizure* 2000; 9(8):544–550.

Chaplan SR, Malmberg AB, Yaksh TL. Efficacy of spinal NMDA receptor antagonism in formalin hyperalgesia and nerve injury evoked allodynia in the rat. *J Pharmacol Exp Ther* 1997; 280(2):829–838.

Chen HS, Pellegrini JW, Aggarwal SK, et al. Open-channel block of *N*-methyl-D-aspartate (NMDA) responses by memantine: therapeutic advantage against NMDA receptor-mediated neurotoxicity. *J Neurosci* 1992; 12(11):4427–4436.

Choi DW, Peters S, Viseskul V. Dextrorphan and levorphanol selectively block *N*-methyl-D-aspartate receptor-mediated neurotoxicity on cortical neurons. *J Pharmacol Exp Ther* 1987; 242(2):713–720.

Christensen MD, Everhart AW, Pickelman JT, Hulsebosch CE. Mechanical and thermal allodynia in chronic central pain following spinal cord injury. *Pain* 1996; 68:97–107.

Clements JA, Nimmo WS, Grant IS. Bioavailability, pharmacokinetics, and analgesic activity of ketamine in humans. *J Pharm Sci* 1982; 71(5):539–542.

Coughenour LL, Barr BM. Use of trifluoroperazine isolates a [(3)H]ifenprodil binding site in rat brain membranes with the pharmacology of the voltage-independent ifenprodil site on *N*-methyl-D-aspartate receptors containing NR2B subunits. *J Pharmacol Exp Ther* 2001; 296(1):150–159.

Davidson EM, Carlton SM. Intraplantar injection of dextrorphan, ketamine or memantine attenuates formalin-induced behaviors. *Brain Res* 1998; 785(1):136–142.

Debono MW, Le Guern J, Canton T, Doble A, Pradier L. Inhibition by riluzole of electrophysiological responses mediated by rat kainate and NMDA receptors expressed in *Xenopus* oocytes. *Eur J Pharmacol* 1993; 235(2–3):283–289.

Doble A, Hubert JP, Blanchard JC. Pertussis toxin pretreatment abolishes the inhibitory effect of riluzole and carbachol on D-[3H]aspartate release from cultured cerebellar granule cells. *Neurosci Lett* 1992; 140(2):251–254.

Ebert B, Mikkelsen S, Thorkildsen C, Borgbjerg FM. Norketamine, the main metabolite of ketamine, is a non-competitive NMDA receptor antagonist in the rat cortex and spinal cord. *Eur J Pharmacol* 1997; 333(1):99–104.

Eide PK, Stubhaug A. Relief of glossopharyngeal neuralgia by ketamine-induced *N*-methyl-aspartate receptor blockade. *Neurosurgery* 1997; 41(2):505–508.

Eide PK, Jørum E, Stubhaug A, Bremmes J, Breivik H. Relief of post-herpetic neuralgia with the *N*-methyl-D-aspartic acid receptor antagonist ketamine: a double-blind, cross-over comparison with morphine and placebo. *Pain* 1994; 58:347–354.

Eide K, Stubhaug A, Oye I, Breivik H. Continuous subcutaneous administration of the *N*-methyl-D-aspartic acid (NMDA) receptor antagonist ketamine in the treatment of post-herpetic neuralgia. *Pain* 1995; 61(2):221–228.

Eisenberg E, Pud D. Can patients with chronic neuropathic pain be cured by acute administration of the NMDA receptor antagonist amantadine? *Pain* 1998; 74(2–3):337–339.

Eisenberg E, LaCross S, Strassman AM. The clinically tested *N*-methyl-D-aspartate receptor antagonist memantine blocks and reverses thermal hyperalgesia in a rat model of painful mononeuropathy. *Neurosci Lett* 1995; 187:17–20.

Eisenberg E, Kleiser A, Doertort A, Haim T, Yarnitsky D. The NMDA receptor antagonist memantine in the treatment of postherpetic neuralgia: a double-blind, placebo-controlled study. *Eur J Pain* 1998; 2:321–327.

Enarson MC, Hays H, Woodroffe MA. Clinical experience with oral ketamine. *J Pain Symptom Manage* 1999; 17(5):384–386.

Felsby S, Juelsgaard P. Combined spinal and epidural anesthesia. *Anesth Analg* 1995; 80(4),821–826.

Felsby S, Nielsen J, Arendt-Nielsen L, Jensen TS. NMDA receptor blockade in chronic neuropathic pain: a comparison of ketamine and magnesium chloride. *Pain* 1996; 64(2):283–291.

Fisher K, Hagen NA. Analgesic effect of oral ketamine in chronic neuropathic pain of spinal origin: a case report. *J Pain Symptom Manage* 1999; 18(1):61–66.

Ghoneim MM, Hinrichs JV, Mewaldt SP, Petersen RC. Ketamine: behavioral effects of subanesthetic doses. *J Clin Psychopharmacol* 1985; 5:70–77.

Grant IS, Nimmo WS, Clements JA. Pharmacokinetics and analgesic effects of i.m. and oral ketamine. *Br J Anaesth* 1981; 53(8):805–810.

Grant KA, Colombo G, Grant J, Rogawski MA. Dizocilpine-like discriminative stimulus effects of low-affinity uncompetitive NMDA antagonists. *Neuropharmacology* 1996; 35:1709–1719.

Haines DR, Gaines SP. *N* of 1 randomised controlled trials of oral ketamine in patients with chronic pain. *Pain* 1999; 83(2):283–287.

Hao JX, Xu XJ. Treatment of a chronic allodynia-like response in spinally injured rats: effects of systemically administered excitatory amino acid receptor antagonists. *Pain* 1996; 66:279–285.

Hao JX, Xu XJ, Aldskogius H, Seiger A, Wiesenfeld-Hallin Z. Allodynia-like effects in rat after ischaemic spinal cord injury photochemically induced by laser irradiation. *Pain* 1991; 45:175–185.

Hays SJ, Bigge CF, Novak PM, et al. New and versatile approaches to the synthesis of CPP-related competitive NMDA antagonists. Preliminary structure-activity relationships and pharmacological evaluation. *J Med Chem* 1990; 33:2916–2924.

Hoffmann V, Coppejans H, Vercauteren M, Adriaensen H. Successful treatment of postherpetic neuralgia with oral ketamine. *Clin J Pain* 1994; 10(3):240–242.

Hollander D, Pradas J, Kaplan R, et al. High-dose dextromethorphan in amyotrophic lateral sclerosis: Phase I safety and pharmacokinetic studies. *Ann Neurol* 1994; 36(6):920–924.

Ilkjaer S, Peterson KL, Brennum J, et al. Effects of systemic *N*-methyl-D-aspartate receptor antagonist (ketamine) on primary and secondary hyperalgesia in humans. *Br J Anaesth* 1996; 76:829–834.

Ilkjaer S, Dirks J, Brennum J, Wernberg M, Dahl JB. Effect of systemic *N*-methyl-D-aspartate receptor antagonist (dextromethorphan) on primary and secondary hyperalgesia in humans. *Br J Anaesth* 1997; 79(5):600–605.

Jeanmonod D, Magnin M, Morel A. Low-threshold calcium spike bursts in the human thalamus. Common physiopathology for sensory, motor and limbic positive symptoms. *Brain* 1996; 119:363–375.

Karpinski N, Dunn J, Hansen L, Masliah E. Subpial vacuolar myelopathy after intrathecal ketamine: report of a case. *Pain* 1997; 73(1):103–105.

Klepstad P, Borchgrevink PC. Four years' treatment with ketamine and a trial of dextromethorphan in a patient with severe post-herpetic neuralgia. *Acta Anaesthesiol Scand* 1997; 41(3):422–426.

Kornhuber J, Bormann J, Hubers M, Rusche K, Riederer P. Effects of the 1-amino-adamantanes at the MK-801-binding site of the NMDA-receptor-gated ion channel: a human postmortem brain study. *Eur J Pharmacol* 1991; 206(4):297–300.

Kornhuber J, Weller M, Schoppmehyer K, Riedere P. Amantadine and memantine are NMDA receptor antagonists with neuroprotective properties. *J Neural Transm Suppl* 1994; 43:91–104.

Koyama S, Katayama Y, Maejima S, et al. Thalamic neuronal hyperactivity following transection of the spinothalamic tract in the cat: involvement of *N*-methyl-D-aspartate receptor. *Brain Res* 1993; 612:345–350.

Kristensen JD, Svensson B, Gordh T. The NMDA-receptor antagonist CPP abolishes neurogenic 'wind-up pain' after intrathecal administration in humans. *Pain* 1992; 51(2):249–253.

Krystal JH, Karper LP, Seibyl JP. Subanesthetic effects of the noncompetitive NMDA antagonist, ketamine, in humans. Psychotomimetic, perceptual, cognitive, and neuroendocrine responses. *Arch Gen Psychiatry* 1994; 51(3):199–214.

Lehmann J, Schneider J, McPherson S, et al. CPP, a selective *N*-methyl-D-aspartate (NMDA)-type receptor antagonist: characterization in vitro and in vivo. *J Pharmacol Exp Ther* 1987; 240(3):737–746.

Lenz FA, Kwan HC, Martin R, et al. Characteristics of somatotopic organization and spontaneous neuronal activity in the region of the thalamic principal sensory nucleus in patients with spinal cord transection. *J Neurophysiol* 1994; 72:1570–1587.

Leung LY, Baillie TA. Comparative pharmacology in the rat of ketamine and its two principal metabolites, norketamine and (Z)-6-hydroxynorketamine. *J Med Chem* 1986; 29(11):2396–2369.

Levitt M, Levitt JH. The deafferentation syndrome in monkeys: dysaesthesias of spinal origin. *Pain* 1981; 10:129–147.

Louvel E. Riluzole in amyotrophic lateral sclerosis. In: Herrling P (Ed). *Excitatory Amino Acids: Clinical Results with Antagonists.* San Diego: Academic Press, 1997, pp 99–108.

Malhotra AK, Pinals DA, Weingartner H, et al. NMDA receptor function and human cognition: the effects of ketamine in healthy volunteers. *Neuropsychopharmacology* 1996; 14:301–307.

Mathisen LC, Skjelbred P, Skoglund LA, Oye I. Effect of ketamine, an NMDA receptor inhibitor, in acute and chronic orofacial pain. *Pain* 1995; 61(2):215–220.

Maurset A, Skoglund LA, Hustveit O, Oye I. Comparison of ketamine and pethidine in experimental and postoperative pain. *Pain* 1989; 36(1):37–41.

Max MB, Byas-Smith MG, Gracely RH, Bennett GJ. Intravenous infusion of the NMDA antagonist, ketamine, in chronic posttraumatic pain with allodynia: a double-blind comparison to alfentanil and placebo. *Clin Neuropharmacol* 1995; 18:360–368.

McNeill DL, Carlton SM, Hulsebosch CE. Intraspinal sprouting of calcitonin gene-related peptide containing primary afferents after deafferentation in the rat. *Exp Neurol* 1991; 114:321–329.

McQuay HJ, Carroll D, Jadad AR, et al. Dextromethorphan for the treatment of neuropathic pain: a double-blind randomised controlled crossover trial with integral n-of-1 design. *Pain* 1994; 9(1):127–133.

Medrik-Goldberg T, Lifschitz D, Pud D, Adler R, Eisenberg E. Intravenous lidocaine, amantadine, and placebo in the treatment of sciatica: a double-blind, randomized, controlled study. *Reg Anesth Pain Med* 1999; 24(6):534–540.

Melzack R, Loeser JD. Phantom body pain in paraplegics: evidence for a central "pattern generating mechanism" for pain. *Pain* 1978; 4:195–210.

Mercadante S, Lodi F, Sapio M, Calligara M, Serretta R. Long-term ketamine subcutaneous continuous infusion in neuropathic cancer pain. *J Pain Symptom Manage* 1995; 10(7):564–568.

Moscucci M, Byrne L, Weintraub M, Cox C. Blinding, unblinding, and the placebo effect: an analysis of patients' guesses of treatment assignment in a double-blind clinical trial. *Clin Pharmacol Ther* 1987; 41(3):259–265.

Nelson KA, Park KM, Robinovitz E, Tsigos C, Max MB. High-dose oral dextromethorphan versus placebo in painful diabetic neuropathy and postherpetic neuralgia. *Neurology* 1997; 48(5):1212–1218.

Neurobiological Technologies, Inc. Results from phase II neuropathic pain trial: positive data support further clinical development of memantine in patients with painful diabetic neuropathy. January 28, 1998.

Nikolajsen L, Hansen CL, Nielsen J, et al. The effect of ketamine on phantom pain: a central neuropathic disorder maintained by peripheral input. *Pain* 1996; 67(1):69–77.

Nikolajsen L, Hansen PO, Jensen TS. Oral ketamine therapy in the treatment of postamputation stump pain. *Acta Anaesthesiol Scand* 1997; 41(3):427–429.

Olney JW, Labruyere J, Price MT. Pathological changes induced in cerebrocortical neurons by phencyclidine and related drugs. *Science* 1989; 244:1360–362.

Olney JW, Labruyere J, Wang G, et al. NMDA antagonist neurotoxicity: mechanism and prevention. *Science* 1991; 254:1515–1518.

Oye I, Rabben T, Fagerlund TH. Analgesic effect of ketamine in a patient with neuropathic pain. *Tidsskr Nor Laegeforen* 1996; 116(26):3130–3131.

Park KM, Max MB, Robinovitz E, Gracely RH, Bennett GJ. Effects of intravenous ketamine, alfentanil, or placebo on pain, pinprick hyperalgesia, and allodynia produced by intradermal capsaicin in human subjects. *Pain* 1995; 63(2):163–172.

Palmer GC, Hutchinson JB. Preclinical and clinical aspects of remacemide hydrochloride. In: Herrling P (Ed). *Excitatory Amino Acids: Clinical Results with Agonists.* San Diego: Academic Press, 1997, pp 109–120.

Palmer GC, Murray RJ, Wilson TC, et al. Biological profile of the metabolites and potential metabolites of the anticonvulsant remacemide. *Epilepsy Res* 1992; 12:9–20.

Pellegrino RG, Petit WA, Brazg R, et al. Memantine in the treatment of diabetic peripheral neuropathy: a placebo-controlled phase IIB trial. *Neurology* 2000; 54:(Suppl. 7)A82–A82.

Persson J, Axelsson G, Hallin RG, Gustafsson LL. Beneficial effects of ketamine in a chronic pain state with allodynia, possibly due to central sensitization. *Pain* 1995; 60(2):217–222.

Preskorn SH. Clinically relevant pharmacology of selective serotonin reuptake inhibitors: an overview with emphasis of pharmacokinetics and effects on oxidative drug metabolism. *Clin Pharmacokinet* 1997; 32(Suppl 1):1–21.

Price DD, Mao J, Frenk H, Mayer DJ. The *N*-methyl-D-aspartate receptor antagonist dextromethorphan selectively reduces temporal summation of second pain in man. *Pain* 1994; 59(2):165–174.

Pud D, Eisenberg E, Spitzer A, Adler R, Fried G, Yarnitsky D. The NMDA receptor antagonist amantadine reduces surgical neuropathic pain in cancer patients: a double blind, randomized, placebo controlled trial. *Pain* 1998; 75(2-3):349–354.

Richens A, Mawer G, Crawford P, Harrison B. A placebo-controlled, double-blind cross-over trial of adjunctive one month remacemide hydrochloride treatment in patients with refractory epilepsy. *Seizure* 2000; 9(8):537–543.

Rogawski MA. Therapeutic potential of excitatory amino acid antagonists: channel blockers and 2,3-benzodiazepines. *Trends Pharmacol Sci* 1993; 14:325–331.

Sang CN, Parada S, Booher S, Robinovitz E, Max MB. A double-blinded randomized controlled trial of dextromethorphan versus memantine versus active placebo in patients with painful diabetic neuropathy and post-herpetic neuralgia. American Pain Society, 1997.

Sang CN, Dobosh L, Miller VA, Brown R. Combination therapy for refractory pain following spinal cord injury using the low affinity N-methyl-D-aspartate (NMDA) receptor antagonist dextromethorphan and gabapentin. *Anesthesiology* 2002; in press.

Scheyer. Remacemide elimination after initial and chronic dosing. *Clin Pharmacol Ther* 1992; 51(2):121–194.

Shimoyama M, Shimoyama N, Gorman AL, Elliott KJ, Inturrisi CE. Oral ketamine is antinociceptive in the rat formalin test: role of the metabolite, norketamine. *Pain* 1999; 81(1-2):85–93.

Stannard CF, Porter GE. Ketamine hydrochloride in the treatment of phantom limb pain. *Pain* 1993; 54(2):227–230.

Steinberg GK, Bell T. Clinical dose-escalation safety study of the NMDA antagonist, dextromethorphan in neurosurgical patients. *Stroke* 1991; 22:141.

Steinberg GK, Bell TE, Yenari MA. Dose escalation safety and tolerance study of the *N*-methyl-D-aspartate antagonist dextromethorphan in neurosurgery patients. *J Neurosurg* 1996; 84(5):860–866.

Stubhaug A, Breivik H, Eide PK, Kreunen M, Foss A. Mapping of punctuate hyperalgesia around a surgical incision demonstrates that ketamine is a powerful suppressor of central sensitization of pain following surgery. *Acta Anaesthesiol Scand* 1997; 41:1124–1132.

Subramaniam S, Donevan SD, Rogawski MA. Block of the *N*-methyl-D-aspartate receptor by remacemide and its des- glycine metabolite. *J Pharmacol Exp Ther* 1996; 276:161–168.

Suzuki T, Kato J, Saeki S, Ogawa S, Suzuki H. Analgesic effect of dextromethorphan for postherpetic neuralgia [Japanese]. *Masui* 1996; 45(5):629–633.

Taira T. Comments on Eisenberg and Pud, *Pain* 74:337–339. *Pain* 1998; 78:221–226.

Tal M, Bennett GJ. Dextrorphan relieves neuropathic heat-evoked hyperalgesia in the rat. *Neuroscience Lett* 1993; 151(1):107–110.

Tal M, Bennett GJ. Extra-territorial pain in rats with a peripheral mononeuropathy: mechano-hyperalgesia and mechano-allodynia in the territory of an uninjured nerve. *Pain* 1994; 57(3):375–382.

Taniguchi K, Shinjo K, Mizutani M, et al. Antinociceptive activity of CP-101,606, an NMDA receptor NR2B subunit antagonist. *Br J Pharmacol* 1997; 122(5):809–812.

Tortella F, Pellicano M, Bowery N. Dextromethorphan and neuromodulation: old drug coughs up new activities. *Trends Pharmacol Sci* 1989; 10:501–507.

Tverskoy M, Oz Y, Isakson A, et al. Preemptive effect of fentanyl and ketamine on postoperative pain and wound hyperalgesia. *Anesth Analg* 1994; 78(2):205–209.

Virani A, Mailis A, Shapiro LE, Shear NH. Drug interactions in human neuropathic pain pharmacotherapy. *Pain* 1997; 73:3–13.

Warncke T, Stubhaug A, Jørum E. Ketamine, an NMDA receptor antagonist, suppresses spatial and temporal properties of burn-induced secondary hyperalgesia in man: a double-blind, cross-over comparison with morphine and placebo. *Pain* 1997; 72:99–106.

Willis WD. Central neurogenic pain: Possible mechanisms. In: Nashold, Ovelmen-Levitt (Eds). *Deafferentation Pain Syndromes: Pathophysiology and Treatment.* New York: Raven Press, 1991.

Wong BY, Coulter DA, Choi DW, Prince DA. Dextrorphan and dextromethorphan, common antitussives, are antiepileptic and antagonize *N*-methyl-D-aspartate in brain slices. *Neurosci Lett* 1988; 85(2):261–266.

Woolf CJ, Thompson SW. The induction and maintenance of central sensitization is dependent on *N*-methyl-D-aspartic acid receptor activation; implications for the treatment of post-injury pain hypersensitivity states. *Pain* 1991; 44:293–299.

Xu XJ, Hao JX, Seiger A, et al. Systemic mexiletine relieves chronic allodynialike symptoms in rats with ischemic spinal cord injury. *Anesth Analg* 1992; 74;649–652.

Xu XJ, Hao JX, Seiger A, Wiesenfeld-Hallin Z. Systemic excitatory amino acid receptor antagonists of the a-amino-3-hydroxy-5-methyl-4-isoxazolepropionic acid (AMPA) receptor and of the *N*-methyl-D-aspartate (NMDA) receptor relieve mechanical hypersensitivity after transient spinal cord ischemia in rats. *J Pharmacol Exp Ther* 1993; 267:140–144.

Yezierski RP. Pain following spinal cord injury: the clinical problem and experimental studies. *Pain* 1996; 68:185–194.

Yezierski RP, Park SH. The mechanosensitivity of spinal sensory neurones following intraspinal injections of quisqualic acid in the rat. *Neurosci Lett* 1993; 115–119.

Zhang Y, Britto MR, Valderhaug KL, Wedlund PJ, Smith AR. Dextromethorphan: enhancing its systemic availability by way of low-dose quinidine-mediated inhibition of cytochrome P4502D6. *Clin Pharmacol Ther* 1992; 51:647–655.

Correspondence to: Christine N. Sang, MD, MPH, Department of Anaesthesia, Harvard Medical School, 55 Fruit Street, Clinics 3, Boston, MA 02114, USA. Tel: 617-724-0330; Fax: 617-734-6210; email: csang@partners.org.

Spinal Cord Injury Pain: Assessment, Mechanisms, Management. Progress in Pain Research and Management, Vol. 23, edited by Robert P. Yezierski and Kim J. Burchiel, IASP Press, Seattle, © 2002.

23

Examples of the Use of Gabapentin in the Treatment of Spinal Cord Injury Pain

Timothy J. Ness,[a] John D. Putzke,[b] Hong-Gang Liu,[c] and James M. Mountz[c]

[a]*Department of Anesthesiology, Pain Treatment Center,* [b]*Department of Physical Medicine and Rehabilitation, and* [c]*Division of Nuclear Medicine, Department of Radiology, University of Alabama at Birmingham, Birmingham, Alabama, USA*

When examining data related to new therapeutic agents for the treatment of pain, basic scientists, clinical researchers, and clinicians ask different questions. The basic scientist wants to know how the drug acts, the clinical researcher wants to know if there is evidence for the effect of the drug on a specific clinical entity, and the clinician wants to know if the patient will not only *receive* benefit, but *perceive* benefit. More importantly, the clinician wants to know if the patient will *continue* to receive and to perceive benefit. Methodologies to address these different questions are diverse, and debates related to the "validity" of different sources of information will continue to be unresolved until the participants agree on the questions being asked. Sources of information influencing therapeutic decisions come in five main forms, which are listed in decreasing order of academic legitimacy but increasing order of influence on clinical decisions: (1) controlled studies specific to the relevant clinical entity, (2) controlled studies related to similar disease processes, (3) published opinions and anecdotes (reviews, series, or case reports), (4) local institutional practices, and (5) personal anecdotal experience.

Pain in patients with spinal cord injury (SCI) has been the subject of few controlled studies, and the correlation with other frequently studied diseases is unknown. In contrast, there are many published opinions and anecdotal reports. Experienced clinicians and researchers support the use of various pharmacological agents ranging from antidepressants to intravenous anesthetics.

The bewildering array of combinations that are reported as effective, the broad range of mechanisms of action of these different agents, and the lack of "hard" evidence leave the practicing clinician with limited guidance for defining a treatment plan (Kezar and Ness 2001). The relatively new anticonvulsant agent, gabapentin, is one of these agents. In Chapter 22, Sang presents evidence from a controlled study that gabapentin along with dextromethorphan may have benefit in the treatment of SCI pain. This chapter will present one main case example along with other institutional experience in order to summarize the additional sources of information that guide our decisions related to the use of gabapentin in this population.

BACKGROUND INFORMATION

Prior to embarking on a discussion of our own experience, we must acknowledge an extensive published literature related to the perceived analgesic effectiveness of gabapentin. Several excellent reviews have addressed the topic of gabapentin, its long-term benefits, and its tolerability as an anticonvulsant (Handforth and Treiman 1994; Sivenius et al. 1994; Morris 1995; Wong et al. 1999), as well as its more recent role in the treatment of neuropathic pain (Backonja 2000; Laird and Gidal 2000; Mao and Chen 2000; Nicholson 2000). General statements and a more extensive listing of studies will be referenced to those reviews unless otherwise stated. The drug's limited toxicity, simple pharmacokinetics, and long-term tolerability have made it attractive as a "trial" agent in the treatment of many disorders. The number of gabapentin-related clinical reports has increased each year (Fig. 1) since the initial case report of effectiveness by Mellick and Mellick (1995). Case and series evidence for the effectiveness of gabapentin has been reported in the treatment of complex regional pain syndromes, painful peripheral neuropathies of multiple types (e.g., diabetic neuropathy, Guillain-Barré syndrome, and taxane-induced neuropathy), neuralgias of various types (e.g., trigeminal neuralgia, postherpetic neuralgia, and neuralgias associated with cancer), as well as many other disorders including headache, interstitial cystitis, vulvodynia, multiple sclerosis, post-polio syndrome, somatoform disorder, and bipolar affective disorder. Controlled studies have demonstrated significant effectiveness in the treatment of painful diabetic neuropathy, postherpetic neuralgia, and migraine headaches (Backonja et al. 1998; Rowbotham et al. 1998; Backonja 1999; Di Trapani et al. 2000), although other controlled studies have suggested only limited benefit (Gorson et al. 1999; Morello et al. 1999). Gabapentin seems to be useful for every neurological disorder, except perhaps for the control of seizures, for which it may have limited effectiveness as a monotherapy (e.g., De Toledo et al. 2000).

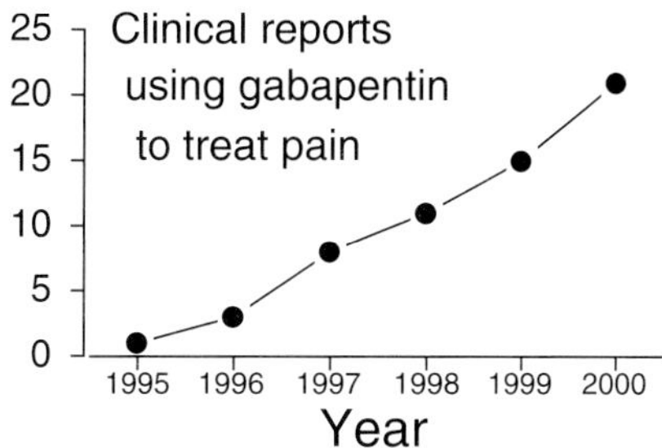

Fig. 1. Results of a MEDLINE search for the keyword "gabapentin." Excluding review articles, all reports of clinical use of gabapentin for the treatment of painful conditions were tabulated by year. Most reports are open trials and case reports.

Gabapentin is a clinical pharmacologist's ideal drug in that it has few interactions with other medications: it has minimal protein binding, does not induce metabolic enzymes, and has simple renal clearance with no known active metabolites (McLean 1994). With the possible exception of patients with myasthenia gravis (Boneva et al. 2000), it is safe for most populations and only requires formal dose adjustment based on renal function. It can be hemodialyzed. Perhaps gabapentin's most important characteristic, from a clinical standpoint, is that it has well-tolerated side effects. Common side effects include somnolence, dizziness and fatigue, and less common complications include ataxia, tremors, peripheral edema, nystagmus, diplopia, and multiple nonspecific gastrointestinal or neurological symptoms. Case examples have associated polyneuropathy, gynecomastia, renal allograft rejection, and anorgasmia with gabapentin use. Large-scale studies of the use of gabapentin as an anticonvulsant demonstrate that few subjects stop the medication due to side effects and that they continue to tolerate the side effects for years.

The effects of gabapentin have also been examined in animal models of pain and analgesia, including the formalin test, the sciatic nerve constriction model, various SCI pain models (Hao et al. 2000; Hulsebosch et al. 2000), diabetic neuropathy models, incisional pain models, inflammatory models including arthritic models, post-thermal injury models, anti-GD2 ganglioside-related neuropathy models, and neuronal models (cultured neurons and electrophysiological dorsal horn models). These models have consistently demonstrated antinociceptive effects of gabapentin, although typically the effects are seen on the portion of the nociceptive response that is increased by the experimental manipulation (the presumed hyperalgesic or allodynic response) and not on basal nociceptive responses. Gabapentin is believed to act on the $\alpha_2\delta$ subunit of voltage-sensitive calcium channels (e.g., Field et al. 2000), to which it binds selectively, although the precise effects of this binding are unknown.

Two case reports describe the effectiveness of gabapentin in the treatment of SCI-related pain, one of which is reviewed here (Ness et al. 1998a).

Other reports include the study by Sang described in Chapter 22 and several individual examples reported along with other series (e.g., Ness et al. 1998b). Kapadia and Harden (2000) reported on a 30-year-old woman who had pain following a gunshot wound who responded favorably to a trial of gabapentin, obtaining an 80% improvement in her pain within the first week of treatment on a regimen of 300 mg p.o. t.i.d. Her dose was increased and she continued to report improved pain control in a daily pain diary, with global daily ratings of 3 on a 0–10-point scale. She was also taking an antidepressant and an opioid, so it would appear that although beneficial, gabapentin was not adequate as a pain monotherapy and did not abolish the patient's pain. That has been our experience in a broader sample of patients, one of whom was Perry G.

ANECDOTAL EXPERIENCE: A CASE HISTORY

In 1981 a mining accident converted Perry G. from a working man with normal activities to a paraplegic. His T12/L1 fracture-dislocation resulted in a T11–12 incomplete Frankel B neurological level. It is difficult for nonparaplegics to fully comprehend the life changes that occur after such an injury. Although Perry's back was stabilized with Harrington rods, he became wheelchair bound, required digital stimulation for bowel evacuation, and needed intermittent urinary bladder catheterization. He developed contractures at both knees. To add insult to injury, he began to experience burning pain in his insensate left foot arch shortly after injury. The episodic bursts of pain, which he described as "searing," lasted for 8–10 seconds and sometimes longer. These crescendos would be followed by a rapid diminution of pain for a period of minutes. The cycle repeated itself with varying intensity and frequency over the day, every day. This cycling of his pain was particularly apparent when Perry was asked to rate his pain on a minute-by-minute basis. He was able to quantify his pain intensity using a verbal 10-point scoring system (0 = absence of pain, 10 = maximal pain), which is reported here as his "pain rating." An example of the cyclic nature of his baseline pain state is demonstrated in Fig. 1A. Perry rated his "global" daily pain rating as 9–10 out of 10.

Despite his ongoing pain, Perry continued to be active and worked at an auto salvage store. He could temper his pain using behavioral methods. He found that if he physically "strained" against the pain by contracting his truncal musculature he could prevent searing episodes. He found the searing episodes so aversive that he strained all day. At night, he would allow a high-intensity episode to occur so that he could experience a sufficiently long interval of minimal pain to be able to go to sleep. After nearly two decades of effort, Perry was approaching exhaustion and conceded the need for pharmacological or procedural interventions.

As a first step, we redefined Perry's injuries by additional imaging. Because of the cyclic nature of his pain, we asked him whether we might examine the effects of his sensations on regional cerebral blood flow (rCBF), and he agreed. We performed single positron emission computed tomography (SPECT) scans of his brain when he was experiencing high-intensity pain (Baseline-PAIN state in Table I) and when his pain was at its lowest intensity (Baseline-NON-PAIN state in Table I). We have previously reported

Table I
Regional cerebral blood flow (rCBF) changes during different pain states in subject Perry G.

	rCBF Ratio			
ROI	Baseline PAIN	Baseline NON-PAIN	Follow-up PAIN	Normal Resting Value
Caudate				0.90 ± 0.04
Right	0.79	0.93	0.86	
Left	0.68	0.90	0.82	
Thalamus				0.95 ± 0.03
Right	0.99	0.92	1.02	
Left	0.99	0.93	1.00	
Putamen				0.90 ± 0.04
Right	0.89	0.86	0.94	
Left	0.84	0.89	0.91	
Somatosensory				
Median				0.86 ± 0.03
Right	0.90	0.87	0.86	
Left	0.85	0.84	0.81	
Parasagittal				0.82 ± 0.03
Right	0.92	0.85	0.89	
Left	0.81	0.81	0.82	
Lateral				0.81 ± 0.03
Right	0.87	0.80	0.83	
Left	0.80	0.81	0.84	
Cingulate gyrus	0.97	0.87	0.99	0.84 ± 0.03

Note: Regional cerebral blood flow (rCBF) ratios were measured as the top 10% counts/pixel in the region of interest (ROI) to the top 10% counts/pixel of the cerebellum in PAIN, NON-PAIN, and Follow-up PAIN states in the SCI subject. ROI for the thalamus was constructed from four transverse sections, for the caudate and putamen from three transverse sections, and for the cingulate and somatosensory cortices from two coronal sections. Baseline measures were reported by Ness et al. (1998a), and normal resting values are those of Liu et al. (1997).

this information (Ness et al. 1998a) in a paper that discusses technical data more fully. Briefly, we acquired two separate rCBF brain SPECT scans 2 weeks apart. During the PAIN state scan, we injected the rCBF tracer ^{99m}Tc HMPAO immediately after a high-intensity (9.0) pain rating was reported. We performed the NON-PAIN scan during the second study while the subject reported a low-intensity pain rating (0.5). Studies using brain SPECT to capture epileptic seizure activity during the ictal state suggest that >90% of the lipophilic tracer ^{99m}Tc HMPAO uptake occurs within 10–15 seconds following i.v. bolus injection and that it correlates with regional cerebral blood flow, without redistribution for several hours (Laich et al. 1997). Transverse and coronal brain sections (as in Fig. 2) were reconstructed as defined by the Mountz reference system method (Mountz et al. 1994), and the rCBF value for each region of interest (ROI) was then calculated. These rCBF values, as well as normal control data (Liu et al. 1997), are shown in Table I.

The brain SPECT scan demonstrated low and asymmetric caudate rCBF, the left (ipsilateral to spontaneous pain) caudate rCBF being lower than the right (contralateral to spontaneous pain). During the PAIN state there was a bilateral reduction in caudate rCBF when compared to the NON-PAIN state. This finding is consistent with previously published data on a patient with familial painful restless leg syndrome (San Pedro et al. 1998). The thalamic nuclei show bilaterally increased rCBF during the PAIN state compared to the NON-PAIN state. This finding is again similar to that found in the report by San Pedro et al. (1998). There was significant activation (increased rCBF) of the right (contralateral) somatosensory cortex during the PAIN state compared to the NON-PAIN state. These findings are in accord with those observed during pain state changes in patients with fibromyalgia syndrome, who demonstrated activation of the cingulate gyrus during the PAIN state as compared to the NON-PAIN state (Mountz et al. 1998).

After his baseline imaging, Perry underwent trials of amitriptyline, carbamazepine, intravenous lidocaine, mexiletine, fluphenazine, and chlorpromazine, all without perceived benefit or with unacceptable side effects. He was then started on a dose of gabapentin 300 mg p.o. t.i.d. and experienced an initial decrease in the rate of cycling of his pain to 5–6 episodes per day and an average subjective pain rating of 2–3 on a scale of 10. Subsequently, he required a stepwise advancement in dose of the gabapentin. His pattern remained stable for more than 6 months, and a repeat formal assessment of pain intensity and pattern demonstrated a reduction in peak pain intensity and frequency (Fig. 2B).

Despite what would appear to an observer as obvious evidence of benefit (a comparison of Fig. 2A and 2B), on several occasions Perry stated that he felt as though he were doing no better or even worse than before initiation

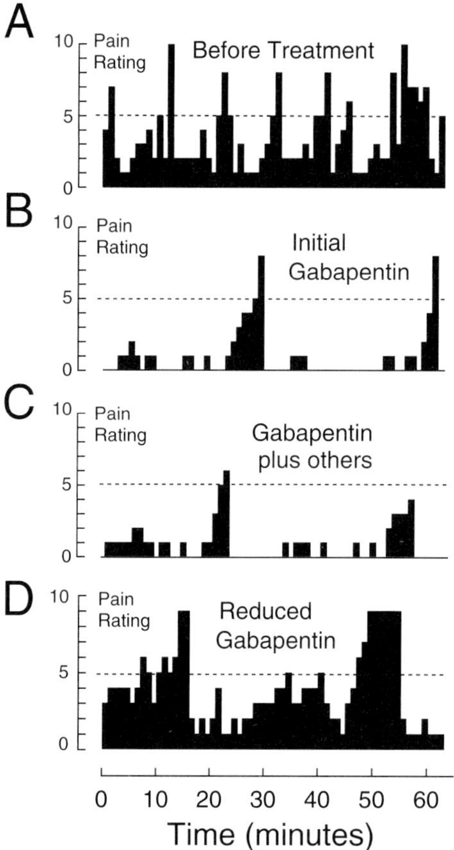

Fig. 2. Verbal reports by Perry G. of pain intensity (Pain Rating) plotted against time, with intensity scaled 0–10 (0 = no pain; 10 = maximal pain). The subject reported the presence and intensity of pain every minute during a 60-minute monitoring on four separate occasions: A, at baseline, prior to the initiation of any pharmacological therapy; B, after being stabilized on 2400 mg/day of gabapentin; C, 4 years after initiation of gabapentin therapy with the addition of clonazepam 0.5 mg p.o. t.i.d., tramadol 100 mg p.o. t.i.d., and dextromethorphan 60 mg p.o t.i.d.; and D, during a controlled taper of gabapentin as described in the text and in Fig. 4. Both the frequency and severity of his periodic pain have decreased with treatment but have not been abolished. With a reduction of his gabapentin dose the pain increased.

of his gabapentin treatment. He discontinued gabapentin treatment twice because he felt the side effects (tremors, somnolence, and an inability to concentrate) outweighed the "minimal" benefit he was receiving. On both occasions, his pain returned to its original pattern over a period of 2 days and at one follow-up visit Perry stated that he had "forgotten how bad it was!" On both occasions, the gabapentin therapy was reinitiated, with prompt improvement in his pain. Due to a perceived limit to the analgesic efficacy of his gabapentin treatment, we added other medications to his regimen. Institution of clonazepam therapy abolished his occasional tremors and slightly reduced his global pain rating. Tramadol improved his global pain rating further, but addition of propoxyphene increased his pain and disturbed his bowel regimen and so was discontinued. Additional trials of opioids were not attempted. Finally, the addition of dextromethorphan resulted in the best pain control he had experienced in the 20 years since his spinal injury.

Now 5 years following initiation of gabapentin therapy, Perry reports his average daily subjective pain rating as 2 or 3 on a 0–10 point scale. There continues to be a cyclic nature to his pain intensity (Fig. 2C). What is somewhat striking in the examination of the various minute-by-minute pain ratings displayed in Fig. 2 is the *lack* of difference between panels B and C despite a huge difference in the perception of well-being on the part of the patient. At the time of panel B, Perry thought he was doing poorly and at the time of panel C, he felt his pain was well controlled and at an acceptable level. The only apparent difference is the level of the peak intensities of the pain, but overall the mean score was similar at these two times. A repeat SPECT scan performed in March 2001 while Perry was on his current regimen of gabapentin (900 mg p.o. t.i.d.), clonazepam (0.5 mg p.o. t.i.d.), tramadol (100 mg p.o. q.i.d.), and dextromethorphan (60 mg p.o. t.i.d.) demonstrated a "normalization" of many of his previous rCBF values. Obtained while approaching a peak pain intensity episode (rating 4–5/10), the rCBF measures for most sites were within two standard deviations of values obtained from subjects not in pain (Table I: Follow-up PAIN versus Normal Resting Values). The left versus right differences in rCBF were minimal. The anterior cingulate cortex rCBF continued to be elevated—in fact, it was more elevated than on the initial measures. Following the SPECT scan, Perry reported that he had been "straining" in order to stop his pain from peaking too soon prior to administration of the ^{99m}Tc HMPAO tracer agent. On his previous measures he had "just let them happen."

INSTITUTIONAL EXPERIENCE: LONGITUDINAL OBSERVATIONS

The case of Perry is but one component of a broader experience with gabapentin and SCI-related pain at the University of Alabama at Birmingham. Now with well over 100 patients with SCI pain who have been given a trial of gabapentin, our best (and least biased) data come from 27 patients who were contacted and recontacted as part of a longitudinal observational study (Putzke et al., in press), which we present here in a summarized form.

In the summer of 1997, we performed a structured interview of 27 subjects with the diagnosis of pain due to traumatic SCI who had received a trial of gabapentin as part of their treatment for pain. Six subjects reported unacceptable side effects and had immediately discontinued the drug. Fourteen subjects reported perceived benefits sufficient to continue the medication for at least 6 months prior to their interview, and seven subjects reported no benefit despite a trial of 900 mg of gabapentin per day or greater. All subjects rated their pain before and after institution of gabapentin treatment, and the 14 subjects reporting benefit had a mean 4.9-point reduction in their 0–10 point scale pain rating (0 = no pain; 10 = maximal pain; Fig. 3). Only two of these subjects used gabapentin as a monotherapy. Of the subjects who could tolerate the medicine, 79% of those with thoracolumbar sensory levels (n = 14) reported benefit compared to only 43% of those with cervical sensory levels (n = 7). Pains localized above the subjects' sensory level, which would have been classified as "mechanical" using the classification of Donovan et al (1982), failed to respond to gabapentin. Pains localized at

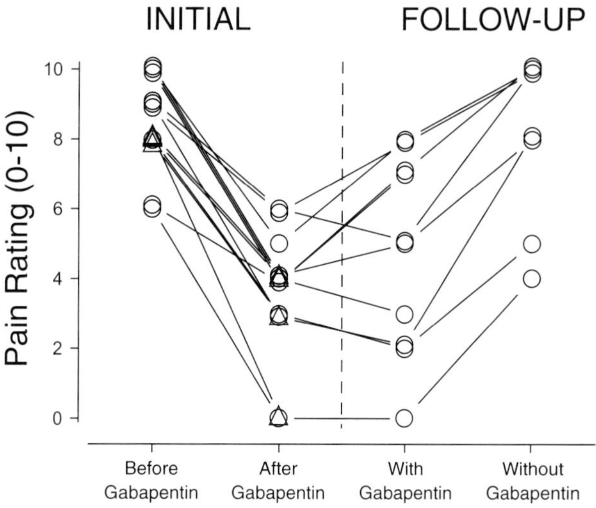

Fig. 3. Reported drop in pain ratings in 14 subjects with SCI pain given an open trial of gabapentin. As described in the text, 13 other subjects reported no benefit. Data are from structured interviews in the summers of 1997 (INITIAL) and 2000 (FOLLOW-UP). Pain was rated on a 10-point scale (0 = no pain; 10 = maximal pain.) Open circles indicate data from 10 subjects reporting long-term benefit from gabapentin at 3-year follow-up; open triangles indicate three subjects lost to follow-up and one subject who at follow-up had discontinued the gabapentin. At follow-up, eight subjects had attempted to discontinue their gabapentin and could report pain ratings with and without therapy.

or below the subjects' sensory levels had equally positive responses to gabapentin; 71% of "at-level" pains and 67% of "below-level" pains were reportedly reduced by gabapentin treatment. Neither gender nor the completeness of subjects' sensory levels appeared to be predictive of reported benefit of gabapentin. Interestingly, if subjects used the descriptor "burning" to characterize their pain, they were more likely to have a favorable response to gabapentin; 69% of subjects with burning pain versus 38% of subjects with nonburning pain reported a reduction of pain with gabapentin.

In the summer of 2000, we attempted to recontact the 14 subjects who reported initial benefit with gabapentin treatment and administered the same structured interview. Two subjects could not be located (one of these had been discharged from care due to noncompliance), one subject was deceased, and one female subject had discontinued gabapentin due to perceived inefficacy of the drug in the treatment of her pain; she had been on a very low daily dose of 300 mg gabapentin. The remaining 10 subjects were all still on gabapentin. Like Perry, 8 of the 10 subjects had missed doses or tried discontinuing gabapentin due to its perceived inefficacy, but an increase in their pain (Fig. 3) prompted them to restart their medication. At the 3-year follow-up, four subjects were on higher doses of gabapentin, four subjects were on the same dose, and two subjects were on lower doses. Although half of the subjects had side effects, they did not find them problematic. All 10 subjects also were treated with other analgesics (70% were taking opioids) because gabapentin alone was not sufficient to control their pain.

ASSESSMENT OF ONGOING BENEFIT OF GABAPENTIN

Anecdotal reports such as those given above, although of value when they are consistent, still have limits when one wishes to extrapolate their findings to a broader population. Current methodologies for the assessment of analgesics (i.e., double-blind, placebo-controlled, randomized, crossover trials) establish the initial effects of a medication but do not typically assess ongoing benefit except in an unblinded fashion or as a retrial following a discontinuation of the medication. Because of Perry G.'s and other patients' experiences where the discontinuation of their medication led to increased pain, we have been experimenting with a method to assess ongoing benefit that we call a sham-controlled, double-blind taper of medications. Similar to placebo-controlled, double-blind trials, in our sham-controlled, double-blind taper of medications both the investigators and the subjects are unaware of which medications are being issued by the pharmacy. Rather than recruiting medication-naive subjects, we recruited subjects who were being treated for their SCI-related pain with gabapentin. Two sets of blister-packed, dated drug packets were issued. One set contained 12–15 days' worth of gabapentin at identical doses to the subjects' ongoing treatment (e.g., 600 mg t.i.d.), but repackaged inside nondescript gelatin capsules. This set of medications was termed the Sham Taper because no actual taper of medications occurs when this packet is used. The other set of medications also contained disguised gabapentin, but in a tapering dose beginning on the third day of treatment. Decreasing by 25–33% at two-day intervals, this Real Taper set of medications reduces the dose of gabapentin to zero after 5–7 days, remains at zero dose for a few days, and then increases the dose back to the pre-trial level. A schematic of the Real Taper and Sham Taper dosing regimen is given in Fig. 4B. The order of Real versus Sham Taper presentation is randomized. We collected daily pain measures (visual analogue scale drawings, word selector lists, and verbal pain reports) throughout the two trial arms. Between trials, subjects were allowed to take their own medications and at any point in either trial, if pain increased to an unacceptable level, subjects could opt to discontinue participation. At the end of the study we asked subjects which medication arm provided better pain control. In this way, this study is effectively an *n* of 1 trial in an enriched population.

To test out this methodology, we first turned to our friend Perry. He was quite agreeable to a blinded trial to taper the gabapentin because he was still

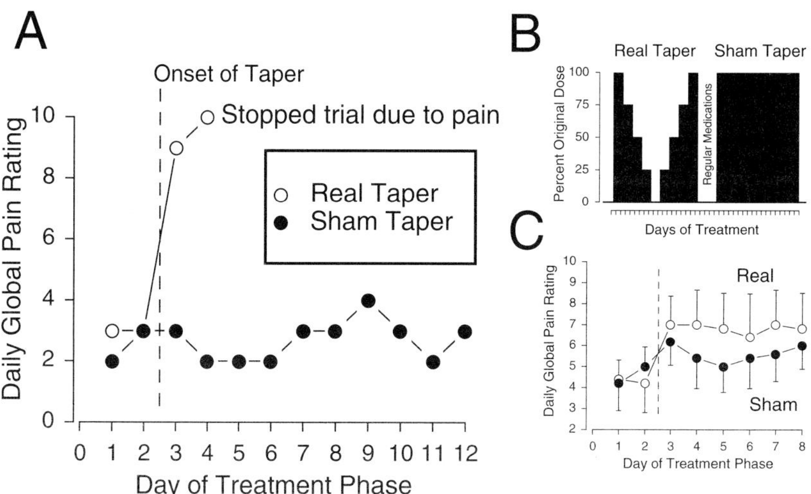

Fig. 4. Effects of a double-blind, sham-controlled taper of gabapentin in subject Perry G. (A) and mean data from five subjects (C). Panel B presents a schematic of the study drug dosing. Scales in A and C are 10-point scales (0 = no pain; 10 = maximal pain) gathered from daily telephone contacts.

not certain whether his improved pain control on four medications had any relation to this first drug. Perry's experience can be visualized in Fig. 4A. On the first day that his gabapentin dose was reduced as part of the Real Taper (Day 3), Perry noted a marked increase in his pain. By the second day of the Real Taper he was convinced that the increase was "real" and he terminated that arm of the study. A return to the use of his normal medications resulted in a resolution of his pain "flare." While he was taking the lowered dose of gabapentin and before he started his regular medications, we performed a minute-by-minute pain assessment, presented in Fig. 2D. It is visually apparent that both the pain intensity and the cycling of his pain increased with just this small decrease in his daily dose of gabapentin (reduced 33%). During the Sham Taper trial, his pain score remained stable.

Perry's "controlled" experience in which the taper of gabapentin resulted in an increase in ongoing pain provided evidence of the long-term effect of gabapentin and perhaps finally convinced him of this effect. His experience was similar to that of four other subjects with SCI-related pain whose experiences are summarized with Perry's in Fig. 4C. The Real Taper of medications resulted in higher pain scores. These findings must be viewed as only preliminary, however, because the changes were not statistically significant, and some alteration in protocol will be necessary to limit novelty effects because all five subjects noted some increase in pain during their first trial, whether it was the Sham or Real Taper arm.

SUMMARY

Gabapentin, in our clinic, has shown long-term utility in the treatment of SCI-related pain. Its low side-effect profile and simple pharmacokinetics have given it long-term tolerability as an analgesic agent, as demonstrated by increases in pain when discontinued on either an open basis or as part of a controlled trial. However, gabapentin does not have proven utility as a monotherapy in the experience of our patients. The best combination of medications taken with gabapentin for the treatment of SCI-related pain is yet to be determined.

ACKNOWLEDGMENT

Resources for production of this manuscript were provided by the University of Alabama at Birmingham Model Spinal Cord Injury System of Care grant from NIDRR (#H133N50009.)

REFERENCES

Backonja MM. Gabapentin monotherapy for the symptomatic treatment of painful neuropathy: a multicenter, double-blind, placebo-controlled trial in patients with diabetes mellitus. *Epilepsia* 1999; 40(Suppl 6):S57–S59.

Backonja MM. Anticonvulsants (antineuropathics) for neuropathic pain syndromes. *Clin J Pain* 2000; 16(Suppl 2):S67–72.

Backonja M, Beydoun A, Edwards KR, et al. Gabapentin for the symptomatic treatment of painful neuropathy in patients with diabetes mellitus: a randomized controlled study. *JAMA* 1998; 280:1831–1836.

Boneva N, Brenner T, Argov Z. Gabapentin may be hazardous in myasthenia gravis. *Muscle Nerve* 2000; 23:1204–1208.

De Toledo JC, Ramsay RE, Lowe MR, Greiner M, Garofalo EA. Increased seizures after discontinuing carbamazepine: results from the gabapentin monotherapy trial. *Ther Drug Monit* 2000; 22:753–756.

Di Trapani G, Mei D, Marra C, Mazza S, Capuano A. Gabapentin in the prophylaxis of migraine: a double-blind randomized placebo-controlled study. *Clin Ter* 2000; 151:145–148.

Donovan WH, Dimitrijevic MR, Dahm L, Dimitri M. Neuropsychological approaches to chronic pain following spinal cord injury. *Paraplegia* 1982; 20:135–146.

Field MJ, Hughes J, Singh L. Further evidence for the role of the alpha-2-delta subunit of voltage dependent calcium channels in models of neuropathic pain. *Br J Pharmacol* 2000; 1331:282–286.

Gorson KC, Schott C, Herman R, Ropper AH, Rand WM. Gabapentin in the treatment of painful diabetic neuropathy: a placebo controlled, double blind, crossover trial. *J Neurol Neurosurg Psychiatry* 1999; 66:251–252.

Handforth A, Treiman DM. Efficacy and tolerance of long-term, high-dose gabapentin: additional observations. *Epilepsia* 1994; 35:1032–1037.

Hao JX, Xu XJ, Urban L, Wiesenfeld-Hallin Z. Repeated administration of systemic gabapentin alleviates allodynia-like behaviors in spinally injured rats. *Neurosci Lett* 2000; 280:211–214.

Hulsebosch CE, Xu GY, Perez-Polo JR, et al. Rodent model of chronic central pain after spinal cord contusion injury and effects of gabapentin. *J Neurotrauma* 2000; 17:1205–1217.

Kapadia NP, Harden N. Gabapentin for chronic pain in spinal cord injury: a case report. *Arch Phys Med Rehabil* 2000; 81:1439–1441.

Kezar LB, Ness TJ. Systemic medications for SCI pain. *Topics SCI Rehabil* 2001; 7:57–72.

Laich E, Kuzniecky R, Mountz JM, et al. Supplementary sensorimotor area epilepsy: seizure localization, propagation and subcortical activation pathways using ictal SPECT. *Brain* 1997; 120:855–864.

Laird MA, Gidal BE. Use of gabapentin in the treatment of neuropathic pain. *Ann Pharmacother* 2000; 34:802–807.

Liu H-G, Mountz JM, San Pedro EC, Inampudi C, Deutsch G. A semi-quantitative cortical circumferential normalization method for clinical evaluation of rCBF brain SPECT. *Clin Nucl Med* 1997; 22:596–604.

Mao J, Chen LL. Gabapentin in pain management. *Anesth Analg* 2000; 91:680–687.

McLean MJ. Clinical pharmacokinetics of gabapentin. *Neurology* 1994; 44(Suppl 5):S17–S22.

Mellick GA, Mellick LB. Gabapentin in the management of reflex sympathetic dystrophy. *J Pain Symptom Manage* 1995; 10:265–266.

Morello CM, Leckband SG, Stoner CP, Moorhouse DF, Sahagian GA. Randomized double-blind study comparing the efficacy of gabapentin with amitriptyline on diabetic peripheral neuropathy pain. *Arch Intern Med* 1999; 159:1931–1937.

Morris GL III. Efficacy and tolerability of gabapentin in clinical practice. *Clin Ther* 1995; 17:891–899.

Mountz JM, Zhang B, Liu H-G, Inampudi C. A reference method for correlation of anatomic and functional brain images: validation and clinical application. *Semin Nucl Med* 1994; 24:256–271.

Mountz JM, Bradley LA, Alarcon GS. Abnormal functional activity of the central nervous system in fibromyalgia syndrome. *Am J Med Sci* 1998; 315:385–396.

Ness TJ, San Pedro EC, Richards JS, et al. A case of spinal cord injury-related pain with baseline rCBF brain SPECT imaging and beneficial response to gabapentin. *Pain* 1998a; 78:139–143.

Ness TJ, Crimaldi JC, McDanal J. Case report on gabapentin. *Reg Anesth Pain Med* 1998b; 23:110–111.

Nicholson B. Gabapentin use in neuropathic pain syndromes. *Acta Neurol Scand* 2000; 101:359–371.

Putzke JD, Richards JS, Hicken B, Ness TJ. Long-term use of Neurontin for treatment of pain following traumatic spinal cord injury. *Clin J Pain* 2002; in press.

Rowbotham M, Harden N, Stacey B, Bernstein P, Magnus-Miller L. Gabapentin for the treatment of postherpetic neuralgia. *JAMA* 1998; 280:1837–1842.

San Pedro EC, Mountz, JM, Mountz JD, et al. Familial painful restless legs syndrome correlates with pain dependent variation of blood flow to the caudate, thalamus and anterior cingulate gyrus. *J Rheumatol* 1998; 25:2270–2275.

Sivenius J, Ylinen A, Kalviainen R, Riekkinen P. Long-term study with gabapentin in patients with drug-resistant epileptic seizures. *Arch Neurol* 1994; 51:1047–1050.

Wong ICK, Chadwick PBC, Fenwick PBC, et al. The long-term use of gabapentin, lamotrigine, and vigabatrin in patients with chronic epilepsy. *Epilepsia* 1999; 40:1439–1445.

Correspondence to: Timothy J. Ness, MD, PhD, Department of Anesthesiology, University of Alabama at Birmingham, 619 19th Street South, JT 845, Birmingham, AL 35233-6810, USA. Tel: 205-975-9643; Fax: 205-934-7437; email: tim.ness@ccc.uab.edu.

Spinal Cord Injury Pain: Assessment, Mechanisms, Management. Progress in Pain Research and Management, Vol. 23, edited by Robert P. Yezierski and Kim J. Burchiel, IASP Press, Seattle, © 2002.

24

Topiramate in the Management of Spinal Cord Injury Pain: A Double-Blind, Randomized, Placebo-Controlled Pilot Study

R. Norman Harden,[a] Ephraim Brenman,[b] Samuel Saltz,[a] and Timothy T. Houle[c]

[a]*Center for Pain Studies, Rehabilitation Institute of Chicago, Chicago, Illinois, USA;* [b]*Spine and Rehabilitation Center, Austin, Texas, USA;* [c]*Illinois Institute of Technology, Chicago, Illinois, USA*

The pharmacotherapy of neuropathic conditions has progressed over the past 20 years, yet we still lack an agent that is both uniformly tolerated and effective (Max et al. 1988; McQuay et al. 1996). The treatment of spinal cord injury (SCI) pain is a particularly understudied and underserved area in pain management and rehabilitation, and there is very little evidence to guide clinicians. Only eight randomized controlled clinical pharmacological trials have been published; all used small samples and most have methodological flaws (see Chapter 20). The opioids, as the principal, and arguably most effective class of analgesics in use today, are notoriously ineffective in neuropathic conditions (Arner and Meyerson 1988; Kupers and Gybels 1995; Harden and Bruehl 1997) and have not been properly studied in SCI pain. Nonsteroidal anti-inflammatory drugs, although good analgesics in nociceptive conditions, are virtually useless in the management of neuropathic pain (Bowsher 1991); again, they have not been studied in SCI pain. Tricyclic antidepressants, and especially the "tricyclic" antiepileptic carbamazepine, are traditionally the drugs of choice in managing nerve damage pain (McQuay et al. 1996), but embarrassingly, they have not been studied in SCI pain. Although various older antiepileptic drugs (AEDs) such as phenytoin have been tried in neuropathic conditions, the results have been disappointing (McQuay et al. 1995). More recently, some of the newer AEDs targeting

GABAergic systems have received increased clinical attention for use in neuropathic pain. For example, gabapentin has been the subject of recent scrutiny after empirical and anecdotal reports of excellent analgesia (Mellick et al. 1995; Attal et al. 1999). Large multicenter, double-blind, randomized controlled trials of this medication have been conducted for diabetic peripheral neuropathy and postherpetic neuralgia (Backonja et al. 1998; Rowbotham et al. 1998). These trials showed statistically significant improvement, not only in subjective pain reports but also in other outcomes such as sleep and quality of life measures (Backonja et al. 1998; Rowbotham et al. 1998). One case report describes the successful use of gabapentin in SCI (Kapadia and Harden 1999), and other anecdotes appear in this volume (see Chapter 23). In addition to GABAergic drugs, certain sodium channel blockers have been described in favorable anecdotal reports in various neuropathic conditions (Simpson et al. 1998; Edwards et al. 1999), but nothing has been published specific to SCI pain (however, see Chapter 20 for a report of a randomized, double-blind, controlled trial of lamotrigine). NMDA and non-NMDA antagonists have also shown early promise in the management of neuropathic pain (Yamamoto and Yaksh 1992; Elliot et al. 1994; see Chapter 22).

The AED topiramate hydrochloride is effective in diabetic neuropathy pain (Edwards et al. 1999), and our clinical experience indicates that it may be useful in other types of neuropathic pain. Integration of these empirical and anecdotal data provided the theoretical rationale for testing topiramate in the control of SCI pain. As a GABA agonist, a sodium and N-type calcium channel blocker, and a non-NMDA (kainate) antagonist (Faught et al. 1996), this compound seems promising for use in neuropathic pain in general, and for SCI pain at or below the level of the lesion in particular. We proposed that topiramate may suppress ectopic neuropathic activity (and pain) in SCI by stabilizing Na^+ channels at the site of injury, by blocking conduction of nociceptive transmission at non-NMDA excitatory kainate receptors, or by blocking Ca^+ transmission at N-type Ca^+ channels. GABAergic effects may also be involved in decreasing pain transmission at the dorsal horn (Backonja et al. 1998; Rowbotham et al. 1998).

This chapter describes the results of a pilot study we conducted to test the efficacy of topiramate in neuropathic pain. The study had a prospective, double-blind, randomized, placebo-controlled, parallel design and incorporated a mixed/within-subject approach. Subjects included 35 patients aged between 18 and 70 years. The subjects had experienced neuropathic pain for 6 months or longer. The sample included patients with four neuropathic pain diagnoses as determined by history and physical examination using criteria published by the International Association for the Study of Pain (IASP; Merskey and Bogduk 1994). The first category was pain at or below the level of a spinal cord lesion (n = 14). The other diagnoses were pain due to stroke, residual limb pain and/or phantom limb pain, and complex regional pain syndrome (aggregate n = 21). None of these other diagnoses had a sufficient number of subjects to develop statistical trends, and this chapter will only discuss the results for SCI pain.

Potential subjects were accepted with the following inclusion criteria: the ability to read and speak English and provide written consent, no hepatic or renal impairment, no history of kidney stones, and no use of carbonic anhydrase inhibitors. We screened for hepatic impairment during the initial washout period, testing levels of serum glutamic-oxaloacetic transaminase (SGOT), serum glutamic-pyruvic transaminase (SGPT), γ-glutamyltransferase (GGT), total bilirubin, and indirect bilirubin. Patients with significantly abnormal results on any test were excluded from the study and were referred to their local physician. The protocol was approved by the Institutional Review Board of the Office for Protection of Research Subjects of Northwestern University.

MEASURES

Daily monitoring diary. Subjects completed a daily pain diary and presented it to the study monitors at each scheduled visit. The diary included daily pain intensity using a visual analogue scale (VAS) and the Present Pain Intensity (PPI) of the McGill Pain Questionnaire–Short Form (Melzack 1987). The diary also measured the subjects' emotional state using an abbreviated version of the Emotional Assessment Scale (Carlson et al. 1989), and monitored their stress level using a VAS of daily stress. The average VAS pain rating by dose level served as the primary outcome measure for between-group analyses.

McGill Pain Questionnaire (MPQ): Short Form. The short form of the MPQ (Melzack 1987) was administered at each clinic visit to assess weekly changes in overall pain intensity.

Pain Disability Index (PDI). The PDI (Tait et al. 1987) was administered at each clinic visit to assess overall disability in seven areas of function (family/home, recreation, social activity, occupation, sexual behavior, self-care, and life-support activity).

Multidimensional Pain Inventory (MPI). The MPI (Kerns et al. 1985) was administered at baseline (prior to washout) and at study termination. It assesses a number of pain-related factors, including pain intensity, cognitive response to pain, perceived control over pain, overall emotional distress, activity levels in a variety of areas, and pain-related social support.

This measure was used as an index to overall improvement in adaptation to chronic pain.

Side effects checklist. Side effects were recorded using a questionnaire in checklist format. The study physician completed this form at each visit.

Beck Depression Inventory (BDI). The BDI (Beck et al. 1979) was used to assess depressive symptoms at baseline and at study termination. The measure was used in secondary analyses to determine whether topiramate or the pain relief it provided improved depressive symptoms, and whether the drug's effectiveness was affected by the extent of depressive symptoms.

Trait form of the State-Trait Anxiety Inventory (STAI). The STAI (Spielberger et al. 1970), which assesses anxiety-related symptoms, was completed at baseline and at the end of the study for use in secondary analyses similar to those described for the BDI.

In addition to the instruments described above, subjects also used a VAS to indicate their perception of the overall efficacy of the medication they received and their willingness to continue taking it.

PROCEDURES

Once subjects provided informed consent, they were taken off all antidepressants or AEDs used for pain for a 1-week washout period. They were also detoxified from daily opioids. We prescribed 5 mg hydrocodone bitartrate/325 mg acetaminophen (Vicodin; Knoll Laboratories) as a "rescue agent" to be taken throughout the study, beginning with the washout period, in doses of up to 1–2 pills every 8 hours as needed. We took a pill count at each visit and at the conclusion of the study. Patients were required to drink at least 48 ounces of fluid a day.

We assigned subjects randomly to topiramate or placebo groups. Dosages in the topiramate group were titrated upward over a period of up to 10 weeks, and the maximum attainable dose was maintained for 4 weeks. Throughout the study, subjects in the placebo group (n = 5) received placebo at the same "dosage" (the same number of pills) and on the same schedule (twice daily) as the topiramate group. Patients taking topiramate (n = 9) started with a total daily dosage of 25 mg, which was increased after 1 week to 50 mg (25 mg b.i.d.), with an increase to 100 mg (50 mg b.i.d.) 1 week later. Subsequent titration was carried at a rate of 50–100 mg weekly to either the maximum tolerable dose or a total of 800 mg daily (400 mg b.i.d.). Dose escalation was halted and the dose reduced to the previously tolerated level if signs of toxicity or intolerable side effects occurred. Dose escalation was also discontinued if the subject recorded a 75% or greater reduction in pain as reflected in the weekly average VAS pain ratings. After subjects maintained the maximum dose for 4 weeks, they received a final evaluation using the same measures given at baseline (see Table I).

Subjects had weekly scheduled clinic visits or telephone calls to monitor their progress and side effects. Clinic visits were scheduled at baseline, at the end of the washout period, and at the end of weeks 3, 6, 10, 12, and 14. Between clinic visits we contacted the subjects by telephone on a weekly basis. To permit accurate pain and functional measures, we asked subjects to stop all rescue medication 8 hours before each clinic visit and also asked

Table I
Schedule of topiramate dosage titration and study events

Time	Dosage	Study Events
Baseline	Washout from current medications	Clinic visit: conducts laboratory tests, baseline measures; provide rescue medications
End of washout	Begin 25 mg	Clinic visit: assess pain, functioning, side effects; take pill count
End of Week 1	Increase to 50 mg (25 mg b.i.d.)	Telephone contact: assess side effects
End of Week 2	Increase to 100 mg (50 mg b.i.d.)	Telephone contact: assess side effects
End of Week 3	Increase to 200 mg (100 mg b.i.d.)	Clinic visit: assess pain, functioning, side effects; take pill count
End of Week 4	Increase to 300 mg (150 mg b.i.d.)	Telephone contact: assess side effects
End of Week 5	Increase to 400 mg (200 mg b.i.d.)	Telephone contact: assess side effects
End of Week 6	Increase to 500 mg (250 mg b.i.d.)	Clinic visit: assess pain, functioning, side effects; take pill count
End of Week 7	Increase to 600 mg (300 mg b.i.d.)	Telephone contact: assess side effects
End of Week 8	Increase to 700 mg (350 mg b.i.d.)	Telephone contact: assess side effects
End of Week 9	Increase to 800 mg (400 mg b.i.d.)	Telephone contact: assess side effects
End of Week 10	Continue 800 mg (400 mg b.i.d.)	Clinic visit: conduct laboratory tests; assess pain, functioning, side effects; take pill count
End of Week 11	Continue 800 mg (400 mg b.i.d.)	Telephone contact: assess side effects
End of Week 12	Continue 800 mg (400 mg b.i.d.)	Clinic visit: assess pain, functioning, side effects; take pill count
End of Week 13	Continue 800 mg (400 mg b.i.d.)	Telephone contact: assess side effects
End of Week 14	End of study	Clinic visit: re-administer baseline measures; assess pain, functioning, side effects; take final pill count

them not to take any rescue medication for 8 hours before completing their pain diaries at home. At each clinic visit we provided the study medication, took a pill count of rescue medication, and monitored side effects. We also assessed pain (MPQ) and functioning (PDI) at each visit (see Table I). After subjects reached their maximum stable dosage, we screened for renal and hepatic impairment, and we also took a routine urinalysis at the highest dosage achieved.

STATISTICAL ANALYSES

For statistical analysis we used SPSS for Windows. We used nonparametric tests (χ^2) to examine differences in rates of side effects across study groups. As a broad measure of effectiveness, we used analysis of covariance (ANCOVA) to examine the degree of change from baseline pain ratings to study termination between study groups. To analyze this change while controlling for the possible effects of baseline pain levels on drug effectiveness, we included pain at termination as the dependent measure, the study group as the independent measure, and pain at baseline as the covariate. A significant group main effect would indicate that topiramate resulted in significant overall reductions in pain relative to placebo when both groups were equalized for baseline pain. Differences in use of rescue medications were compared across groups using *t* tests, and if significant, this variable was used as a covariate in all primary analyses.

For a more detailed analysis of whether increased dosage had a significant effect on pain levels, we conducted repeated-measures ANOVAs using each of the primary outcome measures described above as dependent measures (the repeated measure is the outcome at different dosage levels). A significant overall dosage by group (topiramate vs. placebo) interaction would indicate a linear dose-response relationship. We completed detailed ANOVAs of each dosage interval (0–25 mg, 25–50 mg, 50–100 mg, 100–200 mg, 200–300 mg, 300–400 mg, 400–500 mg, 500–600 mg, 600–700 mg, and 700–800 mg) and examined mean pain scores at each interval to determine which dosage provided optimal effectiveness. We used *t* tests to compare across groups the patients' ratings of overall efficacy and their willingness to continue taking the medication.

Secondary analyses examined whether the effectiveness of topiramate was altered by the presence of depressive or anxiety symptoms. We studied the effects of the drug on mood using analyses similar to those described in the primary analyses above. Finally, ANCOVAs (controlling for baseline values) and repeated-measures ANOVAs examined the impact of the drug on degree of change in the weekly PDI ratings, as well as the change from baseline to study termination on the MPI (as a measure of improved adaptation to chronic pain).

RESULTS

Table II displays the demographic characteristics of the sample. The placebo and drug groups were similar on most characteristics including age, gender, race, other diagnoses, pain intensity, anxiety, and symptoms of depression. On average, the drug group had pain for a longer period of time (12.4 years) than the placebo group (8.5 years).

SIDE EFFECTS

The drug group reported a significantly higher proportion of overall symptoms that are commonly considered to be side effects at baseline (difference in proportions, $P < 0.05$). Therefore, newly reported drug group symptoms (side effects) are better indexed against the drug group at baseline than against the placebo group at a similar dose level.

Table II
Demographic characteristics by treatment group

	Placebo (n = 5)		Topiramate (n = 9)	
Age (years)	37.2 (10.7) (range 27–49)		41.0 (11.3) (range 24–54)	
Gender	2 female 3 male		3 female 6 male	
Race	1 white 3 black 1 Hispanic		1 white 6 black 1 Asian Islander 1 "other"	
Pain chronicity (years)	8.5 (3.1)		12.4 (5.1)	
Baseline pain				
VAS	60.8	(5.5)	58.2	(20.4)
Present Pain Intensity	3.4	(1.1)	3.1	(1.3)
Beck Depression Inventory	14.0	(9.6)	13.4	(5.7)
Pain Disability Index	28	(18.5)	22.8	(10.1)
State-Trait Anxiety Inventory	47.4	(7.1)	45.8	(7.7)
McGill Pain Questionnaire				
Sensory	16.0	(4.9)	15.6	(5.9)
Affective	0.80	(1.3)	1.6	(1.8)

No single side effect increased significantly over the course of treatment ($P > 0.05$). New cases of overall side effects peaked at the 200-mg dose and declined throughout further increases in dose. In fact, the highest proportion of total side effects occurred at baseline, before the drug was administered. The most common newly reported side effects were dry mouth and somnolence (three cases of each); and asthenia, nausea, constipation, memory difficulties, and mood difficulties (two cases of each). Interestingly, the symptom that changed the most during treatment was back pain, which decreased by four cases during treatment. Fig. 1 displays the compliance rates of the drug group using the placebo group's compliance rates as a reference. The drug group complied more with the drug regimen than did the placebo group until the final weeks at the 800-mg dose level. The compliance rates support the tolerability of the drug because rates were very similar for both groups, with no significant differences being observed at any dose level (Group, $F_{1,26} < 2.2$; Group × Dose, $F_{4,104} < 2.2$; $P > 0.17$). The greatest discrepancy in compliance occurred between the 200-mg and 500-mg dose level, with compliance becoming remarkably similar with increases in dose.

PAIN REDUCTION

Groups did not significantly differ on pain intensity during the baseline period (see Table I). However, the drug group did have slightly lower pain scores on both the VAS and PPI, so we used baseline pain as a covariate in all analyses. During the 2-week baseline period the placebo group consumed an average of 17.6 tablets of Vicodin, compared with 29.4 tablets for the drug group. Although this difference was not significant, the direction of this trend would intuitively enhance the drug group's analgesic response, so we also controlled rescue medication usage in all analyses.

The primary outcome measures were the VAS and the PPI, for which we conducted separate analyses. Because medication compliance and rescue medication information were available and differed by dose level, we conducted separate ANCOVAs at the 25-mg, 200-mg, 500-mg, 800-mg, 800-mg, and 800-mg dose intervals using drug (placebo vs. topiramate) as a fixed factor, with baseline pain, rescue medication usage, and compliance with study medication as covariates.

Fig. 2 displays the adjusted means for the placebo and drug groups by dose level on the pain intensity VAS. Although both groups' mean levels slightly decreased with increases in dose, none of the ANCOVAs resulted in significant differences between groups ($F_{1,16} < 3.68$, $P > 0.07$). However, the largest effect size between groups was $\chi^2 = 0.122$ in the final week of the

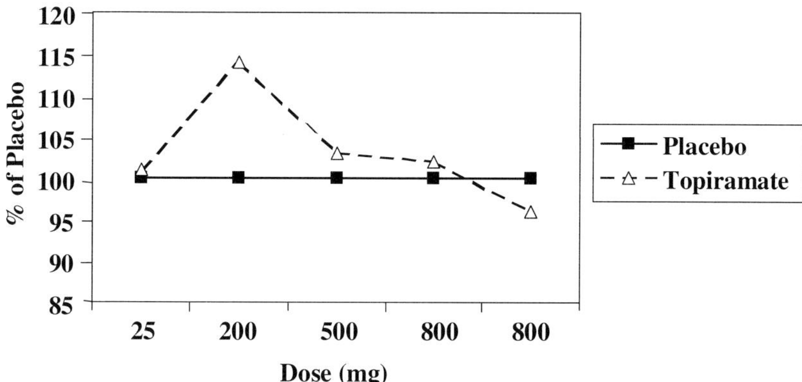

Fig. 1. Compliance with medication regime as a function of dose, using the placebo group as a reference.

800-mg dose level (see Fig. 2). This effect size is still considered small by convention (Cohen 1988), but is large enough to promise significance with modest increases in sample size.

Fig. 3 displays the adjusted means for the placebo and drug groups by dose level on the PPI. Both groups' mean levels slightly decreased with increases in dose. However, unlike the VAS scores, the PPI scores showed that the topiramate subjects had significantly less pain than their placebo counterparts during the final weeks of the 800-mg dose level ($F_{1,6} = 7.73$, $P = 0.032$; see Fig. 3). The difference between VAS and PPI results could be explained by a greater degree of random variation with VAS scores.

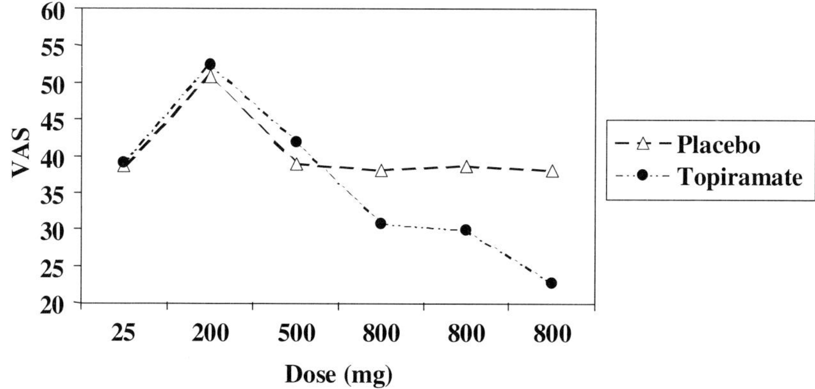

Fig. 2. Adjusted means for the visual analogue scale (VAS) of perceived pain intensity as a function of drug group and dose.

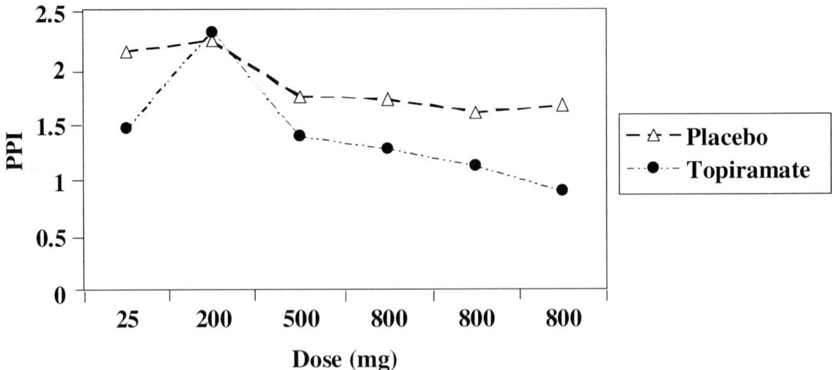

Fig. 3. Adjusted means for the Present Pain Index (PPI) as a function of drug group and dose.

INDIVIDUAL EFFECTS

To identify the comparative effects of the drug over time, we modeled the VAS ratings from each subject's daily diary using a time-series analysis, summarized in Table III. To better ensure the validity of the inferential statistics, we identified potential autocorrelation using Durbin-Watson (*d*) and included a first-order autoregressive process to correct for the dependency in the residuals. As can be seen in the notes column in Table III, we corrected 11 of the 12 models by this method. To ensure that the residuals were white noise, we evaluated the corrected models, including the time parameters, using the modified Box-Pierce Q^*. Also signified in the notes column are 4 of 12 models where the use of rescue medication played a significant role in pain reporting. In these models, we controlled for the effects of rescue medication on pain report before we evaluated the effect of time. Three of the four subjects for whom rescue medication played a major role in pain reporting were in the placebo group. Data from two of the topiramate subjects could not be properly modeled because too many observations were missing.

We evaluated change in pain report during all dose levels of treatment versus baseline, and the *P* values are displayed in Table III. No subjects in the placebo group had significantly less pain while on the placebo versus at baseline, and one subject had significantly more, while two subjects in the topiramate group had significantly less pain on the drug versus at baseline (see Table III).

To examine the effect of increases in dose over time, we regressed pain intensity on time in each model, and Table III presents the *y* intercepts (pain at time = 0), regression coefficients (change in pain over 1 day, b_t), standardized

Table III
Individual pain as a function of time: placebo group versus drug group

Subject	Notes 1, 2	Baseline Change	*Y* Intercept	b_t	B_t	*P*
Placebo						
106	1	0.687	26.14	–0.136	–0.291	*0.001
107	1, 2	0.481	9.37	–0.143	–0.118	0.053
109	1	0.408	54.73	–0.03	–0.119	0.269
116	1, 2	+0.002	4.12	0.165	0.383	+0.014
132	1, 2	0.718	23.06	–0.008	–0.015	0.869
Topiramate						
104	1	0.391	9.91	–0.089	–0.11	0.114
110		0.596	51.08	0.042	0.132	0.183
114	1	*0.028	54.22	–0.195	–0.341	*0.001
117	1	*0.005	24.5	0.04	0.167	0.066
118	1	0.44	67.1	–0.651	–0.61	*0.001
122	1, 2	0.307	2.65	0.012	0.034	0.695
130	1	0.851	34.37	–0.155	–0.319	*0.001
Average: Placebo					–0.032	
Average: Topiramate					–0.150	

Notes: 1 = first-order autoregressive process; 2 = control for rescue medication.
* Significant decrease in pain over time ($P < 0.05$).
+ Significant increase in pain over time ($P < 0.05$).

regression coefficients (B_t), and significance of time in the model (*P*). In the placebo group, time (and corresponding increases in "dose") predicted significantly less pain in one case, while the opposite relationship of increasing pain with increasing "dose" was observed in one case (see Table III). Subject 107 of the placebo group also displayed a trend of decreasing pain ($P = 0.053$). In the topiramate group, three subjects had significantly less pain with increases in dose, and no subjects had significant increases in pain (see Table III).

We also evaluated the aggregate effect of topiramate using a time-series analysis. The topiramate group had a standardized average rate of change of $B_t = -0.150$, while the placebo group had a standardized rate of change of $B_t = -0.032$. This decrease in pain in the topiramate group is 4.7 times higher than that experienced in the placebo group.

PSYCHOMETRICS

No group differences or interactions with topiramate were observed for the BDI, PDI, or STAI instruments throughout the course of treatment.

DISCUSSION

The antiepileptic class of medications has come to the fore in the treatment of postherpetic neuralgia and diabetic peripheral neuropathy, and many doctors have begun to use these compounds to treat other neuropathies, such as radiculopathy and postamputation pain. Pain after SCI is most akin to "central pain" by the IASP criteria; it is not particularly similar to poststroke pain, but it is often considered in the same taxonomy (Merskey and Bogduk 1994). It is likely that the pathophysiology and pathoanatomy are quite different, and it would be reasonable to expect that the optimal pharmacotherapy may also differ. The first-generation AEDs have been only marginally effective for the treatment of SCI pain, yet they have a significant side-effect profile and long-term toxicity (McQuay et al. 1995). We have had some success using some of the newer antiepileptic compounds such as gabapentin in central SCI pain (Kapadia and Harden 1999).

SCI pain above the area of the lesion is usually musculoskeletal or myofascial, and would not be expected to respond particularly well to anticonvulsive therapy. Pain at the level of the lesion is similar in some respects to radiculopathy, and as such may be responsive to both peripherally and centrally acting anticonvulsant drugs. There may be a role for sodium (and perhaps calcium) channel-blocking agents regarding "peripheral" generators. Pain at or near the zone of injury may also involve some central components, and may respond to AEDs that inhibit transmission cells via GABA or to drugs that have an effect on excitatory amino acids or block N-type calcium channels.

AEDs may also be effective for pain sensations experienced below the level of the lesion, or the "classic" SCI pain syndrome. Ectopic activity at the injured area may stimulate spinothalamic pathways and cause cortical sensation below the lesion. If this ectopic activity is due to damaged and "leaky" sodium channels, sodium channel blockers may lack efficacy for this type of pain. Calcium channel dysfunction may also provide a rationale for drugs that either block or normalize calcium levels. The AEDs that are GABA agonists or that enhance natural GABA metabolism may directly inhibit transmission cells at the dorsal horn or may take effect at higher levels. GABA cells originating in the brainstem may have an inhibitory effect at this level or in the thalamus, limbic system, or even the cortex. Central pain phenomena of spinal cord origin may be the most challenging to treat of all the pain types associated with SCI.

In our pilot study, treatment effects began at the 800-mg dose level. Until that time, the placebo and topiramate groups were nearly identical, except that the drug group usually had slightly less pain (after we controlled for baseline pain, rescue medication use, and compliance with the treatment regime). The first 2 weeks at the 800-mg dose level produced a small treatment effect and the middle 2 weeks on the 800-mg dose produced greater effects (showing a trend for significance, which might be attained with 5–10 more patients in each group). The final 2 weeks produced the greatest effects, which were statistically significant.

Interestingly, compliance rates were a large factor in the significant findings: a small change in compliance played a large role in the significance of the results because subjects who complied to a greater extent had better results, for both the topiramate and placebo groups. It is difficult to determine the role of compliance on treatment outcome, as the placebo group perhaps artificially added to compliance effects.

We created an individual model for each SCI subject so that we could assess the effects that topiramate or placebo had on the individual, and we addressed several primary statistical issues for each subject. We addressed the problem of dependency in the residuals using first-order autoregressive processes where needed, so that each model met the necessary regression assumptions. Also included in each model was the role that rescue medication played on pain intensity recording.

We conducted two different analyses were conducted: baseline versus treatment and the effect of time (and dose increases). In general, the individual topiramate subject had greater pain reduction, both in terms of change from baseline and over time, than did placebo subjects. Four of the topiramate subjects had decreased pain, either from baseline or over time. This effect contrasts with the placebo group, where participants did not reliably improve over time, with one subject displaying improvement and one getting significantly worse. On aggregate, topiramate was 4.7 times more effective than placebo.

Unfortunately, in this small sample, the drug group reported significantly more side effects at baseline than did the placebo group. Thus, the drug group had to be compared to itself at baseline in terms of side effects. There were no significant differences in the frequency (or presence) of any particular side effect, which might be a function of the small sample size in the drug group (n = 9). If the observed trends continued, somnolence and dry mouth probably would be reported to a significant extent above and beyond baseline levels.

Aggregating the more than 100 possible symptoms gives us a picture of topiramate as a very tolerable drug. The highest number of symptoms reported at any given time point was at baseline, and the next highest was at the 200-mg dose. Even at this treatment peak, the total side effects reported were around 80% of baseline levels.

Topiramate hydrochloride may represent a viable treatment option in SCI pain. We lack sufficient data to assess whether it would be more effective for pain at the level of injury or for pain experienced below the lesion (central pain). The drug may also be useful for visceral dysesthesia. Although small, this pilot study was randomized and controlled. We hope that a reproduction of this type of study with more subjects will prove whether or not topiramate represents a reasonable option. It appears to be safe and well tolerated in this population; the principal concern in terms of side effects and toxicity would be the development of uric acid stones in patients who would not be able to report the associated pain or bladder distension. Careful attention to bladder hygiene, urine output, and hydration are indicated.

ACKNOWLEDGMENT

Ortho-McNeil provided a grant to R.N. Harden.

REFERENCES

Arner S, Meyerson B. Lack of analgesic effect of opioids on neuropathic and idiopathic forms of pain. *Pain* 1988; 33:11–23.

Attal N, Brasseur L, Chauvin M, Bouhassira D. Effects of single and repeated applications of a eutectic mixture of local anaesthetics (EMLA) cream on spontaneous and evoked pain in post-herpetic neuralgia. *Pain* 1999; 81:203–209.

Backonja M, Beydoun A, Edwards KR, et al. Gabapentin for the symptomatic treatment of painful neuropathy in patients with diabetes mellitus: a randomized controlled trial. *JAMA* 1998; 280(21):1831–1836.

Beck AT, Rush AJ, Shaw BF, Emery G. *Cognitive Therapy of Depression*. New York: Guilford Press, 1979.

Bowsher D. Neurogenic pain syndromes and their management. *Br Med Bull* 1991; 47(3):644–666.

Box GE, Pierce DE. Distribution of residual autocorrelations in autoregressive-integrated moving average time series models. *J Am Statistical Assoc* 1970: 65:1509–1526.

Carlson CR, Collins FL, Stewart JF, et al. The assessment of emotional reactivity: a scale development and validation study. *J Psychopath Behav Assess* 1989; 11:313–325.

Cohen J. *Statistical Power Analysis for the Behavioral Sciences.* Hinsdale, NJ: Lawrence Erlbaum, 1988.

Durbin J, Watson G. Testing for serial autocorrelation in least squares regression, II. *Biometrika* 1951; 38:159–179.

Edwards K, Glantz M, et al. The evaluation of topiramate in the management of painful diabetic neuropathy. The 18th Annual Meeting of the American Pain Society. Fort Lauderdale, FL, 1999.

Faught E, Wilder BJ, Ramsay RE, et al. Topiramate placebo-controlled dose-ranging trial in refractory partial epilepsy using 200-, 400-, and 600-mg daily dosages. *Neurology* 1996; 46:1684–1690.

Elliott K, Minami N, Kolesnikov YA, Pasternak GW, Inturrisi CE. The NMDA receptor antagonists, LY274614 and MK-801, and the nitric oxide synthase inhibitor, NG-nitro-L-arginine, attenuate analgesic tolerance to the mu-opioid morphine but not to kappa opioids. *Pain* 1994; 56:69–75.

Harden RN, Bruehl S. Point/counterpoint: the use of opioids in treatment of chronic pain: an examination of the ongoing controversy. *J Back Musculoskel Rehabil* 1997; 9:155–180.

Kapadia NP, Harden NR. Gabapentin for chronic pain in spinal cord injury: case report. Association of Academic Physiatrists, Annual Meeting. Orlando, FL, 1999.

Kerns RD, Turk DC, Rudy TE. The West Haven-Yale Multidimensional Pain Inventory (WHYMPI). *Pain* 1985; 23:345–356.

Kupers R, Gybels R. The consumption of fentanyl is increased in rats with nociceptive but not neuropathic pain. *Pain* 1995; 60:137–141.

Max MS, Schafer SC, Culnane M, Dubner R, Gracely RH. Association of pain relief with drug side effects in postherpetic neuralgia: a single-dose study of clonidine, codeine, ibuprofen, and placebo. *Clin Pharmacol Ther* 1988; 43(4):363–371.

McQuay HJ, Tramer M, Nye BA, et al. A systematic review of antidepressants in neuropathic pain. *Pain* 1996; 68:217–227.

Mellick GA, Mellicy LB, Mellick LB. Gabapentin in the management of reflex sympathetic dystrophy. *J Pain Symptom Manage* 1995; 10:265–266.

Melzack R. The short form of the McGill Pain Questionnaire. *Pain* 1987; 30:191–197.

Merskey H, Bogduk N. *Classification of Chronic Pain: Descriptions of Chronic Pain Syndromes and Definitions of Pain Terms,* 2nd ed. Seattle: IASP Press, 1994.

Rowbotham M, Harden N, Stacey B, Bernstein P, Magnus-Miller L. Gabapentin for the treatment of postherpetic neuralgia: a randomized controlled trial. *JAMA* 1998; 280(21):1837–1842.

Simpson R, Olney J, McArthur A, et al. A placebo-controlled study of lamotrigine in the treatment of painful sensory polyneuropathy associated with HIV infection. *J Neurovirol* 1998; 4:366.

Spielberger CD, Gorsuch RL, Lushene RE. *Manual for the State-Trait Anxiety Inventory*. Palo Alto: Consulting Psychologists Press, 1970.

Tait RC, Pollard CA, Margolis RB, Duckro PN, Krause SJ. The Pain Disability Index: psychometric and validity data. *Arch Phys Med Rehabil* 1987: 68:438–441.

Yamamoto T, Yaksh TL. Studies on the spinal interaction of morphine and the NMDA antagonist MK-801 on the hyperesthesia observed in a rat model of sciatic mononeuropathy. *Neurosci Lett* 1992; 135:67–70.

Correspondence to: R. Norman Harden, MD, Center for Pain Studies, Rehabilitation Institute of Chicago, 1030 North Clark, Suite 320, Chicago, IL 60610, USA.

Spinal Cord Injury Pain: Assessment, Mechanisms, Management. Progress in Pain Research and Management, Vol. 23, edited by Robert P. Yezierski and Kim J. Burchiel, IASP Press, Seattle, © 2002.

25

Dorsal Root Entry Zone Coagulation in the Management of Spinal Cord Injury Pain

John P. Gorecki

Wichita Surgical Specialists, Wichita, Kansas, USA

The dorsal root entry zone (DREZ) of the spinal cord consists of part of the dorsal gray column, Lissauer's tract, the substantia gelatinosa, and the portion of the sensory root immediately adjacent to the spinal cord. The DREZ includes the five most superficial layers of the dorsal horn and contains Rexed's laminae 1–5. Sindou and colleagues (1974) were the first authors to describe making a surgical lesion in the DREZ. Surgical lesions can be made in the DREZ with radiofrequency coagulation (Samii and Moringlane 1984), microdissection (Sindou 1995), ultrasonic coagulation (Dreval 1993), or LASER (Powers et al. 1988). Indications for DREZ lesioning include the pain of brachial or lumbosacral plexus avulsion, end zone pain of spinal cord injury (SCI), and phantom pain. The pain of SCI includes both nociceptive pain related to the anatomical changes to the spine and central pain related to injury of the spinal cord itself. SCI pain is either spontaneous or induced. Following SCI it is possible to distinguish pain in a dermatomal pattern, usually located at the level of the injury, from diffuse pain. DREZ lesioning is useful for the intermittent induced SCI pain located in a dermatomal pattern, which is usually nociceptive in character and is called end zone pain. This chapter describes the anatomy of the DREZ, surgical technique, and results from DREZ surgery. In addition, this chapter briefly describes an animal model designed to study both the induced and spontaneous pain of SCI.

ANATOMY

The anatomy of the DREZ has been previously documented (Iacono et al. 1988; Ovelmen-Levitt 1996). Sensory input enters the spinal cord through the dorsal root. The primary sensory cell body is located in the dorsal root ganglion, and sensory fibers terminate in the dorsal gray of the spinal cord. Laminae I–IV are the main receiving areas for cutaneous primary afferent terminals, and lamina V receives fine afferents from the skin, muscle, and viscera. Many complex polysynaptic reflex paths originate from this region. Facilitatory and inhibitory effects due to simultaneous activity in various converging afferents modify transmissions to and through the dorsal appendage, where complex transformation of input occurs. The spinothalamic tract is a crossed pathway made up of second-order neurons. The origin of the spinothalamic tract is largely from Rexed's laminae 1 and 5. The spinothalamic tract crosses ventral to the central canal and travels up the cord in the ventral quadrant. The anatomical goal of DREZ coagulation is the elimination of all of the segmental input to the spinothalamic tract. The pain of SCI may be generated in the DREZ, as neurons in the dorsal horn become hyperactive following denervation (Loeser and Ward 1967).

OVERVIEW OF THE DREZ COAGULATION TECHNIQUE

DREZ coagulation is performed under general anesthesia with the patient positioned prone. The spinal cord must be exposed. A laminectomy is performed to expose the appropriate segments of the spinal cord. The operation can be performed through a bilateral laminectomy or hemilaminectomy. Few surgeons employ a laminoplasty for exposure. Lesions are planned to cover the segments involved with pain and to extend the lesions at least two segments above the highest dermatome involved in pain. Planning the exposure to accomplish lesioning at the appropriate segmental levels is important. Localization is accomplished with X-ray or fluoroscopy. The disparity between the cord level and the vertebral body level must be taken into account. DREZ lesions are made along the dorsolateral sulcus of the spinal cord. Additional localizing information is obtained by recording dorsal root somatosensory evoked potentials (SSEPs) directly from the spinal cord. Stimulating peripheral sensory nerves at a known dermatomal level triggers the SSEPs. Electrophysiological mapping of the cord has been described previously (Fazl et al. 1995).

In the technique I am describing, lesions are performed with an electrode energized by the current from a radiofrequency generator. The current passed through the electrode is controlled to maintain a constant temperature for a set period of time. Temperature is measured using a thermistor. The parameters used for DREZ coagulation require a temperature of 75°C for 15 seconds. The electrode is 0.25 mm in diameter and has a 2-mm exposed tip with a small shoulder of insulation that acts both as an electrical insulator and as a mechanical stop to prevent excessively deep penetration of the spinal cord. The intent is to produce a lesion that extends from the surface of the cord to Rexed's lamina 5. Lesions are oval or cylindrical in shape and are spaced 1 mm apart, measured from the center of each lesion. The end result is that the lesions overlap and produce a longitudinal destruction of the DREZ. Typically lesions are made over a segment of the cord measuring 7–10 centimeters in length, so 70–100 lesions are required. Small vessels along the surface of the cord are protected from coagulation and are carefully dissected free if necessary.

The size of a lesion created with radiofrequency energy depends upon the size and shape of the electrode, the temperature, and the length of time the assigned temperature is maintained. Experimental work (Cosman and Cosman 1974, 1996) shows that the size of the lesion increases with time until a maximum is reached at about 60 seconds, so that in theory, a stable lesion would require 60 seconds or more. However, clinical experience demonstrates that parameters of 75°C and 15 seconds result in an adequate lesion.

Structures adjacent to the DREZ include the dorsal columns and the corticospinal or pyramidal tract. Appropriate caution is used to protect these structures while creating lesions. Electrophysiological monitoring helps the surgeon protect these adjacent axonal tracts. It is possible to define the lateral edge of the dorsal column by seeking the loss of SSEPs recorded from an electrode in the cord. High-amplitude SSEPs can be recorded from the dorsal column in response to stimulation of the median or peroneal nerve. The amplitude of these SSEPs is much lower outside the dorsal column. Alternatively, the threshold for the stimulus required to generate the SSEPs is significantly higher when the recording electrode is located outside the dorsal column. Proximity to the corticospinal tract (CST) is defined by recording electromyography (EMG) from muscles in dermatomes distal to the lesioning target. The stimulus is passed through the DREZ electrode. If an EMG response is obtained with a threshold of less than 1 V it is assumed that the electrode is too close to the CST to safely make a lesion. The 1-V threshold is somewhat arbitrary, having been extrapolated from experience with the smaller spinal cords of animals. Anecdotal evidence in humans suggests that a lesion made through an electrode placed in a position that results in an EMG response with a threshold of less than 1 V is likely to result in motor deficit or loss of strength below the level of the lesion.

The laminectomy usually does not result in instability. Instrumentation or spinal fusion is not normally required as an adjunct to DREZ lesioning. The dura must be closed in a watertight fashion. The postoperative course is typical for intradural spinal surgery. The patient is usually ambulated the following day. Perioperative steroids are typically administered to reduce the risk of new neurological deficit due to SCI adjacent to the DREZ lesion. The dose for steroids is the same as that used for acute traumatic SCI.

Syringomyelia is found in some patients with SCI pain. Whenever an associated syringomyelia is identified it is treated at the same surgery (Nashold et al. 1990).

RISKS AND BENEFITS OF DREZ COAGULATION

Complications following DREZ lesions include general complications of anesthesia, general complications of intradural spinal surgery, and specific complications of the DREZ coagulation. The most common specific complication is a failure to achieve the expected pain relief. All patients experience more profound sensory loss, and the sensory loss usually involves a larger dermatomal area. SCI is a potential complication, with effects ranging from deficits in dorsal column function or corticospinal tract function up to complete paralysis. Dorsal column deficit is described in 10% of patients, and new motor weakness resulting in trouble walking is described in 10%. Bladder dysfunction is recognized in 5% of patients following DREZ coagulation. New pain can occur due to the effects of the laminectomy. Leaking of cerebrospinal fluid (CSF) is a potential complication. Spinal deformity has been described. Infection and hemorrhage are rare complications.

Bullitt and Friedman (1996) conducted a retrospective review in patients with SCI pain who underwent DREZ lesions at Duke University Medical Center between 1978 and 1993. Of the more than 800 patients who received DREZ coagulation, 105 patients were operated upon for SCI pain. These 105 patients underwent 127 procedures; some of them had bilateral operations, while others underwent repeat surgery. Follow-up reports are available for 45 patients. Demographics are consistent with those of SCI; 36 patients were men, and 9 were women. The patients varied in age between 26 and 71 years, with a median age of 45 years. The length of follow-up ranged from 1 to 16 years, with a median of 9 years. The injury to the spinal cord was caused by blunt trauma in 50 patients, penetrating trauma in 35, tumor in 4, Chiari malformation in 1, and unknown causes in 15. The location of the injury varied along the spine as follows: 44% of cases involved the conus, 35% the thoracic cord, 17% the lumbar cord, and 4% the cervical cord.

The results were measured by the number of patients experiencing significant pain reduction. At the time of hospital discharge 62% of patients were free of pain, and at the most recent follow-up 37% of patients were pain free. Other patients experienced partial pain relief. Another measure of pain relief is based on the patients' use of opioids. Prior to surgery 94% of patients were using opioids on a daily basis, but following DREZ surgery, at the time of most recent follow-up only 15% of patients were using opioids.

The benefit of DREZ surgery for pain can also be measured indirectly by evaluating the level of function or the extent of participation in daily activities before and after surgery. Each patient was asked to subjectively rate the extent to which the pain limited his or her activity. Prior to DREZ coagulation 85% of patients were unable to work, 76% said their ability to participate in recreation was limited, and 62% said the pain interfered with self-care. After DREZ surgery pain interfered with the ability to work in 45% of patients, with recreation in 45% of patients, and with self-care in only 40% of patients.

Complications in the form of pain, instability, or neurological deficit were recognized in 16 patients out of this group of 45 patients. Leaking of CSF occurred in only 2 of the 105 operated patients, new motor deficit was recognized in 6 patients, and sensory deficit due to DREZ surgery occurred in 7 patients.

The benefits of DREZ surgery on pain are limited to end zone pain. In a retrospective study of 56 paraplegics who underwent DREZ coagulation 74% with end zone pain did well, while only 20% with diffuse pain had good results (Friedman and Nashold 1986: Sindou and Daher 1988).

Although all the outcome data available for DREZ surgery come from retrospective reviews, it is remarkable that the results reported by Sindou et al. (2001) are similar to those reported from Duke (Nashold and Ostdahl 1979). This fact is even more remarkable given that different techniques were used and that the patient populations came from two very different communities, France and the United States. Similar outcomes have been substantiated by several retrospective reports from other centers (Friedman et al. 2001; Gorecki 2002).

An analysis of treatment failure can give some insight into the pathophysiology of the pain or the mechanisms for potential benefit from the procedure. Postprocedure pain can be classified as residual pain, recurrent pain, or new pain. Potential causes of postprocedure pain include incomplete procedure, incorrect procedure, disease progression, neuronal regeneration and new pathways development, new pain or deafferentation pain, external factors, and drug withdrawal. Experience shows that if the original DREZ surgery is done properly and an appropriate number of lesions were created, then repeat DREZ coagulation is of limited benefit. A typical example of the incorrect procedure leading to postprocedure pain is attempting to treat diffuse, constant, spontaneous pain of SCI with DREZ surgery.

THALAMIC TRACT LESIONING IN RATS AS A MODEL OF SCI PAIN

Under sponsorship of the Veterans Affairs Hospital we developed an animal model to allow the evaluation of SCI pain (Ovelmen-Levitt et al. 1995). This model will allow the testing of hypotheses relative to the physiology of SCI pain and will allow prospective analysis of potential therapeutic interventions. It is critical that the model be able to represent both spontaneous pain as well as induced pain. In developing this model we assumed that chronic compulsive self-directed behavior (CSDB) in an experimental animal accurately reflects spontaneous pain. Careful sensory examination of animals allows the demonstration of induced pain. It is not possible to test the assumption that CSDB represents spontaneous pain, but years of animal experimentation support this assertion (Levitt et al. 1992). In addition, a recent report describes similar behavior in humans who are able to verbalize the presence of spontaneous pain (Rossitch et al. 1992; Mailis 1996). Also key to this model is the assumption that a lesion involving the spinothalamic tract is sufficient and necessary for the initiation of SCI pain.

Our experiment consisted of a randomized, controlled prospective analysis of 40 Sprague-Dawley rats. The experimental rats underwent survival surgery to produce selective lesions within the spinal cord. Lesions were produced in the lateral column, dorsolateral column, dorsal column, and dorsal column plus lateral column. The spinothalamic tract was transected with lateral column lesions. We wanted to compare the effects of dorsal column lesions to those of spinothalamic tract lesions. We also wanted to analyze the effects of dorsal column lesions superimposed on spinothalamic lesions. Experimental subjects were compared to control animals that did not receive a spinal cord lesion. The animals were observed for 1 year following surgery. We were able to recognize CSDB, which was used as an endpoint for the experiment. The exact lesion was confirmed by histological examination after the rats were killed at the conclusion of the experiment. Some animals did not demonstrate the expected lesion. Some lesions were classified as supramaximal hemisection and some as less than hemisection of the spinal cord. In addition, each animal underwent careful sensory examination at biweekly intervals following survival surgery. We identified hyperpathia based on an abnormal withdrawal response to tactile stimulation. The observer documenting the presence of CSDB and performing the sensory examination was blinded to the lesion in the spinal cord, although it was possible to recognize control animals as having received no surgery. We also subjected each rat to electrophysiological analysis of the thalamus with microelectrodes using the techniques of Tasker and Lenz (Gorecki et al. 1989; Radhakrishnan et al. 1999), under modified anesthesia.

Behavior suggesting spontaneous pain was observed only in animals with lesions of the spinothalamic tract. Each of these animals demonstrated the expected contralateral analgesia and thermalgesia. The addition of dorsal column lesions to lateral column lesions still allowed the expression of CSDB. Dorsal column lesions alone (Table I) did not cause CSDB. Hyperpathia occurred in some of the animals demonstrating CSDB, but did not occur in animals with dorsal column lesions, i.e., dorsal column lesions abolished hyperpathia. CSDB was associated with spontaneous and induced hyperactivity in the ventral posterior lateral (VPL) thalamus. Microrecording from the thalamus demonstrated displaced receptive fields only in animals with dorsal column lesions. Animals with isolated dorsal column lesions did not demonstrate CSDB and did not have spontaneous or induced hyperactivity in the sensory thalamus (Table II). Thalamic reorganization only occurred in animals with dorsal column lesions. An unexpected observation was that CSDB was not expressed by animals with extensive lesions that included part of the central gray matter. It may be that lesions involving the central gray are somehow protective, and hence prevent the expression of spontaneous pain following SCI even when the spinothalamic tract is severed (cf. Chapters 8 and 9, this volume).

Table I
Summary of behavioral observation and sensory examination of animals with experimental spinal cord lesions

Behavioral Observation	*N*	Lesion	Sensory Examination
CSDB	6	Lateral column	Hyperpathia
CSDB	4	Dorsal column plus lateral column	Hypoalgesia
CSDB	6	Less than hemisection	Hyperpathia
No CSDB	6	Dorsal column	No hypoalgesia, no hyperpathia
No CSDB	6	Dorsolateral fasciculus	No hypoalgesia, no hyperpathia
No CSDB	12	Supramaximal hemisection	Hypoalgesia, no hyperpathia

Abbreviation: CSDB = compulsive self-directed behavior.

Table II
Results of microrecording from the thalamus of animals with experimental spinal cord lesions

N	Lesion	Spontaneous Hyperactivity	Evoked Afterdischarge	Receptive Field
Animals Demonstrating CSDB				
4	Lateral column	+++	+++	Not displaced
2	Dorsal column plus lateral column	++	+	Displaced
1	Hemisection	+	+	Not displaced
Animals not Demonstrating CSDB				
3	Dorsal column	No	No	Displaced
3	Dorsolateral fasciculus	No	No	Normal
1	Hemisection	No	No	Displaced

Abbreviation: CSDB = compulsive self-directed behavior.

SUMMARY

Based on this animal model of SCI pain it appears that injury to the spinothalamic tract is critical for the initiation of spontaneous pain. Injury to the dorsal column does not result in spontaneous pain, but contributes to the induction of hyperpathia. Both spontaneous pain and injury to the spinothalamic tract are associated with changes in spontaneous and induced cellular hyperactivity in the sensory thalamus. These results are consistent with the clinical finding that both SST cordotomy and cordectomy are ineffective treatments for SCI pain. The next step will be to demonstrate whether the DREZ operation can alter the behavioral and electrophysiological findings in this model, given that the operation can help roughly 70% of patients with end zone pain associated with SCI.

REFERENCES

Bullitt E, Friedman AH. DREZ lesions in the treatment of pain following spinal cord injury. In: Nashold BS, Pearlstein RD (Eds). *The DREZ Operation.* Park Ridge, IL: American Association of Neurological Surgeons, 1996, pp 125–137.

Cosman BJ, Cosman ER. *Guide to Radiofrequency Lesion Generation in Neurosurgery.* Radionics Procedure Technique Series Monographs. Burlington, MA: Radionics, Inc., 1974.

Cosman ER, Cosman BJ. Radiofrequency lesion-making in the nervous system. In: Wilkins RH, Rengachary SS (Eds). *Neurosurgery,* 2nd ed, Vol. III. New York: McGraw-Hill, 1996.

Dreval ON. Ultrasonic DREZ: operations for treatment of pain due to brachial plexus avulsion. *Acta Neurochir* 1993, 122:76–81.

Fazl M, Houlden DA, Kiss Z. Spinal cord mapping with evoked responses for accurate localization of the dorsal root entry zone. *J Neurosurg* 1995; 82:57–59.

Friedman AH, Nashold BS Jr. DREZ lesions for relief of pain related to spinal cord injury. *J Neurosurg* 1986; 65:465–469.

Friedman AH, Gorecki JP, Wellons JC. Stump phantom and avulsion pain. In: Burchiel K (Ed). *Textbook of Pain Surgery.* Stuttgart: Thieme, 2001.

Gorecki JP. Neurosurgical management of intractable pain: dorsal root entry zone. In: Winn R (Ed). *Youman's Neurological Surgery.* Orlando, FL: W.B. Saunders, 2002.

Gorecki J, Hirayama T, Dostrovsky JO, Tasker RR, Lenz FA. Thalamic stimulation and recording in patients with patients with deafferentation and central pain. *Stereotact Funct Neurosurg* 1989; 52(2–4):219–226.

Iacono RP, Aguirre ML, Nashold Jr BS. Anatomic examination of human dorsal root entry zone lesions. *Appl Neurophysiol* 1988; 51(2-5):225–229.

Levitt M, Ovelmen-Levitt J, Rossitch Jr E, Nashold Jr BS. On the controversy of autotomy: a response to L. Kruger. *Pain* 1992; 51(1):120–121.

Loeser JD, Ward AA Jr. Some effects of deafferentation on neurons of the cat spinal cord. *Arch Neurol* 1967; 17:629–633.

Mailis A. Compulsive targeted self-injurious behavior in humans with neuropathic pain: a counterpart of animal autotomy? Four case reports and literature review. *Pain* 1996; 64(3):569–578.

Nashold BS Jr, Ostdahl RH. DREZ lesions for pain relief. *J Neurosurg* 1979; 51(1) 59–69.

Nashold BS Jr, Vieira J, El Naggar AO. Pain and spinal cysts in paraplegia: treatment by drainage and DREZ operation. *Br J Neurosurg* 1990; 4(4)327–335.

Ovelmen-Levitt J. The neurobiology of the spinal cord dorsal horn and pathophysiology of neuropathic pain. In: Nashold BS, Pearlstein RD (Eds). *The DREZ Operation.* Park Ridge, IL: American Association of Neurological Surgeons, 1996, pp 13–26.

Ovelmen-Levitt J, Gorecki J, Nguyen KT, Iskandar B, Nashold Jr BS. Spontaneous and evoked dysesthesias observed in the after spinal cordotomies. *Stereotact Funct Neurosurg* 1995; 65(1-4):157–160.

Powers SK, Barbaro NM, Levy RM. Pain control with laser produced dorsal root entry zone lesions. *Appl Neurophysiol* 1988; 51:243–254.

Radhakrishnan V, Tsoukatos J, Davis KD, et al. A comparison of the burst activity of lateral thalamic neurons in chronic pain and non-pain patients. *Pain* 1999; 80(3):567–575.

Rossitch E Jr, Oaks WJ, Ovelmen-Levitt J, Nashold BS Jr. Self-mutilation following brachial plexus injury sustained at birth. *Pain* 1992; 50(2):209–211.

Samii M, Moringlane JR. Thermocoagulation of the dorsal root entry zone for the treatment of intractable pain. *Neurosurgery* 1984; 15(6):953–955.

Sindou M. Microsurgical DREZotomy (MDT) for pain, spasticity, and hyperactive bladder: a 20 year experience. *Acta Neurochir (Wien)* 1995; 137:1–5.

Sindou M, Daher A. Spinal cord ablation procedures for pain. In: Dubner R, Gebhart GF, Bond MR (Eds). *Proceedings of the Vth World Congress on Pain.* Elsevier Science, 1988, pp 477–495.

Sindou M, Fischer G, Goutelle A, Mansuy L. Selective surgery of posterior nerve roots: first results of surgery for pain. *Neurochirurgie* 1974; 20(5):391–408.

Sindou M, Mertens P, Wael M. Microsurgical DREZotomy for pain due to spinal cord and/or cauda equina injuries: long term results in a series of 44 patients. *Pain* 2001; 92(1–2):159–171.

Correspondence to: John P. Gorecki, MD, FRCS, FACS, Wichita Surgical Specialists, 818 North Emporia Street, Suite 200, Wichita, KS 67214-3788, USA. Tel: 316-263-0296, 800-362-3130; Fax: 316-263-9523; email: GOREC001@hotmail.com.

Part V

The Future

Spinal Cord Injury Pain: Assessment, Mechanisms, Management. Progress in Pain Research and Management, Vol. 23, edited by Robert P. Yezierski and Kim J. Burchiel, IASP Press, Seattle, © 2002.

26

Future Directions for the Study and Treatment of Spinal Cord Injury Pain

Robert P. Yezierski[a] and Kim J. Burchiel[b]

[a]Departments of Orthodontics and Neuroscience, College of Dentistry, and the McKnight Brain Institute, University of Florida, Gainesville, Florida, USA; [b]Department of Neurological Surgery, Oregon Health Sciences Center, University of Oregon, Portland, Oregon, USA

Recent years have seen a heightened awareness of secondary consequences associated with spinal cord injury (SCI) (Widerström-Noga et al. 1999). Although SCI research has traditionally focused on the restoration of motor function, we now realize that important strides can be made to improve quality of life for individuals with SCI by addressing bladder and bowel dysfunction, compromised sexual function, spasticity, and altered sensation, including pain. This realization led in 1997 to the development of a new initiative by the International Association for the Study of Pain (IASP). The charge of the Task Force on Pain following Spinal Cord Injury was to develop a strategy to evaluate this condition systematically and to provide a vehicle to coordinate research focusing on the clinical characteristics, central mechanisms, and treatment strategies of various SCI pain syndromes.

The collaborative effort of task force members, combined with that of clinical and basic researchers around the world, has significantly increased our understanding of different SCI pain syndromes (Siddall et al. 2000; Vierck et al. 2000; Finnerup et al. 2001). The increased number of relevant published reports, presentations, symposia, and international workshops reflects the success of this initiative, as does increased funding for clinical and basic science research programs focusing on SCI pain. Most importantly, the pain research community and scientists focusing on SCI research are now sharing their expertise in a cooperative effort to better understand the underlying mechanisms of SCI pain. The 3rd IASP Research Symposium brought these two groups together and represents the first time the SCI and pain communities have collaborated on a meeting devoted exclusively to SCI pain.

The past 5 years have seen enormous progress in defining the clinical characteristics of different SCI pain syndromes and in understanding the many variables influencing the development of at-level and below-level pain (see Chapters 1, 3 ,4, 5). A major step in this process was the development of a new taxonomy that effectively classifies SCI pain conditions (Chapter 2). Recently, Bryce and Ragnarsson (2001) described a comprehensive classification scheme similar in many respects to that proposed in Chapter 2 (see also Chapter 3). A universal taxonomy will enable us to compare results from a wide spectrum of basic and clinical studies. In developing a new taxonomy, the task force aimed not only to facilitate the interpretation of results from experimental studies and clinical trials, but also to guide the application of new therapeutic interventions for specific pain conditions. The hallmark of the new taxonomy is a user-friendly, comprehensive classification scheme that is consistent with current clinical concepts of pain types and terminology. Still a work in progress, the new taxonomy will undergo further refinements as efforts continue toward understanding the clinical characteristics and mechanisms of different SCI pain syndromes.

Despite progress toward finding effective treatments for SCI-related pain states, many unanswered questions remain. This book helps define the state of the art in SCI pain research and treatment and highlight areas of clinical and basic research requiring further investigation.

SCI pain arises from ischemic and/or traumatic injury to the spinal cord. Events initiated by insult to the cord parenchyma are critical in altering the structural and functional integrity of spinal circuits responsible for processing sensory information. To better understand the nature and scope of these changes and their role in pain-generating mechanisms in the spinal cord, it is important to study different cellular and molecular events influencing the survival and excitability of spinal sensory neurons. Accomplishing this goal will require a multidisciplinary effort utilizing the expertise of researchers in the fields of both SCI and pain. Present animal models all produce specific histopathological changes as well as changes in the excitability of spinal sensory neurons, and all result in evoked and/or spontaneous pain-like behaviors (Chapters 6, 7). Through a systematic comparison of existing and new models of SCI pain we must determine whether there are common changes across all models, and if so, how such changes relate to human pain syndromes. We must also determine whether these changes suggest targets for future therapeutic intervention. Important to this comparison will be a determination of the temporal characteristics of histological and physiological changes and their relationship to the onset and progression of at-level and below-level pain behaviors.

One of the most significant advances in understanding the secondary events associated with SCI has been the application of molecular biology to identify changes in gene expression that may affect the functional properties of spinal and supraspinal neurons (Brewer et al. 1997; Abraham et al. 2000, 2001). Several different cascades are initiated following spinal injury, and although many of them influence cell signaling and survival, much emphasis in recent years has been placed on the inflammatory, immunological, and excitotoxic processes. Continued study of these secondary responses to injury and of the glial contribution to the injury process (Watkins et al. 2001) promises to provide additional insights into the central mechanism of SCI pain states.

Continued progress in understanding the clinical characteristics as well as the central mechanisms related to SCI pain allows us to be optimistic about developing effective treatment strategies. Important efforts are underway to understand the spinal pathophysiological, cellular, and molecular changes that contribute to the central mechanism responsible for at-level and below-level pain (Vierck et al. 2000; Yezierski 2000; Chapters 10, 11). In addition to the historical emphasis on changes occurring in the spinal cord, a new appreciation is emerging for the anatomical, functional, and chemical changes initiated by SCI on cortical and subcortical structures (Chapters 12, 13, 15, 16, 17). Studies related to these changes will provide further insight into the location of sites contributing to pain mechanisms (Chapters 6, 14). For example, functional imaging and magnetic resonance spectroscopy will help unravel changes in the anatomical, functional, and chemical organizations of structures involved in sensory processing (Chapters 15–18). The design of these studies should include a comparison of data from groups of subjects with different pain states. Additionally, we cannot overlook the profile of pathophysiological and chemical changes in SCI subjects who do *not* develop pain. These studies are equally important in providing further insights into the interaction and temporal profile of spinal and supraspinal mechanisms responsible for at-level and below-level pain conditions.

Clearly we still need to gain a full appreciation for the complement of varied therapeutic targets that will serve as the cornerstone for the development of novel treatment strategies. Continued progress in the development of new multidisciplinary approaches must rely on the expertise of investigators not only in the field of pain, but also in the field of SCI.

While there are many topics for future studies related to the basic components of SCI pain, much also remains to be learned about the characteristics of the human condition (Yezierski 1996; Richards and Ragnarsson 2001;

Chapters 1, 3, 4). Perhaps the most glaring omission in the study of SCI pain is the lack of carefully designed longitudinal studies focusing on the evolution of altered sensation, on the specific location and descriptors of pain, and on relating clinical characteristics to the results of imaging studies that correlate the pathological characteristics of the injured cord with the clinical signature of sensory changes (Chapter 18). Time course studies provide a valuable account of the dynamic nature of altered sensation following SCI (Siddall et al. 1999).

Well-designed longitudinal studies, while difficult to implement, could have a critical impact on our understanding of this condition. Accomplishing these goals will require standard imaging protocols and behavioral assessment strategies that can be shared in multicenter studies. Compilation and analysis of data from such studies will require the creation of national and international databases.

There is a continuing need to develop novel interventions for SCI pain. "SCI pain" is, after all, a surrogate term for the constellation of pains that occur after SCI. One of our most important challenges is the development of multi-component strategies for the treatment of different pain conditions (Chapter 20). In designing much-needed controlled, randomized, multicenter clinical trials, researchers must use standardized terminology in creating homogeneous populations of subjects with specific clinical conditions (Chapters 19, 24). An easily accessible central repository of results from clinical trials would be a valuable resource for health practitioners.

Chronic SCI pain is a complex condition, typically associated with psychosocial issues that further complicate the design of effective therapies (Richards and Ragnarsson 2001; Widerström-Noga et al. 2001a,b). To better design effective treatment paradigms it is essential to establish the range of factors in patients' daily activities that exacerbate or alleviate specific pain conditions. Although pharmacotherapy is the first line of treatment, and invasive surgical procedures offer hope to a select few patients, we must develop and test novel treatment protocols, including behavioral-cognitive approaches and complementary strategies such as acupuncture, massage, and relaxation, along with established medical approaches. Important in the assessment of this multi-component approach is the reporting of successful treatments as well as those that produce less-than-desirable results.

Intrathecal delivery of agents is another approach requiring evaluation, especially using combinations of agents such as morphine, clonidine, and baclofen (Chapters 20–22). The promise of developing novel routes of administration for established drugs such as gabapentin should also be explored (Chapter 23). Furthermore, technologies such as gene therapy and molecular neurosurgery, which targets specific populations of chemically identified neurons relevant to pain generation, should be evaluated (Chapter 7), as should results from surgical interventions (Chapter 25). The success of ablative techniques in identifying possible sites of pain-generation in the brain and spinal cord will enhance understanding of the central mechanisms of specific types of SCI pain.

Results obtained from studies designed to restore function to the injured cord are vital to understanding SCI pain. Presently, investigators are making significant progress in overcoming the obstacles surrounding successful regeneration of damaged pathways. These methods, while offering potential restoration of motor function, could exacerbate pain. For this reason it is essential to assess the sensory consequences of strategies designed to restore function to the injured cord.

Although SCI pain was first described over 100 years ago, there is still no consistently effective long-term treatment. Continued progress in understanding central pain following SCI requires a commitment to using clinically relevant experimental models that produce pathological changes paralleling those associated with injury in humans and that lead to relevant pain behaviors. The development of new treatments should extend beyond conventional pharmacological manipulations of transmitter systems to include novel approaches targeting cell survival and signaling pathways. Recent progress in developing cellular transplant approaches to treat chronic pain (Sagen et al. 2002) increases the likelihood that cellular therapy may have a place in the arsenal of treatments for SCI pain.

In summary, efforts to standardize the terminology used in defining different types of spinal injury pain will assist in determining the prevalence of different pain syndromes and in promoting effective communication concerning the diagnosis and treatment of specific injury-related pains. The multidisciplinary focus of this volume has the potential to enhance the developing bridge between clinical and basic researchers in the fields of SCI and pain. These bench-to-bedside ties represent our best hope of finding effective treatments for SCI pain and improving the quality of life of patients.

REFERENCES

Abraham KE, Brewer KL, McGinty JF. Opioid peptide messenger RNA expression is increased at spinal and supraspinal levels following excitotoxic spinal cord injury. *Neuroscience* 2000; 99:189–197.

Abraham KE, McGinty JF, Brewer KL. Spinal and supraspinal changes in opioid mRNA expression are related to the onset of pain behaviors following excitotoxic spinal cord injury. *Pain* 2001; 90:181–190.

Brewer K, Yezierski RP, Bethea JR. Excitotoxic spinal cord injury induces diencephalic changes in gene expression. *Soc Neurosci Abstracts* 1997; 23:438.

Bryce TN, Ragnarsson KT. Epidemiology and classification of pain after spinal cord injury. In: Richards JS, Ragnarsson KT (Eds). *Topics in Spinal Cord Injury Rehabilitation: Pain Management,* Vol. 7(2). St. Louis: Thomas Land, 2001, pp 1–17.

Finnerup NB, Yezierski RP, Sang CN, Burchiel K, Jensen TS. Treatment of chronic pain following spinal cord injury. *Pain: Clin Updates* 2001; IX(2):1–6.

Richards JS, Ragnarsson KT (Eds). *Topics in Spinal Cord Injury Rehabilitation: Pain Management,* Vol. 7(2). St. Louis: Thomas Land, 2001.

Sagen J, Lewis-Cullinan C, Goddard M, Burgess FW. Encapsulated cell implants for pain surgery. In: Burchiel K (Ed). *Surgical Management of Pain.* New York: Thieme Medical, 2002, pp 958–972.

Siddall PJ, Taylor DA, McClelland JM, et al. Pain report and the relationship of pain to physical factors in the first 6 months following spinal cord injury. *Pain* 1999; 81:187–197.

Siddall PJ, Yezierski RP, Loeser JD. Pain following spinal cord injury: clinical features, prevalence and taxonomy. *IASP Newsletter* 2000; 3:3–7.

Vierck CJ, Siddall P, Yezierski RP. Pain following spinal cord injury: animal models and mechanistic studies. *Pain* 2000; 89:1–5.

Widerström-Noga EG, Cuevo EF, Broton JG, Duncan RC, Yezierski RP. Perceived difficulty in dealing with consequences of SCI. *Arch Phys Med Rehab* 1999; 80:580–586.

Widerström-Noga EG, Felipe-Cuervo E, Yezierski RP. Chronic pain following spinal cord injury: interference with sleep and daily activities. *Arch Phys Med Rehab* 2001a; 82:1571–1577.

Widerström-Noga EG, Felipe-Cuervo E, Yezierski RP. Relationships among clinical characteristics of chronic pain following traumatic spinal cord injury. *Arch Phys Med Rehab* 2001b; 82:1191–1197.

Watkins LR, Milligan ED, Maier SF. Glial activation: a driving force for pathological pain. *Trends Neurosci* 2001; 124:450–455.

Yezierski RP. Pain following spinal cord injury: the clinical problem and experimental studies. *Pain* 1996; 68:185–194.

Yezierski RP. Pain following spinal cord injury: pathophysiology and central mechanisms. In: Sandkühler J, Bromm B, Gebhart GF (Eds). *Prog Brain Res* 2000; Vol. 129, pp 429–448.

Correspondence to: Robert P. Yezierski, PhD Department of Orthodontics, 1600 S.W. Archer Road, Gainesville, FL 32610, USA. Tel: 352-392-4081; Fax: 352-392-3031; email: ryezierski@dental.ufl.edu.

Index

Locators in *italic* refer to figures.
Locators followed by t refer to tables.

N

Progress in Pain Research and Management Series

Spinal Cord Injury Pain: Assessment, Mechanisms, Management, edited by Robert P. Yezierski and Kim J. Burchiel, 2002

Complex Regional Pain Syndrome, edited by R. Norman Harden, Ralf Baron, and Wilfrid Jänig, 2001

Neuropathic Pain: Pathophysiology and Treatment, edited by Per T. Hansson, Howard L. Fields, Raymond G. Hill, and Paolo Marchettini, 2001

Acute and Procedure Pain in Infants and Children, edited by G. Allen Finley and Patrick J. McGrath, 2001

The Child with Headache: Diagnosis and Treatment, edited by Patricia A. McGrath and Loretta M. Hillier, 2001

Pain Imaging, edited by Kenneth L. Casey and M. Catherine Bushnell, 2000

Sex, Gender, and Pain, edited by Roger B. Fillingim, 2000

Proceedings of the 9th World Congress on Pain, edited by Marshall Devor, Michael C. Rowbotham, and Zsuzsanna Wiesenfeld-Hallin, 2000

Psychological Mechanisms of Pain and Analgesia, by Donald D. Price, 1999

Opioid Sensitivity of Chronic Noncancer Pain, edited by Eija Kalso, Henry J. McQuay, and Zsuzsanna Wiesenfeld-Hallin, 1999

Chronic and Recurrent Pain in Children and Adolescents, edited by Patrick J. McGrath and G. Allen Finley, 1999

Assessment and Treatment of Cancer Pain, edited by Richard Payne, Richard B. Patt, and C. Stratton Hill, 1998

Sickle Cell Pain, by Samir K. Ballas, 1998

Measurement of Pain in Infants and Children, edited by G. Allen Finley and Patrick J. McGrath, 1998

Molecular Neurobiology of Pain, edited by David Borsook, 1997

Proceedings of the 8th World Congress on Pain, edited by Troels S. Jensen, Judith A. Turner, and Zsuzsanna Wiesenfeld-Hallin, 1997

Pain Treatment Centers at a Crossroads: A Practical and Conceptual Reappraisal, edited by Mitchell J.M. Cohen and James N. Campbell, 1996

Reflex Sympathetic Dystrophy: A Reappraisal, edited by Wilfrid Jänig and Michael Stanton-Hicks, 1996

Visceral Pain, edited by Gerald F. Gebhart, 1995

Temporomandibular Disorders and Related Pain Conditions, edited by Barry J. Sessle, Patricia S. Bryant, and Raymond A. Dionne, 1995

Touch, Temperature, and Pain in Health and Disease: Mechanisms and Assessments, edited by Jörgen Boivie, Per Hansson, and Ulf Lindblom, 1994

Proceedings of the 7th World Congress on Pain, edited by Gerald F. Gebhart, Donna L. Hammond, and Troels S. Jensen, 1994

Pharmacological Approaches to the Treatment of Chronic Pain: New Concepts and Critical Issues, edited by Howard L. Fields and John C. Liebeskind, 1994